THE COMPLETE AIR FRYER COOKBOOK

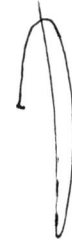

1001 QUICK AND CRISPY RECIPES FOR BEGINNERS TO FRY, GRILL, ROAST, BAKE AND COOK CRUCHY OIL FREE MEALS ON A BUDGET

Elisabeth Dwayne

TABLE OF CONTENTS

Introduction   **29**

What is an Air Fryer?   29

Which Air Fryer Should You Buy?   29

How Do You Use An Air Fryer?   30

Air Fryer Dos and Don'ts   30

Chapter 1: 501 Recipes for Fry   **31**

Recipe 1: Air Fried Calzone   31

Recipe 2: Air Fried Chicken Tenders   31

Recipe 3: Air Fried Churros   31

Recipe 4: Air Fried Cookie Balls   31

Recipe 5: Air Fried Crab Herb Croquettes   31

Recipe 6: Air-Fried Crumbed Fish   31

Recipe 7: Air Fried Oreos   32

Recipe 8: Air Fried Radishes   32

Recipe 9: Air Fried Shirred Eggs   32

Recipe 10: Air Fried Sourdough Sandwiches   32

Recipe 11: Air-Fried Spring Onions   32

Recipe 12: Air Fryer Beef Fajitas   32

Recipe 13: Air Fryer Broccoli and Tofu Scramble   33

Recipe 14: Air Fryer Cheese and Bacon Fries   33

Recipe 15: Air Fryer Empanadas   33

Recipe 16: Air Fryer Fried Pickles   33

Recipe 17: Air Fryer Pork Ribs   33

Recipe 18: Air Fryer Spinach Pakora   33

Recipe 19: Ajillo Mushrooms   34

Recipe 20: Apple Dumplings   34

Recipe 21: Apple Maple Crisp   34

Recipe 22: Apple Rollups   34

Recipe 23: Apricot Glazed Pork Tenderloins   34

Recipe 24: Artichoke Hearts   34

Recipe 25: Asian Halibut   34

Recipe 26: Asparagus and Parmesan   35

Recipe 27: Asparagus Fries   35

Recipe 28: Avocado and Turkey Rolls   35

Recipe 29: Avocado Shrimp   35

Recipe 30: Bacon and Brown Sugar Little Smokies   35

Recipe 31: Bacon and Cheese Stuffed Chicken   35

Recipe 32: Bacon and Ham Burger Patties   36

Recipe 33: Bacon Biscuits   36

Recipe 34: Bacon Cashews   36

Recipe 35: Bacon Cheese Sandwich   36

Recipe 36: Bacon Egg and Cheese Eggroll   36

Recipe 37: Bacon, Lettuce, Tempeh and Tomato Sandwiches   36

Recipe 38: Bacon Lettuce Wraps   37

Recipe 39: Bacon Omelet   37

Recipe 40: Bacon Wings   37

Recipe 41: Bacon Wrapped Brie   37

Recipe 42: Bacon Wrapped Chicken   37

Recipe 43: Bacon Wrapped Filet Mignon   37

Recipe 44: Bacon Wrapped Hot Dogs   38

Recipe 45: Bacon Wrapped Scallops   38

Recipe 46: Bacon Wrapped Stuffed Chicken   38

Recipe 47: Bagel Chips   38

Recipe 48: Balsamic Beef and Veggie Skewers   38

Recipe 49: Balsamic Caprese Hasselback   38

Recipe 50: Balsamic Salmon   39

Recipe 51: Banana Beignets   39

Recipe 52: Banana Chips   39

Recipe 53: Barbecue Drumsticks   39

Recipe 54: Barbeque Chicken Wings   39

Recipe 55: Basil Cod Croquettes   39

Recipe 56: Basil Green Lentil Balls   40

Recipe 57: Bass Fillet in Coconut Sauce   40

Recipe 58: Bavarian Bratwurst with Sauerkraut   40

Recipe 59: Beef and Broccoli   40

Recipe 60: Beef and Spinach Sautee   40

Recipe 61: Beef Burgers   40

Recipe 62: Beef Cheeseburgers   41

Recipe 63: Beef Fajitas   41

Recipe 64: Beef Fillet with Garlic Mayo   41

Recipe 65: Beef Lumpia   41

Recipe 66: Beef Meatballs   41

Recipe 67: Beef Roll-Up   41

Recipe 68: Beef Rolls   41

Recipe 69: Beef Strip with Snow Pea and Mushrooms   42

Recipe 70: Beets Chips   42

Recipe 71: Black Beans and Quinoa   42

Recipe 72: Black Cod with Grapes, Pecans, Fennel and Kale   42

Recipe 73: Bow Tie Pasta Chips   42

Recipe 74: Braised Lamb Shanks   43

Recipe 75: Breaded Artichoke Hearts   43

Recipe 76: Breaded Flounder   43

Recipe 77: Breaded Mushrooms   43

Recipe 78: Breaded Parmesan Perch   43

Recipe 79: Breaded Shrimp with Lemon   43

Recipe 80: Breakfast Beef Chili   44

Recipe 81: Breakfast Buns   44

Recipe 82: Breakfast Cherry and Almond Bars   44

Recipe 83: Breakfast Chicken Hash   44

Recipe 84: Breakfast Coconut Porridge   44

Recipe 85: Breakfast Cod Nuggets   44

Recipe 86: Breakfast Granola   45

Recipe 87: Breakfast Liver Pate   45

Recipe 88: Breakfast Meatloaf Slices   45

Recipe 89: Breakfast Mushroom Cakes   45

Recipe 90: Breakfast Potatoes   45

Recipe 91: Breakfast Sausage Casserole   45

Recipe 92: Breakfast Tuna and Bacon   46

Recipe 93: Broccoli Casserole   46

Recipe 94: Broccoli Cheese Quiche   46

Recipe 95: Broccoli Hash   46

Recipe 96: Broccoli Pesto with Quinoa   46

Recipe 97: Broccoli Stuffed Peppers   46

Recipe 98: Broccoli with Cheese Sauce   47

Recipe 99: Brown Sugar Glazed Salmon   47

Recipe 100: Brussels Sprout Salad with Pancetta   47

Recipe 101: Buffalo Cauliflower   47

Recipe 102: Buffalo Chicken Strips   47

Recipe 103: Buffalo Ranch Chickpeas   47

Recipe 104: Buttermilk Chicken   48

Recipe 105: Cabbage and Sweet Potatoes   48

Recipe 106: Cajun Cheese Sticks   48

Recipe 107: Cajun Chicken Kebabs 48

Recipe 108: Cajun Chicken Livers 48

Recipe 109: Cajun Flounder Fillets 49

Recipe 110: Caramel Apple Crisps 49

Recipe 111: Caribbean Jerk Cod Fillets 49

Recipe 112: Cauliflower Buffalo Bites 49

Recipe 113: Cauliflower Burger 49

Recipe 114: Cauliflower Hash 49

Recipe 115: Cauliflower Patties 50

Recipe 116: Cauliflower with Lime Juice 50

Recipe 117: Cheese and Bacon Filled Sweet Potatoes 50

Recipe 118: Cheese and Egg Breakfast Sandwich 50

Recipe 119: Cheese Cauliflower Mash 50

Recipe 120: Cheese Crusted Brussels Sprouts 50

Recipe 121: Cheese Sticks 51

Recipe 122: Cheesy Bacon Pockets 51

Recipe 123: Cheesy Bell Pepper Eggs 51

Recipe 124: Cheesy Bombs in Bacon 51

Recipe 125: Cheesy Cauliflower Hash Browns 51

Recipe 126: Cheesy Fingerling Potatoes 51

Recipe 127: Cheesy Fried Broccoli 52

Recipe 128: Cheesy Garlic Bread 52

Recipe 129: Cheesy Roasted Sweet Potatoes 52

Recipe 130: Cheesy Spinach Macaroni 52

Recipe 131: Chicken and Pepper Fajitas 52

Recipe 132: Chicken and Vegetable Fried Rice 52

Recipe 133: Chicken Avocado Burgers 53

Recipe 134: Chicken Bites 53

Recipe 135: Chicken Breasts Wrapped in Bacon 53

Recipe 136: Chicken Burgers with Blue Cheese Sauce 53

Recipe 137: Chicken Cheese Dinner Rolls 53

Recipe 138: Chicken Cheese Tortilla 53

Recipe 139: Chicken Cilantro with Beets 54

Recipe 140: Chicken Cordon Bleu Patties 54

Recipe 141: Chicken Drumsticks 54

Recipe 142: Chicken Filled Mushroom Bites 54

Recipe 143: Chicken Fillet with Brie and Ham 54

Recipe 144: Chicken Fillets with Coriander 54

Recipe 145: Chicken Hawaiian Rolls   55

Recipe 146: Chicken Kebabs   55

Recipe 147: Chicken Legs with Pineapple   55

Recipe 148: Chicken Meatballs   55

Recipe 149: Chicken Potatoes and Chickpea   55

Recipe 150: Chicken Scotch Eggs   55

Recipe 151: Chicken Tenders with Basil-Strawberry Glaze   55

Recipe 152: Chicken Thighs with Lemon Garlic   56

Recipe 153: Chicken with Sauce, Vegetables and Rice   56

Recipe 154: Chili Avocado Chimichurri Appetizer   56

Recipe 155: Chili Con Carne   56

Recipe 156: Chili Cheese Toasts   56

Recipe 157: Chili Hash Browns   56

Recipe 158: Chimichurri Skirt Steak   57

Recipe 159: Chinese Style Beef and Broccoli   57

Recipe 160: Chipotle Chicken Drumsticks   57

Recipe 161: Chorizo and Beef Burger   57

Recipe 162: Cilantro and Feta Beef Meatballs   57

Recipe 163: Classic Chicken Wings   58

Recipe 164: Classic Beef Meatballs   58

Recipe 165: Coconut Crusted Chicken Tenders   58

Recipe 166: Coconut-Custard Pie   58

Recipe 167: Cod Fillets and Peas   58

Recipe 168: Cod Fillets with Honey Glazed Greens   58

Recipe 169: Coleslaw Stuffed Wontons   58

Recipe 170: Corn-Crusted Chicken Tenders   59

Recipe 171: Cornflake Chicken Nuggets   59

Recipe 172: Cornflakes Toast Sticks   59

Recipe 173: Cornmeal Coated Catfish   59

Recipe 174: Cowboy Rib Eye Steak   59

Recipe 175: Crab Cakes   59

Recipe 176: Crab Wontons   60

Recipe 177: Cranberry Nutmeg Scones   60

Recipe 178: Crashed Bones with Chips and Ham   60

Recipe 179: Cream Potato   60

Recipe 180: Creamy Chicken Salad   60

Recipe 181: Creamy Pesto Spaghetti Squash   60

Recipe 182: Creole Chicken Drumettes   61

Recipe 183: Creole Turkey with Peppers 61

Recipe 184: Crispy Air Fried Pickles 61

Recipe 185: Crispy and Crunchy Baby Corn 61

Recipe 186: Crispy Banana Bites 61

Recipe 187: Crispy Breakfast Pies 61

Recipe 188: Crispy Breakfast Avocado Fries 62

Recipe 189: Crispy Breakfast Taco Wraps 62

Recipe 190: Crispy Brussels Sprouts 62

Recipe 191: Crispy Cheese Sticks 62

Recipe 192: Crispy Chicken Nuggets 62

Recipe 193: Crispy Chicken Skins 62

Recipe 194: Crispy Chicken Strips 63

Recipe 195: Crispy Coconut Tilapia 63

Recipe 196: Crispy Crabstick Crackers 63

Recipe 197: Crispy Fried Pork Chops the Southern Way 63

Recipe 198: Crispy Lamb 63

Recipe 199: Crispy Mustard Pork Tenderloin 63

Recipe 200: Crispy Nachos Prawns 64

Recipe 201: Crispy Onion Rings 64

Recipe 202: Crispy Paprika Fish Fillets 64

Recipe 203: Crispy Parmesan Crusted Pork Chops 64

Recipe 204: Crispy Popcorn Chicken 64

Recipe 205: Crispy Pork Belly 64

Recipe 206: Crispy Pork Dumplings 64

Recipe 207: Crispy Shrimp 65

Recipe 208. Crispy Shrimp Scampi 65

Recipe 209: Crispy Southwestern Ham Egg Cups 65

Recipe 210: Crispy Sweet-and-Sour Cod Fillets 65

Recipe 211: Crispy Tofu Bites 65

Recipe 212: Crumbed Fish Fillets with Tarragon 65

Recipe 213: Crunchy Canadian Bacon 65

Recipe 214: Crunchy Chicken Strips 66

Recipe 215: Crunchy Fish Taco 66

Recipe 216: Crunchy Golden Nuggets 66

Recipe 217: Crusted Tilapia Coconut Flavor 66

Recipe 218: Curried Cauliflower Florets 66

Recipe 219: Curried Chicken Legs 66

Recipe 220: Delicate Steak with Garlic 67

Recipe 221: Dessert Fries   67

Recipe 222: Dijon Lime Chicken   67

Recipe 223: Dijon Mustard Breaded Chicken   67

Recipe 224: Dill Mashed Potato   67

Recipe 225: Dilly Red Snapper   67

Recipe 226: Duck with Miso Paste   68

Recipe 227: Eggplant Fries   68

Recipe 228: Eggplant Parmesan   68

Recipe 229: Eggplants Satay   68

Recipe 230: Eggs in Zucchini Nests   68

Recipe 231: Fennel and Chicken Ratatouille   68

Recipe 232: Fennel with Shirataki Noodles   69

Recipe 233: Feta and Mushroom Frittata   69

Recipe 234: Feta Orzo and Lamb Chops   69

Recipe 235: Figs with Honey and Mascarpone   69

Recipe 236: Fijian Coconut Fish   69

Recipe 237: Filled Mushrooms with Crab and Cheese   69

Recipe 238: Fish and Cauliflower Cakes   70

Recipe 239: Fish Fillets with Parmesan Cheese   70

Recipe 240: Fish Tortillas with Coleslaw   70

Recipe 241: Five Spice Cream Cheese Chicken   70

Recipe 242: Five Spice Duck Breast   70

Recipe 243: Fluffy Potato Cakes   70

Recipe 244: French Toast Soldiers   71

Recipe 245: French Toast Sticks   71

Recipe 246: Friday Night Cheeseburgers   71

Recipe 247: Fried Bananas   71

Recipe 248: Fried Catfish with Fish Fry   71

Recipe 249: Fried Cheesecake Bites   71

Recipe 250: Fried Chicken Thighs and Legs   72

Recipe 251: Fried Cod and Spring Onion   72

Recipe 252: Fried Hasselback Potatoes   72

Recipe 253: Fried Hot Prawns with Cocktail Sauce   72

Recipe 254: Fried Meatballs in Tomato Sauce   72

Recipe 255: Garlic Chicken Kebab   72

Recipe 256: Garlic Lemon Cod Fillet   73

Recipe 257: Garlic Mozzarella Sticks   73

Recipe 258: Garlic Mussels   73

Recipe 259: Garlic Salmon Balls 73

Recipe 260: Garlicky Rosemary Lamb Chops 73

Recipe 261: Garlicky Sea Bass with Root Veggies 73

Recipe 262: German-Style Pork Patties 74

Recipe 263: Ginger Pork Chops 74

Recipe 264: Gingered Bacon Wrapped Scallops 74

Recipe 265: Glazed Chicken Thighs 74

Recipe 266: Golden Breaded Turkey Schnitzel 74

Recipe 267: Greek Chicken Wings 74

Recipe 268: Greek Eggplant Rounds 75

Recipe 269: Greek Street Tacos 75

Recipe 270: Greek-Style Deviled Eggs 75

Recipe 271: Greek Styles Mini Burger Pies 75

Recipe 272: Greek Veggie with Thyme 75

Recipe 273: Green Bean Crisps 75

Recipe 274: Green Stuffed Peppers 76

Recipe 275: Ground Chicken Meatballs 76

Recipe 276: Guajillo Chile Chicken Meatballs 76

Recipe 277: Guilt Free Vegetable Fries 76

Recipe 278: Halibut with Coleslaw 76

Recipe 279: Ham and Cheese Stuffed Chicken 76

Recipe 280: Ham and Tomatoes Omelet 77

Recipe 281: Ham Breakfast 77

Recipe 282: Ham Breakfast Pie 77

Recipe 283: Ham with Avocado 77

Recipe 284: Hash Browns 77

Recipe 285: Hazelnut-Crusted Fish 77

Recipe 286: Healthy Chicken Tenders 78

Recipe 287: Herbed Zucchini Poppers 78

Recipe 288: Herby Roasted Cherry Tomatoes 78

Recipe 289: Home-Style Fish Sticks 78

Recipe 290: Homemade Ranch Tater Tots 78

Recipe 291: Honey Duck Breasts 78

Recipe 292: Honey Glazed Salmon 79

Recipe 293: Honey Onions 79

Recipe 294: Honey Sea Bass 79

Recipe 295: Horseradish Salmon 79

Recipe 296: Hot Chicken with Mustard 79

Recipe 297: Hot Okra Wedges   79

Recipe 298: Intense Buffalo Chicken Wings   79

Recipe 299: Italian Chicken and Cheese Frittata   80

Recipe 300: Italian Herb Stuffed Chicken   80

Recipe 301: Italian-Style Tomato-Parmesan Crisps   80

Recipe 302: Jalapeno Poppers   80

Recipe 303: Japanese-Inspired Glazed Chicken   80

Recipe 304: Jerk Meatballs   80

Recipe 305: Kale and Potato Nuggets   81

Recipe 306: Kale Chips with White Horseradish Mayo   81

Recipe 307: Kentucky-Style Pork Tenderloin   81

Recipe 308: Kidney Beans in Air Fryer   81

Recipe 309: Lamb Rack with Lemon Crust   81

Recipe 310: Layered Cheese and Ham Casserole   81

Recipe 311: Lemon Drumsticks   82

Recipe 312: Lemon Garlic Chicken Breast   82

Recipe 313: Lemon Garlic Prawns Wrapped in Bacon   82

Recipe 314: Lemon Garlic Scallops   82

Recipe 315: Lemon Pepper Tilapia Fillets   82

Recipe 316: Lemon Pepper Turkey   82

Recipe 317: Lemon Turkey Wings   82

Recipe 318: Lemony Chicken with Barbecue Sauce   83

Recipe 319: Lemony Lamb Chops   83

Recipe 320: Lime Chicken   83

Recipe 321: Lobster Tails with Green Olives   83

Recipe 322: Marinated Scallops with Butter and Beer   83

Recipe 323: Mashed Sweet Potato Tots   83

Recipe 324: Meatballs in Tomato Sauce   84

Recipe 325: Mediterranean Air Fried Veggies   84

Recipe 326: Mexican Cheesy Zucchini Bites   84

Recipe 327: Mexican Chicken Roll-Ups   84

Recipe 328: Mexican Crunchy Cheese Straws   84

Recipe 329: Mexican Taco Chicken Fingers   84

Recipe 330: Mighty Meatballs   85

Recipe 331: Mini Sweet Pepper Poppers   85

Recipe 332: Minced Beef Keto Breakfast Sandwich   85

Recipe 333: Mini Peppers with Goat Cheese   85

Recipe 334: Mini Shrimp Frittata   85

Recipe 335: Mojito Fish Tacos   85

Recipe 336: Molten Sweet Potato Hash   86

Recipe 337: Molten Sweet Purple Potatoes   86

Recipe 338: Mouthwatering Tuna Melts   86

Recipe 339: Mushroom Leek Frittata   86

Recipe 340: Mushroom Turkey Patties   86

Recipe 341: Mustard Air Chicken   86

Recipe 342: Mustard Marina Ted Beef   87

Recipe 343: Mutton Chops   87

Recipe 344: Nutmeg Pork Cutlets   87

Recipe 345: Nutty Asparagus   87

Recipe 346: Old Bay Cod Fish   87

Recipe 347: Old Bay Crispy Chicken Wings   87

Recipe 348: Omelet with Onion and Cheese   88

Recipe 349: Onion Lamb Kebabs   88

Recipe 350: Onion Green Beans   88

Recipe 351: Oregano Chicken Breast   88

Recipe 352: Panko Chicken Tenders   88

Recipe 353: Parmesan Haddock Fillets   88

Recipe 354: Parmesan Sticks   89

Recipe 355: Party Buffalo Chicken Drumettes   89

Recipe 356: Pastrami Onion Wraps   89

Recipe 357: Pecan-Crusted Catfish Fillets   89

Recipe 358: Peppered Garlic Mushroom Caps   89

Recipe 359: Perfect Asparagus   89

Recipe 360: Philadelphia Herby Chicken Breasts   89

Recipe 361: Pickle Fries   90

Recipe 362: Pigs in a Blanket   90

Recipe 363: Pizza Dogs   90

Recipe 364: Pizza Peppers   90

Recipe 365: Pizza Toast   90

Recipe 366: Pork Bacon Bites   90

Recipe 367: Pork Belly with Peanuts   91

Recipe 368: Pork Chops   91

Recipe 369: Pork Chops with Stir-Fried Jalapeno Peppers   91

Recipe 370: Pork Chunks with Sweet and Sour Sauce   91

Recipe 371: Pork Cordon Bleu   91

Recipe 372: Pork Kabobs with Pineapple   91

Recipe 373: Pork Katsu   92

Recipe 374: Pork Satay with Peanut Sauce   92

Recipe 375: Potato Fritters   92

Recipe 376: Potato Gratin   92

Recipe 377: Potato with Crispy Skin   92

Recipe 378: Prawn Paste Chicken Wings   93

Recipe 379: Quick Bacon Hash   93

Recipe 380: Ranch Chips   93

Recipe 381: Raspberry Crumble   93

Recipe 382: Red Wine Turkey Wings   93

Recipe 383: Restaurant-Style Chicken Thighs   93

Recipe 384: Rib Eye Bites with Mushrooms   94

Recipe 385: Rice Wine Chicken Breasts   94

Recipe 386: Risotto with Zucchini and Red Capsicum   94

Recipe 387: Roast Lamb Shoulder   94

Recipe 388: Roasted Butternut Pumpkin with Nuts and Balsamic Vinaigrette   94

Recipe 389: Roasted Citrus Turkey Drumsticks   94

Recipe 390: Roasted Rack of Lamb with Macadamia Crust   94

Recipe 391: Rosemary Citrus Chicken   95

Recipe 392: Rosemary Lemon Chicken   95

Recipe 393: Sage Pork with Potatoes   95

Recipe 394: Salmon Croquettes   95

Recipe 395: Salmon in Papillote with Orange   95

Recipe 396: Salmon Patties   95

Recipe 397: Salmon with Creamy Zucchini   96

Recipe 398: Salt and Vinegar Chickpeas   96

Recipe 399: Salted Lemon Artichokes   96

Recipe 400: Sauce Chicken Thighs   96

Recipe 401: Sausage Balls   96

Recipe 402: Sausage Cheese Burritos   97

Recipe 403: Sausage Egg Cup   97

Recipe 404: Scotch Eggs   97

Recipe 405: Scrambled Pancake Hash   97

Recipe 406: Sea Salted Caramel Cookie Cups   97

Recipe 407: Seafood Tostadas   97

Recipe 408: Seed Porridge   98

Recipe 409: Seedy Rib Eye Steak Bites   98

Recipe 410: Semolina Veggie Cutlets   98

Recipe 411: Sesame-Crusted Tuna Steak ... 98

Recipe 412: Sesame Flavored Chicken Breast ... 98

Recipe 413: Shredded Chicken ... 98

Recipe 414: Shrimps Fried with Celery ... 99

Recipe 415: Simply Fried Chicken Thighs ... 99

Recipe 416: Skirt Steak with Horseradish Cream ... 99

Recipe 417: Smoked Paprika Sweet Potato Fries ... 99

Recipe 418: Smoky Roasted Veggie Chips ... 99

Recipe 419: Spaghetti Squash Fritters ... 99

Recipe 420: Spiced Chicken Breasts ... 99

Recipe 421: Spiced Chicken Wings in Air Fryer ... 100

Recipe 422: Spiced Mexican Stir-Fried Chicken ... 100

Recipe 423: Spicy Cajun Baby Corns ... 100

Recipe 424: Spicy Cheese Lings ... 100

Recipe 425: Spicy Fried Chicken ... 100

Recipe 426: Spicy Sriracha Cauliflower ... 100

Recipe 427: Spicy Sweet Potato Wedges ... 101

Recipe 428: Spinach and Tomato Egg ... 101

Recipe 429: Spinach Pie ... 101

Recipe 430: Squash with Cumin and Chili ... 101

Recipe 431: Steak and Cabbage ... 101

Recipe 432: Steamed Salmon with Dill Sauce ... 101

Recipe 433: Stuffed Cuttlefish ... 102

Recipe 434: Stuffed Peppers with Cheese and Bacon ... 102

Recipe 435: Super Simple Fisherman's Fishcakes ... 102

Recipe 436: Sweet and Sour Sesame Tofu ... 102

Recipe 437: Sweet Cream Cheese Wontons ... 102

Recipe 438: Sweet Mustard Coconut Shrimp ... 102

Recipe 439: Sweet Potato and Tuna Chips ... 103

Recipe 440: Sweet Potato Chips ... 103

Recipe 441: Sweet Potato Crisps ... 103

Recipe 442: Sweet Potato Fries ... 103

Recipe 443: Sweet Potato Hash Browns ... 103

Recipe 444: Sweet Potato Tots ... 103

Recipe 445: Sweets and Treats ... 103

Recipe 446: Taco Dogs ... 104

Recipe 447: Tandoori Chicken with Mint Yogurt ... 104

Recipe 448: Tangy Cod Fillets ... 104

Recipe 449: Tasty Breakfast Cups   104

Recipe 450: Tasty Brussels Sprouts with Guanciale   104

Recipe 451: Tasty Cheesy Omelet   104

Recipe 452: Tasty Cod Patties   105

Recipe 453: Tasty Roasted Kidney Beans and Peppers   105

Recipe 454: Tawa Veggies   105

Recipe 455: Tender Coconut Shrimps   105

Recipe 456: Tender Steak with Salsa Verde   105

Recipe 457: Teriyaki Beef Strips   105

Recipe 458: Teriyaki Glazed Steak   106

Recipe 459: Thyme Sirloin Finger Strips   106

Recipe 460: Thyme Steak Finger Strips   106

Recipe 461: Thyme Sweet Potato Wedges   106

Recipe 462: Thyme Turkey Breast   106

Recipe 463: Truffle Vegetable Croquettes   106

Recipe 464: Tuna Veggie Stir-Fry   107

Recipe 465: Turkey and Avocado Burrito   107

Recipe 466: Turkey and Cheese Calzone   107

Recipe 467: Turkey and Chicken Meatballs   107

Recipe 468: Turkey and Mushroom Sandwiches   107

Recipe 469: Turkey Bacon with Scrambled Eggs   107

Recipe 470: Turkey Breast with Maple Mustard Glaze   108

Recipe 471: Turkey Burrito   108

Recipe 472: Turkey Cordon Bleu   108

Recipe 473: Turkey Curry Samosas   108

Recipe 474: Turkey Hummus Wraps   108

Recipe 475: Turkey Patties   108

Recipe 476: Turkey Sausage Patties   109

Recipe 477: Tuscan Stuffed Chicken   109

Recipe 478: Twisted Deviled Eggs   109

Recipe 479: Vegan Croutons   109

Recipe 480: Vegan French Toast   109

Recipe 481: Vegan Stuffed Bell Peppers   109

Recipe 482: Vegetable Egg Cups   110

Recipe 483: Vegetable Egg Pancake   110

Recipe 484: Vegetable Egg Souffle   110

Recipe 485: Vegetable Quiche   110

Recipe 486: Vegetable Rolls for Lunch   110

Recipe 487: Vegetable Skewers   110

Recipe 488: Vegetarian Hash Browns   111

Recipe 489: Veggie Balls   111

Recipe 490: Veggie Burrito with Tofu   111

Recipe 491: Veggie Casserole with Cashew   111

Recipe 492: Very Berry Breakfast Puffs   111

Recipe 493: Zesty Ranch Fish Fillets   111

Recipe 494: Zucchini and Bell Pepper Stir-Fry   112

Recipe 495: Zucchini, Carrots and Yellow Squash   112

Recipe 496: Zucchini Chips   112

Recipe 497: Zucchini Corn Fritters   112

Recipe 498: Zucchini Cubes   112

Recipe 499: Zucchini Curly Fries   112

Recipe 500: Zucchini Fries and Roasted Garlic Aioli   113

Recipe 501: Zucchini Hash   113

Chapter 2: 250 Recipes for Grill   **113**

Recipe 502: Air Fried Turkey Breast with Basil   113

Recipe 503: Air Fried Whole Chicken   113

Recipe 504: Air Fryer Baby Back Ribs   113

Recipe 505: Air Fryer Grilled Chicken Breasts   113

Recipe 506: Air-Grilled Honey-Glazed Salmon   114

Recipe 507: Almond Pork Bite   114

Recipe 508: Apple Slaw Topped Alaskan Cod Filet   114

Recipe 509: Apricots with Brioche   114

Recipe 510: Aromatic T-Bone Steak with Garlic   114

Recipe 511: Artichoke Turkey Pizza   114

Recipe 512: Artichoke with Red Pepper Pizza   115

Recipe 513: Asian Pork Chops   115

Recipe 514: Asparagus Steak Tips   115

Recipe 515: Authentic Korean Chili Pork   115

Recipe 516: Awesome Korean Pork Lettuce Wraps   115

Recipe 517: Baby Back Rib Recipe from Kansas City   115

Recipe 518: Bacon Cheeseburger Pizza   116

Recipe 519: Bacon Egg Muffins with Chives   116

Recipe 520: Bacon 'n' Bell Pepper Pita Pockets   116

Recipe 521: Balsamic Artichokes   116

Recipe 522: Balsamic-Glazed Pork Chops   116

Recipe 523: Balsamic Mushroom Sliders with Pesto   116

Recipe 524: Banana Skewers   117

Recipe 525: Barbeque Air Fried Chicken   117

Recipe 526: Barley Porridge   117

Recipe 527: Basil Bell Pepper Bites   117

Recipe 528: BBQ Lamb   117

Recipe 529: BBQ Pork Ribs   117

Recipe 530: Beef and Mango Skewers   117

Recipe 531: Beef Bulgogi with Scallions and Sesame   118

Recipe 532: Beef Recipe Texas-Rodeo Style   118

Recipe 533: Beef Strips, Corn and Tomatoes   118

Recipe 534: Beef Wellington   118

Recipe 535: Beef with Cauliflower and Green Peas   118

Recipe 536: Bell Peppers with Potato Stuffing   118

Recipe 537: Black Bean Fajitas   119

Recipe 538: Bourbon-BBQ Sauce Marinated Beef BBQ   119

Recipe 539: Breakfast Grilled Ham and Cheese   119

Recipe 540: Broccoli Chicken   119

Recipe 541: Broccoli Chicken Casserole   119

Recipe 542: Brussel Sprouts, Mango, Avocado Salsa Tacos   119

Recipe 543: Buttermilk Brined Turkey Breast   120

Recipe 544: Buttery Parmesan Broccoli Florets   120

Recipe 545: Buttery Scramble Eggs   120

Recipe 546: Cadienne Chicken Pasta   120

Recipe 547: Caesar Chicken   120

Recipe 548: Caesar Marinated Grilled Chicken   120

Recipe 549: Cajun Sweet-Sour Grilled Pork   121

Recipe 550: Capers 'n Olives Topped Flank Steak   121

Recipe 551: Caprese Grilled Chicken with Balsamic Vinegar   121

Recipe 552: Caraway, Sichuan 'n Cumin Lamb Kebabs   121

Recipe 553: Catfish Fillets with Parsley   121

Recipe 554: Cauliflower, Okra, and Pepper Casserole   121

Recipe 555: Charred Onions and Steak Cube BBQ   122

Recipe 556: Cheddar Pimiento Strips   122

Recipe 557: Cheese Stuffed Chicken   122

Recipe 558: Cheesy BBQ Chicken Pizza   122

Recipe 559: Cheesy Creamy Broccoli Casserole   122

Recipe 560: Cheesy Rice Croquettes   122

Recipe 561: Chicken Cacciatore   122

Recipe 562: Chicken Paillard   123

Recipe 563: Chicken Roast with Pineapple Salsa   123

Recipe 564: Chicken Shawarma   123

Recipe 565: Chicken with Artichoke Hearts   123

Recipe 566: Chicken with Cashew Nuts and Bell Pepper   123

Recipe 567: Chili Chicken Slider   124

Recipe 568: Chili Garlic Chicken Wings   124

Recipe 569: Chili-Rubbed Flank Steak   124

Recipe 570: Citrusy Chicken Breasts   124

Recipe 571: Classic Grilled Cheese   124

Recipe 572: Classic Maple-Glazed Chicken   124

Recipe 573: Classic Spring Chicken   124

Recipe 574: Coconut Battered Fish Fillets   125

Recipe 575: Coconut Fish with a Fine Note   125

Recipe 576: Coconut Pork Chops   125

Recipe 577: Cod Fillet with Hummus   125

Recipe 578: Cod Steaks and Plum Sauce   125

Recipe 579: Cod with Chorizo Potatoes   125

Recipe 580: Creole Fried Tomatoes   126

Recipe 581: Crispy Breakfast Taco Wraps   126

Recipe 582: Crispy Crusted Chicken   126

Recipe 583: Curry Pork Roast in Coconut Sauce   126

Recipe 584: Effortless Pepperoni Pizza   126

Recipe 585: Eggplant Rolls with Quinoa   126

Recipe 586: Espresso-Grilled Pork Tenderloin   127

Recipe 587: Feisty Rum and Pineapple Sundae   127

Recipe 588: Filet Mignon   127

Recipe 589: Fish with Seasonal Herbs in a Packet   127

Recipe 590: Fruity Lime Salad   127

Recipe 591: Garlic Chicken Kebab   127

Recipe 592: Garlic Lamb Shank   128

Recipe 593: Generous Hot Pepper Wings   128

Recipe 594: Ginger, Garlic and Pork Dumplings   128

Recipe 595: Glazed Lamb Chops   128

Recipe 596: Golden Squash Croquettes   128

Recipe 597: Greek Chicken Breasts   128

Recipe 598: Greek Potatoes   129

Recipe 599: Greek Tomato Olive Chicken   129

Recipe 600: Green Beans with Sesame Seeds   129

Recipe 601: Green Bell Pepper with Califlower Stuffing   129

Recipe 602: Grilled Asparagus   129

Recipe 603: Grilled BBQ Turkey   129

Recipe 604: Grilled Broccoli   130

Recipe 605: Grilled Buffalo Chicken Wings   130

Recipe 606: Grilled Cheese and Prawn Sandwiches   130

Recipe 607: Grilled Cheese Fish   130

Recipe 608: Grilled Cheese Sandwich   130

Recipe 609: Grilled Chicken   130

Recipe 610: Grilled Chicken and Sauce   131

Recipe 611: Grilled Chicken Breasts   131

Recipe 612: Grilled Chicken Breasts with Broccoli   131

Recipe 613: Grilled Cod Fillets Mixed with Grapes Salad and Fennel   131

Recipe 614: Grilled Cod with Avocado and Olives Salad   131

Recipe 615: Grilled Cumin Hanger Steak   131

Recipe 616: Grilled Fish and Cheese   132

Recipe 617: Grilled Fish Fillet with Pesto Sauce   132

Recipe 618: Grilled Fruit   132

Recipe 619: Grilled Halibut with Sun Dried Tomatoes   132

Recipe 620: Grilled Hawaiian Chicken   132

Recipe 621: Grilled Hawaiian Chicken Breasts   132

Recipe 622: Grilled High Rib with Spicy Sauce   133

Recipe 623: Grilled Lemony Saba Fish   133

Recipe 624: Grilled Masala Lamb Chops   133

Recipe 625: Grilled Orange Chicken   133

Recipe 626: Grilled Parsley and Thyme Salmon   133

Recipe 627: Grilled Peaches   133

Recipe 628: Grilled Pears with Cinnamon Drizzle   134

Recipe 629: Grilled Pork and Bell Pepper Salad   134

Recipe 630: Grilled Pork Chops with Sweet Potatoes   134

Recipe 631: Grilled Pork in Cajun Sauce   134

Recipe 632: Grilled Pork Shoulder   134

Recipe 633: Grilled Salmon with Capers and Dill   134

Recipe 634: Grilled Scallion Cheese Sandwich   135

Recipe 635: Grilled Skirt Steak with Sauce   135

Recipe 636: Grilled Soy Salmon Fillets   135

Recipe 637: Grilled Stuffed Lobster   135

Recipe 638: Grilled Tofu Sandwich								135

Recipe 639: Grilled Tomato Salsa								135

Recipe 640: Grilled Tomatoes								136

Recipe 641: Grilled Turkey Skewers with Satay Sauce								136

Recipe 642: Grilled Vegetables with Lamb								136

Recipe 643: Grilled Vienna Sausage with Broccoli								136

Recipe 644: Ground Pork and Apple Burgers								136

Recipe 645: Flavorful and Juicy Grilled Chicken								136

Recipe 646: Fruit and Vegetable Skewers								137

Recipe 647: Ham and Pineapple Skewers								137

Recipe 648: Healthy Flapjacks								137

Recipe 649: Herby Tomato Meatloaf								137

Recipe 650: Honey Glazed Pineapple Fries								137

Recipe 651: Honey-Luscious Asparagus								137

Recipe 652: Horseradish Mayo and Gorgonzola Mushrooms								138

Recipe 653: Hot Paprika Potato Wedges								138

Recipe 654: Indian Meatball with Lamb								138

Recipe 655: Italian Chicken Marsala								138

Recipe 656: Juicy Boneless BBQ Ribs								138

Recipe 657: Kale and Cheese Sandwiches								138

Recipe 658: Lamb Gyro								139

Recipe 659: Lamb Meatballs								139

Recipe 660: Legs of Goose Wrapped in Bacon with Parsnips								139

Recipe 661: Leg of Lamb with Smoked Paprika								139

Recipe 662: Lemon Grilled Chicken								139

Recipe 663: Lemon Lamb Rack								139

Recipe 664: Lemon Pepper Chicken								140

Recipe 665: Lemon Pepper Shrimp								140

Recipe 666: Maple Glazed Sausages and Figs								140

Recipe 667: Marinated Beef BBQ								140

Recipe 668: Marshmallow and Banana Boats								140

Recipe 669: Mayonnaise and Rosemary Grilled Steak								140

Recipe 670: Mexican Chicken Lasagna								141

Recipe 671: Mexican Corn Dish								141

Recipe 672: Morning Mini Cheeseburger Sliders								141

Recipe 673: Mozzarella and Smoked Fish Tart								141

Recipe 674: Mustard and Veggie								141

Recipe 675: Mustard Fish Mania								141

Recipe 676: Nugget and Veggie Taco Wraps 142

Recipe 677: Oregano Chicken Legs with Lemon 142

Recipe 678: Original Grilled Cheese Sandwiches 142

Recipe 679: Outstanding Rack of Lamb 142

Recipe 680: Oyster Chicken Breasts 142

Recipe 681: Paprika and Pickles Fritters 142

Recipe 682: Paprika Grilled Shrimp 143

Recipe 683: Pepperoni Grilled Cheese 143

Recipe 684: Perfect Fillet of Beef 143

Recipe 685: Pineapple and Veggie Souvlaki 143

Recipe 686: Pineapple Fish Fillet 143

Recipe 687: Pizza Margherita with Spinach 143

Recipe 688: Pork and Fruit Kebabs 144

Recipe 689: Pork and Mixed Greens Salad 144

Recipe 690: Pork Balls 144

Recipe 691: Pork Burgers with Red Cabbage Salad 144

Recipe 692: Pork Chops in Cream 144

Recipe 693: Pork Ratatouille 144

Recipe 694: Pork Rind Nachos 145

Recipe 695: Potato and Vegetable Strudel 145

Recipe 696: Potatoes with Cottage Cheese 145

Recipe 697: Prosciutto-Wrapped Asparagus 145

Recipe 698: Quick Tuna Tacos 145

Recipe 699: Spicy Honey Mustard Chicken 145

Recipe 700: Quinoa Green Pizza 146

Recipe 701: Ranch Chicken 146

Recipe 702: Roast Beef 146

Recipe 703: Roasted Hamburgers 146

Recipe 704: Roasted Pepper Chicken 146

Recipe 705: Roasted Pumpkin Seeds 146

Recipe 706: Saffron Spiced Rack of Lamb 146

Recipe 707: Salmon Asparagus and Horseradish 147

Recipe 708: Salmon in Puff Pastry Croissants 147

Recipe 709: Salmon with Cream Cheese 147

Recipe 710: Salmon with Herbs 147

Recipe 711: Salmon with Pesto and Roasted Tomatoes 147

Recipe 712: Salt-and-Pepper Beef Roast 147

Recipe 713: Saucy Chicken with Leeks 148

Recipe 714: Seasoned Chicken Breasts   148

Recipe 715: Seasoned Garlic Carrots   148

Recipe 716: Simple Cuban Sandwiches   148

Recipe 717: Sirloin Roast Beef   148

Recipe 718: Slow Roasted Beef Short Ribs   148

Recipe 719: Smoked Shrimp   149

Recipe 720: Soy Chorizo and Spring Onion Toast   149

Recipe 721: Soy Salmon Fillets   149

Recipe 722: Spaghetti Squash Burrito Bowls   149

Recipe 723: Spicy Air Fryer Salmon   149

Recipe 724: Spicy Chicken Drumsticks with Grill Marinade   149

Recipe 725: Spicy Grilled Steak   150

Recipe 726: Spicy Grilled Tomatoes   150

Recipe 727: Steak and Vegetable Kebabs   150

Recipe 728: Stroganoff Short Steak   150

Recipe 729: Stuffed Portabella Mushroom   150

Recipe 730: Stuffed Tomatoes   150

Recipe 731: Super Cheese Sandwiches   151

Recipe 732: Sweet and Sour Pork   151

Recipe 733: Sweet and Spicy Swordfish Kebabs   151

Recipe 734: Sweet Plantains   151

Recipe 735: Taco Beef and Green Chile Casserole   151

Recipe 736: Tasty Caribbean Chicken   151

Recipe 737: Tender and Juicy Chicken   152

Recipe 738: Teriyaki Glazed Salmon   152

Recipe 739. Teriyaki Salmon   152

Recipe 740: Tex Mex Chicken   152

Recipe 741: Thyme Meatless Patties   152

Recipe 742: Toasted Vegetables with Rice and Eggs   152

Recipe 743: Tomato Short Ribs   153

Recipe 744: Tuna and Fruit Kebabs   153

Recipe 745: Tuna Wraps   153

Recipe 746: Turkey Meatballs   153

Recipe 747: Turkey Spring Rolls   153

Recipe 748: Two-Cheese Grilled Sandwiches   153

Recipe 749: Veggies and Halloumi Cheese   154

Recipe 750: Whole Chicken with Prunes and Capers   154

Recipe 751: Zucchini Feta Paws   154

Chapter 3: 250 Recipes for Bake   154

Recipe 752: Almond Nuggets   154

Recipe 753: Almond Orange Butter Cake   154

Recipe 754: Almond Pecan Cookies   154

Recipe 755: Almond-Pumpkin Porridge   155

Recipe 756: Almond Orange Cake   155

Recipe 757: Apricot-Cheese Mini Pies   155

Recipe 758: Apricot Crumble with Blackberries   155

Recipe 759: Aromatic Mushroom Omelet   155

Recipe 760: Asparagus Strata   155

Recipe 761: Avocado and Spinach Melts   156

Recipe 762: Baked Almond Chicken   156

Recipe 763: Baked Apple   156

Recipe 764: Baked Bacon Egg Cups   156

Recipe 765: Baked Cheese Crisps   156

Recipe 766: Baked Cheese 'n Pepperoni Calzone   156

Recipe 767: Baked Chicken Wings   157

Recipe 768: Baked Eggs for Breakfast   157

Recipe 769: Baked Eggs in Avocado Nests   157

Recipe 770: Baked Eggs with Cheese   157

Recipe 771: Baked Eggs and Sausage Muffins   157

Recipe 772: Baked Eggs with Spinach and Basil   157

Recipe 773: Baked Eggplant and Zucchini   158

Recipe 774: Baked Pears with Chocolate   158

Recipe 775: Baked Shrimp Bites   158

Recipe 776: Baked Stuffed Peppers   158

Recipe 777: Baked Sweet Potato with Yogurt Chives Sauce   158

Recipe 778: Baked Tomato   158

Recipe 779: Baked Zucchini Eggplant   159

Recipe 780: Balsamic London Broil   159

Recipe 781: Banana and Walnut Cake   159

Recipe 782: Banana Muffins with Chocolate Chips   159

Recipe 783: Basil Feta Crostini   159

Recipe 784: Basmati Risotto   159

Recipe 785: Battered Chicken Thighs   160

Recipe 786: Beans and Eggs   160

Recipe 787: Beef Casserole   160

Recipe 788: Beef Enchilada Dip   160

Recipe 789: Beefy Bell Pepper 'n Egg Scramble 160

Recipe 790: Berbere Beef Steaks 160

Recipe 791: Berry-Glazed Turkey Breast 160

Recipe 792: Black and White Brownies 161

Recipe 793: Black Bean and Tomato Chili 161

Recipe 794: Black Bean Stuffed Potato Boats 161

Recipe 795: Black Forest Hand Pies 161

Recipe 796: Black Olive and Shrimp Salad 161

Recipe 797: Blueberry Pancakes 161

Recipe 798: Breakfast Blueberry Cobbler 162

Recipe 799: Breakfast Casserole 162

Recipe 800: Breakfast Pocket Pies 162

Recipe 801: Broccoli and Cheese Egg Ramekins 162

Recipe 802: Broccoli and Mushroom Beef 162

Recipe 803: Broccoli Cheddar Quiche 162

Recipe 804: Bruschetta with Basil Pesto 163

Recipe 805: Buffalo Chicken Meatballs 163

Recipe 806: Butter Baked Mussels 163

Recipe 807: Butter Walnut and Raisin Cookies 163

Recipe 808: Caprese Flatbread 163

Recipe 809: Cauliflower and Bacon Bake 164

Recipe 810: Cauliflower Chicken Casserole 164

Recipe 811: Cauliflower Cottage Pie 164

Recipe 812: Cauliflower Poppers 164

Recipe 813: Cheese and Crab Stuffed Mushrooms 164

Recipe 814: Cheese Cauliflower Muffins 164

Recipe 815: Cheesy Bacon and Egg Hash 165

Recipe 816: Cheesy Breakfast Casserole 165

Recipe 817: Cheesy Broccoli Casserole 165

Recipe 818: Cheesy Broccoli Rice 165

Recipe 819: Cheesy Chorizo, Corn, and Potato Frittata 165

Recipe 820: Cheesy Crab Toasts 165

Recipe 821: Cheesy Creamy Broccoli Casserole 166

Recipe 822: Cheesy Garlic Sweet Potatoes 166

Recipe 823: Cheesy Green Wonton Triangles 166

Recipe 824: Cheesy Italian Meatloaf 166

Recipe 825: Cheesy Mushrooms and Spinach Frittata 166

Recipe 826: Cheesy Tuna Tower 166

Recipe 827: Chicken Cheese Taquitos 167

Recipe 828: Chicken Cheese Zucchini Casserole 167

Recipe 829: Chickpea and Bulgur Baked Dinner 167

Recipe 830: Chipotle Pork Chops 167

Recipe 831: Chocolate and Nut Mix Bars 167

Recipe 832: Chocolate Apricot Muffins 167

Recipe 833: Chocolate Peanut Butter Bread Pudding 168

Recipe 834: Chorizo and Garlic Veggie Bake 168

Recipe 835: Chorizo and Vegetable Bake 168

Recipe 836: Cinnamon Banana Bread with Pecans 168

Recipe 837: Cinnamon Pear Oat Muffins 168

Recipe 838: Classic Butter-Bread Pudding 169

Recipe 839: Classic Raisin Bread Pudding 169

Recipe 840: Coated Artichoke Fries 169

Recipe 841: Cocktail Chicken Meatballs 169

Recipe 842: Coconut Chicken Bake 169

Recipe 843: Coconut Cream Roll-Ups 169

Recipe 844: Coconut Mini Tarts 170

Recipe 845: Coconut Orange Cake 170

Recipe 846: Coconut Pie 170

Recipe 847: Corn and Bell Pepper Casserole 170

Recipe 848: Corn Dog Cupcakes 170

Recipe 849: Crab Cake Bites 170

Recipe 850: Cranberry Chicken Curry 171

Recipe 851: Cranberry Crusted Salmon 171

Recipe 852: Creamy Baked Dory 171

Recipe 853: Creamy Cauliflower Casserole 171

Recipe 854: Creamy Horseradish Roast Beef 171

Recipe 855: Creamy Spinach-Broccoli Dip 172

Recipe 856: Croissant Mushroom and Egg 172

Recipe 857: Croissant Mushroom, Tomatoes and Egg 172

Recipe 858: Crunchy Granola Muffins 172

Recipe 859: Crusted Scallops 172

Recipe 860: Crustless Cheesecake 172

Recipe 861: Curried Cauliflower 173

Recipe 862: Date and Hazelnut Cookies 173

Recipe 863: Delicious Clafoutis 173

Recipe 864: Dijon Shrimp Cakes 173

Recipe 865: Effortless Toffee Zucchini Bread 173

Recipe 866: Egg and Bacon Cups 173

Recipe 867: Egg and Bacon Toasts 174

Recipe 868: Eggless Brownies 174

Recipe 869: Eggplant and Bell Peppers with Basil 174

Recipe 870: English Pumpkin Egg Bake 174

Recipe 871: Farfalle with White Sauce 174

Recipe 872: Feta and Mushroom Frittata 175

Recipe 873: Filled Mushrooms with Crab 175

Recipe 874: Fish with Vegetables 175

Recipe 875: Flank Steak with Caramelized Onions 175

Recipe 876: Flavorful Baked Halibut 175

Recipe 877: Fluffy Vegetable Strata 175

Recipe 878: Fruity Baked Oatmeal 176

Recipe 879: Full Baked Trout en Papillote with Herbs 176

Recipe 880: Garlicky Veggie Bake 176

Recipe 881: Ginger Turkey Meatballs 176

Recipe 882: Goat Cheese Stuffed Turkey Roulade 176

Recipe 883: Golden Pork Quesadillas 176

Recipe 884: Greek Cod with Asparagus 177

Recipe 885: Greek Gyros with Chicken and Rice 177

Recipe 886: Greek Pita Pockets 177

Recipe 887: Green Strata 177

Recipe 888: Halibut Quesadillas 177

Recipe 889: Ham and Corn Muffins 177

Recipe 890: Healthy Broccoli Casserole 178

Recipe 891: Herbed Cheddar Cheese Frittata 178

Recipe 892: Herby Cheesy Nuts 178

Recipe 893: Herby Parmesan Pita 178

Recipe 894: Herby Prawn and Zucchini Bake 178

Recipe 895: Honey Oatmeal 178

Recipe 896: Italian Baked Chicken 179

Recipe 897: Italian Baked Grape Tomatoes 179

Recipe 898: Italian Baked Tofu 179

Recipe 899: Italian Chicken Pesto Bake 179

Recipe 900: Italian Sausage Rolls 179

Recipe 901: Italian Stuffed Bell Peppers 179

Recipe 902: Italian Style Stuffed Mushrooms 180

Recipe 903: Lamb Potato Chips Baked   180

Recipe 904: Lamb Tomato Bake   180

Recipe 905: Lava Cakes   180

Recipe 906: Lemon Mini Pies with Coconut   180

Recipe 907: Lemon Pies with Vanilla and Coconut   180

Recipe 908: Lemony Apple Butter   181

Recipe 909: Lentils and Dates Brownies   181

Recipe 910: Low Carb Peanut Butter Cookies   181

Recipe 911: Low Carb Snickerdoodle Cookies   181

Recipe 912: Luscious Triple Berry Cobbler   181

Recipe 913: Marble Cheesecake   181

Recipe 914: Margherita Pizza   182

Recipe 915: Marmalade-Almond Topped Brie   182

Recipe 916: Mascarpone Mushrooms   182

Recipe 917: Mascarpone Mushrooms with Pasta   182

Recipe 918: Matcha Granola   182

Recipe 919: Meatball and Cabbage Bake   182

Recipe 920: Mediterranean Granola   183

Recipe 921: Mini Molten Lava Cakes   183

Recipe 922: Mint Lamb with Roasted Hazelnuts   183

Recipe 923: Mixed Berry Dutch Baby Pancake   183

Recipe 924: Mixed Seed Crackers   183

Recipe 925: Mushroom and Turkey Bread Pizza   183

Recipe 926: Nordic Salmon Quiche   184

Recipe 927: Oat Muffins with Blueberries   184

Recipe 928: Onion Omelet   184

Recipe 929: Orange Chicken Rice   184

Recipe 930: Paprika Mushroom and Buckwheat Pilaf   184

Recipe 931: Parma Ham and Egg Toast Cups   185

Recipe 932: Parmesan Baked Chicken Breast   185

Recipe 933: Parmesan, Garlic, Lemon Roasted Zucchini   185

Recipe 934: Parmesan Sausage Egg Muffins   185

Recipe 935: Parsnip and Potato Bake   185

Recipe 936: Peach Cake   185

Recipe 937: Peach French Toast   186

Recipe 938: Peach Pie   186

Recipe 939: Peanut Butter-Chocolate Bread Pudding   186

Recipe 940: Pecorino Dill Muffins   186

Recipe 941: Pesto Chicken Bake   186

Recipe 942: Pesto Egg and Ham Sandwiches   186

Recipe 943: Pesto Pepperoni Pizza Bread   187

Recipe 944: Philly Cheese Steak Stuffed Peppers   187

Recipe 945: Pinto Bean Casserole   187

Recipe 946: Pistachio Crusted Salmon   187

Recipe 947: Pita and Pepperoni Pizza   187

Recipe 948: Pizza Puffs   187

Recipe 949: Plum Cake   188

Recipe 950: Potato Casserole   188

Recipe 951: Pumpkin Bread with Walnuts   188

Recipe 952: Pumpkin Cake   188

Recipe 953: Pumpkin Empanadas   188

Recipe 954: Pumpkin Pudding and Vanilla Wafers   188

Recipe 955: Quick Paella   189

Recipe 956: Rich Salmon Burgers with Broccoli Slaw   189

Recipe 957: Ricotta and Broccoli Cannelloni   189

Recipe 958: Rosemary Baked Cashews   189

Recipe 959: Russet Potatoes with Yogurt and Chives   189

Recipe 960: Salmon and Greek Yogurt Sauce   190

Recipe 961: Salmon Baked Cheese and Broccoli   190

Recipe 962: Sausage Frittata with Parmesan   190

Recipe 963: Scalloped Potatoes   190

Recipe 964: Sicilian-Style Vegetarian Pizza   190

Recipe 965: Simple Green Bake   190

Recipe 966: Smoked Salmon Croissant Sandwich   191

Recipe 967: Smooth Walnut-Banana Loaf   191

Recipe 968: Spaghetti Squash Lasagna   191

Recipe 969: Spicy Honey Orange Chicken   191

Recipe 970: Spicy Spinach Dip   191

Recipe 971: Spinach Frittata   191

Recipe 972: Sriracha Salmon Melt Sandwiches   192

Recipe 973: Strip Steak with Potatoes   192

Recipe 974: Stuffed Pepper   192

Recipe 975: Stuffed Tomatoes and Broccoli   192

Recipe 976: Sumptuous Turkey and Cauliflower Meatloaf   192

Recipe 977: Sweet Roasted Pumpkin Rounds   192

Recipe 978: Sweet Squares   193

Recipe 979: Sweety Blueberry Muffins   193

Recipe 980: Taco Crunch Wrap   193

Recipe 981: Taco Pie with Meatballs   193

Recipe 982: Tilapia Roast in Garlic and Olive Oil   193

Recipe 983: Tofu Scramble   193

Recipe 984: Tomato and Halloumi Bruschetta   194

Recipe 985: Tomato Mushroom Frittata   194

Recipe 986: Tri-Color Frittata   194

Recipe 987: Tuna Bake   194

Recipe 988: Tuna Melts with English Muffins   194

Recipe 989: Tuna Sandwiches   194

Recipe 990: Turkey and Leek Hamburger   195

Recipe 991: Turkey Cheese Taquitos   195

Recipe 992: Turkey, Mushroom and Egg Casserole   195

Recipe 993: Turkey Taco Casserole   195

Recipe 994: Tuscan Salmon   195

Recipe 995: Vegetarian Quinoa Cups   195

Recipe 996: Vietnamese Gingered Tofu   196

Recipe 997: Viking Toast   196

Recipe 998: Winter Vegetables with Herbs   196

Recipe 999: Yogurt Baked Potatoes   196

Recipe 1000: Zucchini Egg Bake   196

Recipe 1001: Zucchini Manicotti   196

INTRODUCTION

An Air Fryer is a straightforward machine used to fry foods without the use of oil. That's correct, and the machine eliminates the use of oil to fry foods and crisps up ingredients just with the help of a bit of water. Introduced in 2010, the machine has since made its way into millions of kitchens worldwide and is set to grow in popularity in the years to come. The device is easy to use and helps in making nutritious meals using minimal ingredients.

Most people might be thinking that Air Fryers are limited to cooking only, but in reality, it is a multipurpose device as it can fry, roast, grill, and bake delicious, mouth-watery meals. An Air Fryer utilizes "Rapid Air Technology" to cook food that usually requires submerged in a bottomless basket of fat or oil.

WHAT IS AN AIR FRYER?

An Air Fryer is a countertop appliance used to make food crispy on the outside and soft inside. Unlike a deep fryer, Air Fryers use little to no oil and hot air to "fry" food. Air Fryers allow you to enjoy all your favourite fried foods more healthily.

Instead of submerging your food in oil in a deep fryer, you place your food in a tray, basket or bowl inside the Air Fryer. The air is heated to a specific temperature and circulated the meal using fans. The hot air cooks the food quickly for a set time and heats the small amount of oil on the outside, giving it a crispy, fried texture.

Air Fryers are very convenient and easy to use. No time is wasted heating up cooking oil. You can prepare and put your ingredients in the Air Fryer, set the time and temperature, walk away and come back to a tasty fried snack or meal.

Deep-frying food with too much oil adds fat and unnecessary calories to your diet, leading to serious health issues, such as diabetes and obesity. Using very little oil to no oil in an Air Fryer significantly reduces the fat content of your meals. Air fried food will taste slightly different from deep-fried food as much less oil is used. Air fried food tastes like extra-crispy oven-baked food and, in many cases, will taste better. In this book, you will find recipes to help you find creative ways to enjoy fried foods, including meat, fish, and vegetables, to maintain a healthy diet.

Benefits of Using Air Fryers
- Uses little to no oil
- Reduced fat and calories
- Easy to set up and use
- Hands-free cooking
- Safe to use
- Multiple uses
- Easy to clean
- Efficient

WHICH AIR FRYER SHOULD YOU BUY?

Air Fryers have recently exploded in popularity and are quickly becoming a household appliance favourite. If you regularly enjoy fried foods, an Air Fryer is worth having. You can find Air Fryers from all the popular household kitchen appliance brands, varying in price. The cheapest models have the essential functions to manually set the time and temperature and usually have a smaller capacity. The price of an Air Fryer increases with the size and number of extra features. Premium innovative Air Fryers allow you to control the appliance with an app on your phone. Some Air Fryers consist of multiple compartments, giving you the extra space to cook significant cuts of meat or several meals at once.

All Air Fryers function in the same manner as a convection oven by circulating hot air. There are two main types of Air Fryers; Air Fryers with a tray or basket and Air Fryers with a bowl. The first type of Air Fryers includes a tray or basket, typically located in the back of the device that you add food to and slot in. The disadvantage with this type of Air Fryer is it does not allow you to check the progress of your food without pulling out the tray or basket, leading to longer cooking times. Air Fryers with a bowl typically have a viewing window in the lid so you can check on the food without interfering with the cooking process.

If you're looking for an Air Fryer, think about whether you'd benefit from one with a stirring paddle or a spinning basket. Having a paddle that automatically stirs your food saves you from having to stir or turn over the food yourself. This ensures your food is cooked evenly, although not necessary to cook your meal successfully.

Air Fryers are very versatile and can cook a range of meal types, including snacks and desserts. Some Air Fryers give you the option of grilling your food, which can come in handy for meat and fish recipes. Be sure also to check if your Air Fryer is dishwasher safe and wait for the Air Fryer to cool down before cleaning.

The most popular Air Fryers are 3 - 5 litres, well suited for families. A 3-litre Air Fryer is an excellent option if you don't have much counter space available. If you often entertain large numbers of people, a 6-10 litre Air Fryer will give you the capacity to cook more food in fewer batches. Review the size guide below to help you decide which size Air Fryer best suits your needs.

How Do You Use An Air Fryer?

Using an Air Fryer couldn't be easier. Once you have prepared your ingredients with little to no oil, add them to the tray, basket or bowl, load the food into the Air Fryer, set the temperature and time settings, and let the Air Fryer do the rest. Just like any oven, your Air Fryer may need a few minutes to preheat. When the Air Fryer reaches the desired temperature, the digital display will indicate ready to use.

Adding oil to the outside of your food will get you the crispy fried texture. Choose a healthy oil like olive oil, coconut oil or avocado oil. Be sure to spray the food out of the Air Fryer to prevent buildup in the appliance and ensure the food is evenly coated. You may want to add an extra layer of oil halfway through the cooking time to get the extra food crispy. Adding a piece of bread under your food is a simple way to soak up any grease.You mustn't overload your Air Fryer tray, basket or bowl. Giving the food enough space ensures it cooks evenly and thoroughly. To prepare more food, try cooking in batches. Many Air Fryers come with accessories that you can use, such as a grill rack, muffin tins, and fine mesh baskets. Whichever you use, be sure they fit comfortably in the Air Fryer compartment. Having a thermometer handy can help check if your meat has reached the right temperature. To ensure the successful preparation of air fried foods, follow the do's and don'ts listed below.

Air Fryer Dos and Don'ts

Do's
- Preheat your Air Fryer
- Use little to no oil
- Shake basket halfway through cooking time
- Spread food out in a single layer
- Use to reheat food
- Use parchment paper to avoid sticking
- Use a rack to keep lightweight foods down

Don'ts
- Overfill
- Clean whilst still hot
- Scratch non-stick surfaces
- Use higher temperatures to save time

CHAPTER 1: 501 RECIPES FOR FRY

RECIPE 1: AIR FRIED CALZONE

Serve: 4 | Total Time: 20 minutes

4 oz. cheddar cheese, grated.
1 oz. mozzarella cheese
1 oz. bacon, diced.
2 cups cooked and shredded turkey
1 egg, beaten

Pizza dough
4 tbsp. tomato paste
1 tsp. basil
1 tsp. oregano
Salt and pepper, to taste

Preheat your Air Fryer to temperature of 350 degrees F. Divide the pizza dough into 4 equal pieces so you have the dough for 4 small pizza crusts. Combine the tomato paste, basil and oregano in a small bowl. Brush the mixture onto the crusts, just make sure not to go all the way and avoid brushing near the edges on one half of each crust, place 1/2 turkey and season the meat with some salt and pepper. Top the meat with bacon. Divide mozzarella and cheddar cheeses between pizzas. Brush the edges with beaten egg. Fold the crust and seal with a fork. Cook for 10 minutes.

RECIPE 2: AIR FRIED CHICKEN TENDERS

Serve: 4 | Total Time: 20 minutes

1 ½ lb. chicken breasts, cut into strips.
1 cup seasoned breadcrumbs
1 egg, lightly beaten
½ tsp. dried oregano
Salt and ground black pepper
Cooking spray

Preheat your Air Fryer to temperature of 390 degrees F. Season the chicken with oregano, salt and pepper. Take a bowl and, add beaten egg. In a separate bowl, add the crumbs. Dip chicken tenders in the egg wash, then in the crumbs. Roll the strips in the breadcrumbs and press firmly so the breadcrumbs stick well. Spray the chicken tenders with cooking spray and arrange them on the Air Fryer. Cook for 14 minutes.

RECIPE 3: AIR FRIED CHURROS

Serve: 6 | Total Time: 25 minutes

¼ cup butter
½ cup milk
1 pinch salt
½ cup all-purpose flour
2 eggs
¼ cup white sugar
½ tsp ground cinnamon

Add butter to a saucepan and place it over medium-high heat to melt. Stir in salt and milk. Cook until the milk is boiled. Stir in flour and let it cook for 7 minutes with continuous stirring. Add eggs and mix well. Remove the hot frying pan and put it in the pastry bag. Pipe this dough into thick strips in the Air Fryer basket. Cook the churros for 5 minutes at 340 F. Meanwhile, mix cinnamon and sugar. Roll the churros in the cinnamon mixture. Serve.

RECIPE 4: AIR FRIED COOKIE BALLS

Serve: 6 | Total Time: 20 minutes

½ cup all-purpose flour
½ cup all-purpose flour
1 tbsp sugar
½ tbsp brown sugar
½ tsp baking powder
¼ tsp xanthan gum
1 egg, beaten
½ tbsp butter, melted
½ tsp vanilla extract
Pinch of cinnamon (optional)
3 tbsp mini sugar-free chocolate chips
Coconut oil, for frying

Mix all dry ingredients in a bowl. Whisk in egg, vanilla, and melted butter. Mix well until smooth dough forms then fold in chocolate chips. Roll the dough into a ball then refrigerate until Air Fryer is ready. Grease the Air Fryer's Basket with coconut oil and preheat the fryer to 375 F. Divide the dough into small cookie-sized balls and place them in the basket. Return the fryer basket to the Air Fryer and cook them for 3-5 minutes. Serve.

RECIPE 5: AIR FRIED CRAB HERB CROQUETTES

Serve: 6 | Total Time: 18 minutes

1 lb. crab meat
1 cup breadcrumbs
2 egg whites
Salt and black pepper to taste
½ tsp parsley, chopped
¼ tsp chives
¼ tsp tarragon
2 tbsp celeries, chopped
4 tbsp mayonnaise
4 tbsp light sour cream
1 tsp olive oil
½ tsp lime juice
½ cup red pepper, chopped
¼ cup onion, chopped

Preheat your Air Fryer to 355°Fahrenheit. Add breadcrumbs with salt and pepper in a bowl. In another small bowl add the egg whites. Add all the remaining ingredients into another bowl and mix well. Make croquettes from crab mixture and dip into egg whites, and then into breadcrumbs. Place into Air Fryer and cook for 18-minutes.

RECIPE 6: AIR-FRIED CRUMBED FISH

Serve: 4 | Total Time: 25 minutes

1 cup dry bread crumbs
4 flounder fillets
1 egg, beaten
¼ cup vegetable oil
1 lemon, sliced
Ensure that your Air Fryer is preheated to 355 F. Grab a clean bowl and mix the breadcrumbs and the oil in it. Stir until you have a

crumbly and loose mixture. Dip the fish fillets into the egg, and then into the bread crumb mixture. In either case, coat thoroughly and evenly. Place the coated fillets gently in the preheated Air Fryer. Allow cooking until the fish flakes easily with a fork (it takes about 12 minutes). Garnish with lemon slices and serve.

RECIPE 7: AIR FRIED OREOS

Serve: 9 | Total Time: 20 minutes

9 Oreo cookies
½ cup complete pancake mix
⅓ cup water
Cooking spray
1 tbsp confectioners' sugar, or to taste

Whisk pancake mix with water in a bowl until smooth. Layer the Air Fryer's Basket with parchment paper. Grease the parchment paper with cooking spray. Dip each Oreo cookie with the pancake mixture and place them in the prepared basket. Cook the coated Oreos in the Air Fryer at 400 F for 5 minutes. Flip the fried Oreos and cook for 3 minutes more. Drizzle confectioners' sugar over the fried Oreos. Serve fresh.

RECIPE 8: AIR FRIED RADISHES

Serve: 4 | Total Time: 20 minutes

1 pound (454 g) radishes
2 tbsp unsalted butter, melted
1/2 tsp garlic powder
1/2 tsp dried parsley
1/4 tsp dried oregano
1/4 tsp ground black pepper

Detach roots from radishes and cut into quarters. In a small bowl, attach butter and seasonings. Merge the radishes in the herb butter and place into the Air Fryer basket. Adjust the temperature to 350F (180C) and set the timer for 10 minutes. Halfway through the cooking time, merge the radishes in the Air Fryer basket. Serve warm.

RECIPE 9: AIR FRIED SHIRRED EGGS

Serve: 2 | Total Time: 20 minutes

4 slices of ham
4 eggs, divided
2 tbsp. heavy cream
3 tbsp. Parmesan cheese
2 tsp. chopped chives
2 tsp. butter, for greasing
¼ tsp. paprika
¾ tsp. salt
¼ tsp. pepper

Preheat your Air Fryer to temperature of 320 degrees F. Grease a pie pan with the butter. Arrange the ham slices on the bottom of the pan to cover it completely. In a small bowl, combine one egg, heavy cream, salt, and pepper. Pour the mixture over the ham slices. Crack the other eggs over the ham. Sprinkle with Parmesan cheese. Cook for 14 minutes. Season with paprika, garnish with chives and serve.

RECIPE 10: AIR FRIED SOURDOUGH SANDWICHES

Serve: 2 | Total Time: 25 minutes

2 slices ham
4 slices sourdough bread
2 lettuce leaves
1 tomato, sliced.
2 slices mozzarella cheese
2-tbsp. mayonnaise
Cooking spray
Salt and pepper to taste

On a clean board, lay the sourdough slices and spread with mayonnaise. Top 2 of the slices with ham, lettuce, tomato and mozzarella cheese. Season with salt and pepper. Top with the remaining two slices to form two sandwiches. Spray with oil and transfer to the Air Fryer. Cook for 14 minutes at 340 degrees F, flipping once halfway through cooking. Serve hot!

RECIPE 11: AIR-FRIED SPRING ONIONS

Serve: 20 | Total Time: 14 minutes

1 packet spring rolls
1 small onion, diced
3 garlic cloves, minced
1 cup fresh mixed vegetables
1 cup ground beef
2 tbsp hot water
1/3 cup noodles

Add the noodles into hot water. Once the noodles are soft, drain and slice into short lengths. Heat a pan over medium heat with oil. Add the ground beef, soy sauce, mixed vegetables, onion, and garlic. Stir and cook for 3-minutes or until meat is browned. Take the pan away from the heat and add the noodles. Mix well and set aside. Place stuffing on spring roll sheet diagonally across. Fold the sheet from top point, then fold both sides, and brush the last side with water before rolling roll. Repeat for rest of spring rolls and stuffing. Preheat your Air Fryer to 350°Fahrenheit. Brush prepared spring rolls with oil and place inside of Air Fryer. Cook for 8-minutes and serve.

RECIPE 12: AIR FRYER BEEF FAJITAS

Serve: 6 | Total Time: 25 minutes

Beef:
1/8 cup carne aside seasoning
2 pounds beef flap meat
Diet 7-Up

Fajita veggies:
1 tsp chili powder
1-2 tsp pepper
1-2 tsp salt
2 bell peppers, your choice of color
1 onion

Slice flap meat into manageable pieces and place into a bowl. Season meat with carne seasoning and pour diet soda over meat. Cover and chill overnight. Ensure your Air Fryer is preheated to 380 degrees. Place a parchment liner into Air Fryer basket and spray with olive oil. Place beef in layers into the basket. Cook 8-10 minutes. Remove and set to the side. Slice up veggies and spray Air Fryer basket. Add veggies to the fryer and spray with olive oil. Cook 10 minutes at 400 degrees, shaking 1-2 times during cooking process. Serve meat and veggies on wheat tortillas and top with favorite keto fillings!

RECIPE 13: AIR FRYER BROCCOLI AND TOFU SCRAMBLE

Serve: 3 | Total Time: 30 minutes

4 cups broccoli florets
1 block tofu, chopped finely
2 ½ cups red potatoes, chopped
2 tbsp olive oil
2 tbsp tamari
1 tsp turmeric powder
½ tsp garlic powder
½ tsp onion powder
½ cup onion, chopped

Preheat your Air Fryer to 400°Fahrenheit. Mix the potatoes in a bowl with half of the olive oil. Place the potatoes into a baking dish that will fit into your Air Fryer and cook them for 15-minutes. Combine the remaining olive oil, tofu, tamari, turmeric, garlic powder and onion powder. Stir in the chopped onions. Add the broccoli florets. Pour this mixture on top of the air-fried potatoes and cook for an additional 15-minutes. Serve warm.

RECIPE 14: AIR FRYER CHEESE AND BACON FRIES

Serve: 2 | Total Time: 35 minutes

2 medium potatoes, peeled
2 tsp olive oil
4 bacon rashers
Salt and ground black pepper to taste
1 oz cheddar cheese, grated

Ensure that your Air Fryer is preheated to 360 F. Dice the peeled potatoes and transfer them into the Air Fryer. Sprinkle a teaspoon of olive oil over them. Allow cooking

at 360 F for 10 minutes. Dice the fat-free bacon into bits, and add them to the cooked potatoes in the Air Fryer. Allow the combination to cook for another 5 minutes. Shake and add another teaspoon of olive oil. Resume cooking for another 2 minutes but at a higher temperature of 390 F. Withdraw and sprinkle with pepper, salt, and the grated cheese. Serve.

RECIPE 15: AIR FRYER EMPANADAS

Serve: 5 | Total Time: 20 minutes

1 pie crust, refrigerated
3 slices deli Swiss cheese, chopped into small pieces
1/4-pound deli ham, thinly sliced and cut into small pieces
3 small dill pickles, cut into small pieces
1 1/2 tbsp mustard

Preheat Air Fryer to 175°C. Cut 10 circles out of pie crust, and spread mustard onto each. Add a slice of ham, cheese, and pickles. Crease the empty end over to cover the fillings and pleat edges together with a fork. Grease Air Fryer container with cooking oil, place empanadas batters into the bin and splash again with cooking oil. Cook for 8 minutes, flipping part way through. Remove from Air Fryer and enjoy!

RECIPE 16: AIR FRYER FRIED PICKLES

Serve: 4 | Total Time: 20 minutes

1/2 cup crushed pork rinds
3 tbsp parmesan cheese, finely grated
16 sliced dill pickles
1/2 cup almond flour
1 large free-range egg, beaten
1 tsp olive oil

Preheat the Air Fryer to 370F. Mix the pork and parmesan properly in a shallow bowl. Whisk eggs together properly in another bowl. In another bowl, add the almond

flour. Dip the pickle in the almond flour, then the egg, then the pork and parmesan. Cook for 6 minutes. Serve and enjoy.

RECIPE 17: AIR FRYER PORK RIBS

Serve: 2 | Total Time: 27 minutes

1 lb. pork ribs
Salt and pepper to taste
½ cup BBQ sauce
1 tsp liquid Stevia
1 tsp spice mix
1 medium onion, chopped
1 tbsp olive oil

Warm the oil in a medium pan. Add onion to pan and sauté for 2-minutes. Add spice mix, stevia, and BBQ sauce into pan and stir well. Remove pan from heat and set aside. Season pork ribs with salt and pepper and place inside of Air Fryer basket. Air fry the ribs at 320°Fahrenheit for 10-minutes. Brush BBQ sauce on both sides of pork. Air fry pork for an additional 15-minutes, cut into slices and serve.

RECIPE 18: AIR FRYER SPINACH PAKORA

Serve: 4 | Total Time: 35 minutes

4 large handfuls spinach, chopped
1 Onion, chopped, 1 green chilies, chopped
3 small ginger, chopped
1/2 tbsp chickpea and rice flour
1/2 curry powder and salt
Water

Place spinach, onions, green chilies and ginger in a bowl, and include salt and chili powder. Add chickpea flour and rice flour and mix well. Include 1/2 cup water. Spray Air Fryer container with cooking oil and scoop the batter blend into the basket, without covering. Cook at 185°C for 6 to 7 minutes. Flip and press delicately with the back of a spoon. Cook for an additional 8 minutes and serve.

RECIPE 19: AJILLO MUSHROOMS

Serve: 4 | Total Time: 30 minutes

2/3 cup panko bread crumbs
1 cup cremini mushrooms
1/3 cup all-purpose flour
1 egg, beaten
½ tsp smoked paprika
3 garlic cloves, minced
Salt and pepper to taste

Preheat the Air Fryer to 400°F. Put the flour on a plate. Mix the egg and garlic in a shallow bowl. On a separate plate, combine the panko, smoked paprika, salt, and pepper and mix well. Cut the mushrooms through the stems into quarters. Dip the mushrooms in flour, then the egg, then in the panko mix. Press to coat, then put on a wire rack and set aside. Add the mushrooms to the frying basket in a single layer and spray with cooking oil. Air Fry for 6-8 minutes, flipping them once until crisp. Serve warm.

RECIPE 20: APPLE DUMPLINGS

Serve: 8 | Total Time: 40 minutes

2 tbsp sultana raisins
1 tbsp brown sugar
2 sheets puff pastry
2 small apples, peeled and cored
2 tbsp butter, melted

Ensure that your Air Fryer is preheated to 320 F. Apply some aluminum foil as lining for the Air Fryer basket. Get a clean bowl, and in it, combine the sultanas and brown sugar. On a clean work surface, place a soft pastry sheet and with the apple placed on the sheet, fill the core with the sultana mixture. Fold the pastry around the apple such that it is entirely covered. Do the same for the remaining filling, apple, and pastry. Transfer the dumplings into the already- prepared Air Fryer basket. Brush the dumplings with melted butter before cooking for 25 minutes or until you have soft, golden brown apples.

RECIPE 21: APPLE MAPLE CRISP

Serve: 4 | Total Time: 30 minutes

3 cups apples, chopped
1 tbsp pure maple syrup
2 tsp lemon juice
3 tbsp all-purpose flour, divided
1/3 cup quick oats
¼ cup brown sugar
2 tbsp light butter, melted
½ tsp cinnamon

Toss the chopped apples with 1 tbsp all-purpose flour, cinnamon, maple syrup, and lemon juice in a suitable bowl. Spread the apples in a baking dish and set it aside. Whisk oats, brown sugar, and remaining all-purpose flour in a small bowl. Stir in melted butter then spread this mixture over the apples. Return the fryer basket to the Air Fryer and cook for 20 minutes at 350 F. Enjoy fresh.

RECIPE 22: APPLE ROLLUPS

Serve: 2 | Total Time: 15 minutes

8 slices whole wheat sandwich bread
4 ounces Colby Jack cheese, grated
½ small apple, chopped
2 tbsp butter, melted

Remove crusts from bread and flatten the slices with rolling pin. Don't be gentle. Press hard so that bread will be very thin. Top bread slices with cheese and chopped apple, dividing the ingredients evenly. Roll up each slice tightly and secure each with one or two toothpicks. Brush outside of rolls with melted butter. Place in Air Fryer and cook at temperature of 390°F for 5minutes, until outside is crisp and nicely browned.

RECIPE 23: APRICOT GLAZED PORK TENDERLOINS

Serve: 2 | Total Time: 15 minutes

½ tsp salt
1/2 tsp pepper
1-lb pork tenderloin

2 tbsp minced fresh rosemary or 1 tbsp dried rosemary, crushed
2 tbsp olive oil, divided
4garlic cloves, minced

Apricot Glaze:
1 cup apricot
2 garlic cloves, minced
3 tbsp lemon juice

Garlic, oil, pepper, salt, rosemary Brush on pork. If necessary, cut pork in half crosswise. Grease the Air Fryer baking pan with cooking spray. Pork. Brown pork for 3 minutes each side in a 390F Air Fryer. In a small dish, combine all glaze ingredients. 5 min. basting pork. 20 minutes at 330F.

RECIPE 24: ARTICHOKE HEARTS

Serve: 2 | Total Time: 30 minutes

1 cup arrowroot flour (gluten free & easily digestible)
1 tbsp organic herb de provence
1-2 eggs
1 bag of frozen artichoke hearts
Cooking spray

Fill a clean basin with a cup of Arrowroot Flour and Herb de Provence. Mix well. Get another bowl and make an egg wash by whisking 1-2 eggs. Pick each artichoke and dip in the egg mixture before the flour mixture. Ensure generous coating in both instances, while avoiding the contamination of the egg wash by the excess flour mix from your hands. Ensure that our Air Fryer basket remains non-sticky by coating oil. Allow the chips to cook for 15 minutes under the chips feature. Flip the artichokes after about 7 minutes using your thongs.

RECIPE 25: ASIAN HALIBUT

Serve: 3 | Total Time: 40 minutes

1 pound halibut steaks
2/3 cup soy sauce
A ¼ cup of sugar
2 tbsp lime juice

½ cup mirin
¼ tsp red pepper flakes, crushed
A ¼ cup of orange juice
¼ tsp ginger, grated
1 garlic clove, minced
Put soy sauce in a pan, heat up over medium heat, add mirin, sugar, lime and orange juice, pepper flakes, ginger, and garlic, stir well, bring to a boil and take off the heat. Transfer half of the prepared marinade to a mixing bowl, add the halibut, toss to coat, and chill for 30 minutes. Transfer halibut to your Air Fryer and cook at 3900 F. for 10 minutes, flipping once. Divide halibut steaks on plates, drizzle the rest of the marinade all over and serve hot. Enjoy!

RECIPE 26: ASPARAGUS AND PARMESAN

Serve: 2 | Total Time: 16 minutes

1 tsp sesame oil
11 oz asparagus
1 tsp chicken stock
½ tsp ground white pepper
3 oz Parmesan

Wash the asparagus and chop it roughly. Sprinkle the chopped asparagus with the chicken stock and ground white pepper. Then sprinkle the vegetables with the sesame oil and shake them. Place the asparagus in the Air Fryer basket. Cook the vegetables for 4 minutes at 400 F. Meanwhile, shred Parmesan cheese. When the time is over – shake the asparagus gently and sprinkle with the shredded cheese. Cook the asparagus for 2 minutes more at 400 F. After this, transfer the cooked asparagus in the serving plates. Serve and taste it!

RECIPE 27: ASPARAGUS FRIES

Serve: 6 | Total Time: 25 minutes

1 large egg, beaten
1 tsp honey
½ cup Parmesan cheese, grated
1 cup panko bread crumbs

12 asparagus spears, trimmed
1 pinch cayenne pepper, optional
¼ cup Greek yogurt
¼ cup stone-ground mustard

Ensure that your Air Fryer is preheated to 400 F. Get a long, narrow dish, and in it combing egg and honey. Beat together and set aside. In a separate plate, combine the Parmesan cheese and panko. After coating each asparagus stalk in the egg mixture, roll it also in the panko mix and allow thorough coating. Arrange six spears in the Air Fryer and allow cooking to the desired brownness - this takes 4 to 6 minutes. Do the same for the other spears. In a small dish, combine cayenne, yogurt, and mustard. Serve the asparagus spears with the dipping sauce.

RECIPE 28: AVOCADO AND TURKEY ROLLS

Serve: 4 | Total Time: 28 minutes

1 pound (454 g) ground turkey
1 tbsp olive oil
1 avocado, peeled, pitted, and chopped
2 garlic cloves, minced
½ cup bread crumbs
salt and black pepper, to taste
8 small rolls
Mix the turkey, olive oil, avocado, garlic, bread crumbs, salt, and black pepper until everything is well combined. Form the mixture into eight small patties. Cook the patties at 380ºF (193ºC) for about 20 minutes or until cooked through; make sure to turn them over halfway through the cooking time. Serve your patties in the prepared rolls and enjoy!

RECIPE 29: AVOCADO SHRIMP

Serve: 4 | Total Time: 15 minutes

½ cup onion, chopped
2 lb. shrimp
1 tbsp. seasoned salt
1 avocado
½ cup pecans, chopped

Pre-heat the fryer at 400°F. Put the chopped onion in the basket of the fryer and spritz with some cooking spray. Leave to cook for five minutes. After adding the shrimp, set the timer for another five minutes. Sprinkle with some seasoned salt, then allow to cook for an additional five minutes. During these last five minutes, halve your avocado and remove the pit. Cube each half, then scoop out the flesh. Take care when removing the shrimp from the fryer. Place it on a dish and top with the avocado and the chopped pecans.

RECIPE 30: BACON AND BROWN SUGAR LITTLE SMOKIES

Serve: 4 | Total Time: 20 minutes

14 ounces of Little Smokies
2/3 ounce of Bacon
1/3 cup of Brown Sugar Substitute
Toothpicks

Cut Bacon tips into thirds, and put the brown sugar substitute into a shallow dish that is enough to fit the bacon thirds. Coat both of the sides of the bacon with the brown sugar substitute. Wrap one little smokie by a slice of brown sugar-coated bacon and pin it with a Toothpick. Repeat with the rest of the little smokies and then place them inside of the Air Fryer basket. Cook at about a heat of 350 °F for about 10 minutes until the bacon is crisped, flip halfway through the cooking process.

RECIPE 31: BACON AND CHEESE STUFFED CHICKEN

Serve: 4 | Total Time: 25 minutes

1 pound (454 g) chicken breasts
4 tbsp goat cheese
4 tbsp bacon
1 tbsp olive oil
½ tsp garlic powder
1 tsp dried basil
1 tsp dried oregano
1 tsp dried parsley flakes

Flatten the chicken breasts with a mallet. Stuff each piece of chicken with cheese and bacon. Roll them up and secure with toothpicks. Then, sprinkle the chicken with olive oil, garlic powder, basil, oregano, and parsley. Place the stuffed chicken breasts in the Air Fryer basket. Cook the chicken at 400°F (204°C) for about 20 minutes, turning them over halfway through the cooking time. Bon appétit!

RECIPE 32: BACON AND HAM BURGER PATTIES

Serve: 4 | Total Time: 18 minutes

1-lb. ground beef
1/4 cup deli ham, chopped.
1/4 green onions, chopped.
1/4 cup bacon, chopped.
3 tbsp. breadcrumbs
1 tsp. ground nutmeg
1 tsp. Italian seasoning
salt and pepper, to taste

Preheat the Air Fryer to temperature of 400 degrees F. Mix together the ground beef, chopped bacon and ham. In another bowl, mix together the breadcrumbs, ground nutmeg, Italian seasoning, green onions, salt and pepper. Add the meat mixture to the breadcrumbs mixture and knead well to combine. Divide into 4 equal portions and flatten them slightly to form patties. Using the Air Fryer Double Layer Rack, place the patties in the Air Fryer Basket. Cook for 8 minutes or until the meat is cooked through and browned. Serve and enjoy!

RECIPE 33: BACON BISCUITS

Serve: 6 | Total Time: 30 minutes

3 tbsp butter
4 tbsp heavy cream
1 tsp oregano
1 tbsp apple cider vinegar
1 cup almond flour
1/2 tsp baking soda
4 ounces bacon, cooked
1 egg

Start by whisking your eggs. Chop your bacon, adding it into your egg, sprinkling with apple cider vinegar and baking soda. Add in your oregano and heavy cream, stirring well. Add in your almond flour and butter next, and mix well. Once your batter is smooth, and then preheats your Air Fryer to 400. Pour your batter into muffin molds, and then cook for ten minutes. Allow them to cool to room temperature before serving.

RECIPE 34: BACON CASHEWS

Serve: 12 | Total Time: 15 minutes

3 cups raw cashews
2 tbsp blackstrap molasses
3 tbsp liquid smoke
2 tsp salt

In a large dish, combine all the ingredients and cover the cashews liberally and evenly. Transfer the coated cashews into the Air Fryer basket, and allow cooking for 8-10 minutes at 350 F. While cooking, shake the basket at intervals of 2 minutes - this ensures that the cashews cook evenly. Be extra careful at the last 2 minutes and shake/check consistently to avoid burning the cashews. Allow the cooked cashews to cool to room temperature - this takes about 15 minutes. Then transfer the cool cashews into an airtight storage container and serve.

RECIPE 35: BACON CHEESE SANDWICH

Serve: 2 | Total Time: 12 minutes

4 Whole Wheat bread slices
1 tbsp butter melted
2 slices mild cheddar cheese
6 slices cooked bacon
2 slices mozzarella cheese

Melt butter in a microwave-safe bowl by heating it for 15 seconds in the microwave. Spread the melted butter on one side of the bread slices and place 2 of these slices in the Air Fryer Basket with

their buttered side up. Place one slice of cheddar cheese, 3 cooked bacon slices and one slice of mozzarella cheese on top of each bread slice. Finally, stack the remaining bread pieces butter side down on top of the cheese layers. Return the fryer basket to the Air Fryer and cook for 4 minutes at 370 F. Flip the sandwiches and continue cooking for 3 minutes. Serve warm.

RECIPE 36: BACON EGG AND CHEESE EGGROLL

Serve: 4 | Total Time: 25 minutes

4 eggs
4 slices bacon
1/2 cup shredded cheddar cheese
5 egg roll wrappers

Firstly, fry the bacon until crispy and set aside. Drain the bacon fat, but leave a little left behind in the skillet. Using the bacon fat, scramble your eggs. Roll out your eggroll wrappers. In a separate bowl, crumble the bacon into tiny pieces, then mix in the eggs and the cheese. Scoop in equal amounts of the mixture to the center of each wrapper. Pull the bottom left corner of the wrapper over the mixture, then fold each side in. Wet the remaining edge and roll the eggroll shut. Preheat Air Fryer to 360°F and cook eggrolls for 10 minutes, turning midway.

RECIPE 37: BACON, LETTUCE, TEMPEH AND TOMATO SANDWICHES

Serve: 4 | Total Time: 5 minutes

8-ounce package tempeh
1 cup warm vegetable broth
Tomato slices and lettuce, to serve
¼ tsp chipotle chili powder
½ tsp garlic powder
½ tsp onion powder
1 tsp Liquid smoke
3 tbsp soy sauce

Begin by opening the packet of tempeh and slice into pieces about

¼ inch thick. Grab a medium bowl and add the remaining ingredients except for lettuce and tomato and stir well. Place the pieces of tempeh onto a baking tray that will fit into your Air Fryer and pour over the flavor mix. Put the tray in Air Fryer and cook for 5-minutes at 360°Fahrenheit. Remove from Air Fryer and place on sliced bread with the tomato and lettuce and any other extra toppings you desire.

RECIPE 38: BACON LETTUCE WRAPS

Serve: 4 | Total Time: 50 minutes

8 ounces (227 g) (about 12 slices) reduced-sodium bacon
8 tbsp mayonnaise
8 large romaine lettuce leaves
4 Roma tomatoes, sliced
Salt and freshly ground black pepper
Set the bacon in a single layer in the Air Fryer basket. (It's OK if the bacon sits a bit on the sides.) Set the Air Fryer to 350F (180C) and cook for 10 minutes. Check for crispiness and cook for 2 to 3 minutes longer if needed. Cook in batches, if necessary, and drain the grease in between batches. Scatter 1 tablespoon of mayonnaise on each of the lettuce leaves and top with the tomatoes and cooked bacon. Flavor to taste with salt and freshly ground black pepper. Roll the lettuce leaves as you would a burrito, securing with a toothpick if desired.

RECIPE 39: BACON OMELET

Serve: 6 | Total Time: 13 minutes

6 eggs
1 tsp butter
4-ounces bacon
1 tbsp dill, dried
½ tsp salt
½ tsp turmeric
¼ cup almond milk

In a bowl, whisk eggs, then add the almond milk. Add the turmeric,

dried dill, salt and mix well. Slice the bacon. Preheat your Air Fryer to 360°Fahrenheit and place the bacon in the Air Fryer basket tray. Cook the bacon for 5-minutes. Turn the bacon over and pour the egg mixture on top of it. Cook the omelet for 8-minutes. When the omelet is cooked, transfer it to a plate and slice into servings. Serve warm.

RECIPE 40: BACON WINGS

Serve: 12 | Total Time: 85 minutes

12 bacon strips
1 tsp. paprika
1 tbsp. black pepper
1 tsp. oregano
12 chicken wings
1 tbsp. Kosher salt
1 tbsp. brown sugar
1 tsp. chili powder
Celery sticks
Blue cheese dressing

Preheat the Air Fryer at 325 degrees Fahrenheit. Mix sugar, salt, chili powder, oregano, pepper, and paprika. Coat chicken wings with this dry rub. Wrap a bacon strip around each wing. Arrange wrapped wings in the Air Fryer basket. Cook for thirty minutes on each side in the Air Fryer. Let cool for five minutes. Serve and enjoy with celery and blue cheese.

RECIPE 41: BACON WRAPPED BRIE

Serve: 8 | Total Time: 15 minutes

4 slices of sugar-free bacon
1 (8-ounce) round Brie

Put two slices of bacon to form an X. Then place the third slice of bacon parallel across the center of the X. Place the fourth slice of bacon straight up across the X. Then it should look like a plus sign (+) on top of an X. Position the Brie in the middle of the bacon. Wrap the bacon around the Brie, locking with a few toothpicks. Torn a piece of parchment to fit your Air Fryer basket and place the

bacon-wrapped Brie on top. Put it inside the basket of the Air Fryer. Alter the temperature to 400°F, then change the timer for 10 minutes. When 3 minutes keep on the timer, cautiously flip Brie. When cooked, bacon will be crunchy, and cheese will be soft and melty. When serving it, cut into eight slices.

RECIPE 42: BACON WRAPPED CHICKEN

Serve: 2 | Total Time: 25 minutes

1 pound chicken tender, skinless and boneless
4-6 bacon stripes
4 tbsp brown sugar
½ tsp chili powder

In the large bowl mix brown sugar and chili powder. Cut chicken tenders into 2-inch pieces. Wrap chicken pieces into bacon strips and toss with sugar mixture. Preheat the Air Fryer to 390-400°F. Place wrapped chicken into the Fryer and cook for about 10-15 minutes depending on the size of the chicken. Replace the meal from the cooking basket and enjoy crispy bacon and tender, juicy chicken. You may use dipping sauce you prefer.

RECIPE 43: BACON WRAPPED FILET MIGNON

Serve: 2 | Total Time: 25 minutes

2 bacon slices
2 (4-ounce) filet mignon
Salt and ground black pepper, as required
Olive oil cooking spray

Wrap 1 bacon slice around each filet mignon and secure with toothpicks. Season the filets with the salt and black pepper lightly. Arrange the filet mignon onto a coking rack and spray with cooking spray. Place the drip pan in the cooking chamber of the Instant Vortex plus Air Fryer Oven. Choose the "Air Fry" and set the temperature to 375 degrees Fahrenheit. After setting the timer for 15 minutes, press the "Start" button. Place the frying rack in the middle position when the display says "Add Food." Turn the filets when the display says "Turn Food." When cooking time is complete, remove the rack from Vortex and serve hot.

RECIPE 44: BACON WRAPPED HOT DOGS

Serve: 4 | Total Time: 25 minutes

4 strips thick-cut bacon
4 beef hot dogs
4 hot dog buns, slightly toasted

Wrap a piece/slice of bacon around each hot dog, gently overlapping the edges of the bacon. Set aside. Select the Broil function on the Air Fryer, fix the time to 20 minutes, then press Start/Cancel to preheat. Line the food tray with foil, then set the wire rack on top of the food tray. Place the bacon-wrapped hot dogs on the wire rack, then insert the rack and food tray at top position in the preheated Air Fryer toaster oven. Press Start/Cancel. Flip the hot dogs halfway through cooking. Remove when done and place each hot dog in a hot dog bun. Serve with your choice of toppings.

RECIPE 45: BACON WRAPPED SCALLOPS

Serve: 9 | Total Time: 15 minutes

½ cup mayonnaise
2 tbsp Sriracha sauce
1 lb bay scallops
1 pinch coarse salt
1 pinch black pepper
12 slices bacon, cut into thirds
1 serving olive oil cooking spray

Thoroughly mix mayonnaise and Sriracha sauce together in a small bowl. Refrigerate Sriracha mayo in a bowl covered. Preheat your Air Fryer machine to 390 F. Place the scallops onto a plate and blot them

dry with a paper towel. Gently rub them with black pepper and salt for seasoning. Now wrap each scallop with 1/3 slice of bacon and insert a toothpick to secure the wrap. Grease the Air Fryer's basket with cooking spray. Place the wrapped scallops in the basket in a single layer; add them in batches. Cook each batch in the Air Fryer for 7 minutes approximately. Serve warm.

RECIPE 46: BACON WRAPPED STUFFED CHICKEN

Serve: 4 | Total Time: 30 minutes

4 chicken breast fillets
4 slices sharp cheese slices
1/4 cup cream cheese
12 rashers bacon

Preheat the Air Fryer to temperature of 350 degrees F. Slice the chicken fillets almost all the way to the end but leave half an inch uncut. Pound the breasts lightly until flattened. Season with salt and pepper. Place a slice of cheese and a dollop of cream cheese on each chicken. Roll the chicken and wrap each chicken breast with 3 rashers of bacon. Use a toothpick to secure the bacon and chicken in place. Arrange them in the Air Fryer Basket and use the Air Fryer Double Layer Rack if needed. Cook for about at least 15 minutes or until the bacon is golden brown and the chicken is cooked through. Serve and enjoy!

RECIPE 47: BAGEL CHIPS

Serve: 2 | Total Time: 4 minutes

Sweet:
1 large plain bagel
2 teaspoons sugar
1 teaspoon ground cinnamon
butter-flavored cooking spray

Savory:
1 large plain bagel
1 teaspoon Italian seasoning
½ teaspoon garlic powder
oil for misting or cooking spray

Preheat Air Fryer to 390°F. Cut bagel into ¼-inch slices or thinner. Mix the seasonings together. Spread out the slices, mist with oil or cooking spray, and sprinkle with half of the seasonings. Turn over and repeat to coat the other side with oil or cooking spray and seasonings. Place in Air Fryer basket and cook for 2minutes. Shake basket or stir a little and continue cooking for 2 minutes or until toasty brown and crispy.

RECIPE 48: BALSAMIC BEEF AND VEGGIE SKEWERS

Serve: 4 | Total Time: 25 minutes

2 tbsp balsamic vinegar
2 tsp olive oil
½ tsp dried oregano
Salt and pepper to taste
¾ lb round steak, cubed
1 red bell pepper, sliced
1 yellow bell pepper, sliced
1 cup cherry tomatoes

Preheat Air Fryer to 390°F. Put the balsamic vinegar, olive oil, oregano, salt, and black pepper in a bowl and stir. Toss the steak in and allow to marinate for 10 minutes. Poke 8 metal skewers through the beef, bell peppers, and cherry tomatoes, alternating ingredients as you go. Place the skewers in the Air Fryer and Air Fry for 5-7 minutes, turning once until the beef is golden and cooked through and the veggies are tender. Serve and enjoy!

RECIPE 49: BALSAMIC CAPRESE HASSELBACK

Serve: 4 | Total Time: 15 minutes

4 tomatoes
12 fresh basil leaves
1 ball fresh mozzarella
Salt and pepper to taste
1 tbsp olive oil
2 tsp balsamic vinegar
1 tbsp basil, torn

Preheat Air Fryer to 325°F. Remove the bottoms from the

tomatoes to create a flat surface. Make 4 even slices on each tomato, 3/4 of the way down. Slice the mozzarella and the cut into 12 pieces. Stuff 1 basil leaf and a piece of mozzarella into each slice. Sprinkle with salt and pepper. Place the stuffed tomatoes in the frying basket and Air Fry for 3 minutes. Transfer to a large serving plate. Drizzle with olive oil and balsamic vinegar and scatter the basil over. Serve and enjoy!

RECIPE 50: BALSAMIC SALMON

Serve: 2 | Total Time: 13 minutes

2 salmon fillets
1 cup of water
2 tbsp balsamic vinegar
1 1/2 tbsp honey
Salt and Pepper

Season salmon with pepper and salt. Mix together vinegar and honey. Brush fish fillets with vinegar honey mixture. Transfer water into the fryer then place trivet into the basket. Place fish fillets on top of the trivet. Seal fryer and cook on manual high pressure for 3 minutes. As soon as the cooking is done, release pressure using the quick-release method then open the lid. Garnish with parsley and serve.

RECIPE 51: BANANA BEIGNETS

Serve: 6 | Total Time: 8 minutes

1 cup almond flour
1/3 tsp nutmeg, freshly grated
½ tsp lemon juice
3 eggs
½ tbsp baking powder
2 tbsp Truvia for baking
1 tsp ground cloves
1/3 cup milk
1 ½ large-sized over-ripe bananas, peeled and sliced
½ tsp lemon peel, grated
A pinch of turmeric

In a bowl, drizzle banana slices with lemon juice. In another bowl,

combine the dry ingredients. In the second bowl, combine all the wet ingredients. Add the wet mixture to the dry and combine well. Dip each banana slice into the batter. Air-fry for 8-minutes at 335°Fahrenheit working in batches.

RECIPE 52: BANANA CHIPS

Serve: 3 | Total Time: 35 minutes

3-4 raw bananas
½ tsp salt
½ tsp turmeric powder
1 tsp oil
½ tsp chaat masala

After peeling the bananas, keep them. Combine salt, turmeric powder, and water, and in this mixture, cut the bananas into slices. This ensures that the banana doesn't turn black and retains its nice yellow color. Retain the banana slices in the mixture for about 5 to 10 minutes. Withdraw the chips from the mixture and dry. Then add some oil on the chips - this ensures that they do not stick while in the Air Fryer. Ensure that your Air Fryer is preheated to 360 F for 5 minutes. Place the chips in the Air Fryer basket and allow air frying for 15 minutes at 360 F. Add chat masala and salt. Keep the chips in an airtight jar, and serve instantly.

RECIPE 53: BARBECUE DRUMSTICKS

Serve: 2 | Total Time: 45 minutes

4 chicken drumsticks
½ tbsp mustard
1 clove garlic, crushed
1 tsp chili powder
2 tsp brown sugar
1 tbsp olive oil
freshly ground black pepper

Preheat the Air Fryer to 390F. Mix the garlic with the brown sugar, mustard, pinch of salt, freshly ground pepper, chili powder and the oil. Rub the drumsticks with the marinade and allow to marinate

for at least 20 minutes. Put the drumsticks in the Air Fryer basket and set the timer to 10 minutes. Then lower the temperature to 300F and roast the drumsticks for another 10 minutes until done. Serve with French bread and corn salad.

RECIPE 54: BARBEQUE CHICKEN WINGS

Serve: 4 | Total Time: 25 minutes

2 tbsp honey
Salt and ground black pepper to taste
BBQ chicken seasoning
1 tbsp olive oil
1 lb chicken wings

Get a clean bowl and in it, mix the honey, salt, pepper, BBQ chicken seasoning, and the olive oil. Using the BBQ mixture, brush the chicken wings generously. Ensure that your Air Fryer is preheated to 400 F. Transfer the chicken wings into the Air Fryer, while maintaining a single layer. Allow frying for 18 minutes, while turning the wings after 9 minutes. Withdraw when both sides are fried. Serve.

RECIPE 55: BASIL COD CROQUETTES

Serve: 4 | Total Time: 20 minutes

1 ½ cups bread crumbs
1 egg, beaten
2 tbsp lemon juice
2/3 lb cooked cod, chopped
2 green onions, chopped
½ tsp dried basil
Salt and pepper to taste
2 tbsp olive oil

Preheat Air Fryer to 390°F. Mix together ½ cup bread crumbs, egg, and lemon juice in a bowl. Then add the chopped cod, green onions, basil, salt, and pepper. Set aside. In a shallow plate, combine the 1 cup of bread crumbs and olive oil until well mixed. Take the cod mixture and form 1½-inch round, compact balls. Roll the croquettes into the bread crumb mixture. Place the croquettes into the frying basket, without overcrowding and Air Fry until brown and crisp, 6-8 minutes. Serve.

RECIPE 56: BASIL GREEN LENTIL BALLS

Serve: 6 | Total Time: 20 minutes

½ cup cooked green lentils
2 garlic cloves, minced
¼ white onion, minced
¼ cup parsley leaves
5 basil leaves
1 cup cooked millet
1 tbsp lime juice
1 tbsp olive oil
½ tsp salt

Preheat Air Fryer to 380°F. Blitz the cooked lentils with the garlic, onion, parsley, and basil in your food processor until mostly smooth. Transfer the lentil mixture into a large bowl, and stir in millet, lime juice, olive oil, and salt. Stir until well combined. Form the lentil mixture into balls. Arrange the rice balls in a single layer in the frying basket. Air Fry for 10-12 minutes, turning once until the balls are browned on all sides. Serve and enjoy!

RECIPE 57: BASS FILLET IN COCONUT SAUCE

Serve: 4 | Total Time: 35 minutes

¼ cup of coconut milk
½ pound bass fillet
1 tbsp olive oil
2 tbsp jalapeno, chopped
2 tbsp lime juice, freshly squeezed
3 tbsp parsley, chopped
Salt and pepper to taste

Preheat the Air Fryer for 5 minutes. Season the bass with salt and pepper to taste. Brush the surface with olive oil. Place in the Air Fryer and cook for 15 minutes at 3500F. Meanwhile, place in a saucepan, the coconut milk, lime juice, jalapeno, and parsley. Heat

over medium flame. Serve the fish with coconut sauce.

RECIPE 58: BAVARIAN BRATWURST WITH SAUERKRAUT

Serve: 4 | Total Time: 30 minutes

1 lb pork bratwurst, pierced with a fork
1 (12-oz) bottle lager beer
½ onion, sliced
2 cups drained sauerkraut
2 bay leaves
2 tbsp ketchup

Place bratwurst, beer, onion, bay leaves and 2 cups of water in a saucepan over high heat and bring it to a boil. Low the heat to and simmer for 15 minutes. Drain. Preheat Air Fryer at 400ºF. Place cooked bratwurst and onions in the greased frying basket and Air Fry for 3 minutes. Turn bratwurst, add in sauerkraut and cook for 3 more minutes. Serve with ketchup on the side.

RECIPE 59: BEEF AND BROCCOLI

Serve: 4 | Total Time: 20 minutes

1 minced garlic clove
1 sliced ginger root
1 tbsp. olive oil
1 tsp. almond flour
1 tsp. sweetener of choice
1 tsp. low-sodium soy sauce
1/3 C. sherry
2tsp. sesame oil
1/3 C. oyster sauce
1 pounds of broccoli
3/4 pound round steak

Remove stems from broccoli and slice into florets. Slice steak into thin strips. Combine sweetener, soy sauce, sherry, almond flour, sesame oil, and oyster sauce together, stirring till sweetener dissolves. Put strips of steak into the mixture and allow to marinate 45 minutes to 2 hours. Add broccoli and marinated steak to Air Fryer. Place garlic, ginger, and olive oil on top. Cook 12 minutes

at 400 degrees. Serve with cauliflower rice!

RECIPE 60: BEEF AND SPINACH SAUTEE

Serve: 4 | Total Time: 30 minutes

2 tomatoes, chopped
2 tbsp crumbled Goat cheese
½ lb ground beef
1 shallot, chopped
2 garlic cloves, minced
2 cups baby spinach
2 tbsp lemon juice
1/3 cup beef broth

Preheat Air Fryer to 370°F. Crumble the beef in a baking pan and place it in the Air Fryer. Air Fry for 3-7 minutes, stirring once. Drain the meat and make sure it's browned. Toss in the tomatoes, shallot, and garlic and Air Fry for an additional 4-8 minutes until soft. Toss in the spinach, lemon juice, and beef broth and cook for 2-4 minutes until the spinach wilts. Top with goat cheese and serve.

RECIPE 61: BEEF BURGERS

Serve: 4 | Total Time: 10 minutes

1 lb. ground beef
1 tsp parsley, dried
½ tsp oregano, dried
½ tsp ground black pepper
½ tsp salt
½ tsp onion powder
½ tsp garlic powder
1 tbsp Worcestershire sauce
Olive oil cooking spray

In a mixing bowl, mix the seasonings. Add the seasoning to beef in a bowl. Mix well to combine. Divide the beef into four patties, put an indent in the middle of patties with your thumb to prevent patties from bunching up in the middle. Place burgers into the Air Fryer and spray the tops with olive oil. Cook for 10-minutes at 400°Fahrenheit; no need to flip patties. Serve on a bun with a side dish of your choice.

RECIPE 62: BEEF CHEESEBURGERS

Serve: 4 | Total Time: 30 minutes

1 lb ground beef
Salt, to taste
2 cloves garlic, minced
1 tbsp low-sodium soy sauce
Black pepper, to taste
4 slices American cheese
4 hamburger buns
Mayonnaise, to serve
Lettuce, to serve
Sliced tomatoes, to serve
Thinly sliced red onion, to serve

Mix beef with soy sauce, and garlic in a large bowl. Make 4 patties of 4 inches of diameter. Rub them with salt and black pepper on both sides. Place the prepared patties in the Air Fryer basket and cook for 4 minutes at 375 F, then flip the half-cooked patties and cook for another 4. For small-sized Air Fryers, cook the patties in batches. Add each patty in the hamburger buns along with mayo, tomatoes, onions, and lettuce. Serve.

RECIPE 63: BEEF FAJITAS

Serve: 2 | Total Time: 15 minutes

8 oz sliced mushrooms
½ onion, cut into half-moons
1 tbsp olive oil
Salt and pepper to taste
1 strip steak
½ tsp smoked paprika
½ tsp fajita seasoning
2 tbsp corn

Preheat Air Fryer to 400°F. Combine the olive oil, onion, and salt in a bowl. Add the mushrooms and toss to coat. Spread in the frying basket. Sprinkle steak with salt, paprika, fajita seasoning and black pepper. Place steak on top of the mushroom mixture and Air Fry for 9 minutes, flipping steak once. Let rest onto a cutting board for 5 minutes before cutting in half. Divide steak, mushrooms, corn, and onions between 2 plates and serve.

RECIPE 64: BEEF FILLET WITH GARLIC MAYO

Serve: 8 | Total Time: 50 minutes

3 lb. beef fillet
1 cup mayonnaise
4 tbsp. Dijon mustard
1/3 cup sour cream
1/4 cup chopped tarragon
2 tbsp. chopped chives
2 cloves garlic (minced)
Salt and black pepper, to taste

Preheat the Air Fryer to 3700F. Season beef using salt and pepper, transfer to the Air Fryer, and cook for 20 minutes. Remove and set aside. In a bowl, whisk the mustard and tarragon. Add the beef and toss, return to the Air Fryer and cook for 20 minutes. In a separate bowl, mix the garlic, sour cream, mayonnaise, chives, salt, and pepper. Whisk and set aside. Serve the beef with the garlic-mayo spread.

RECIPE 65: BEEF LUMPIA

Serve: 10 | Total Time: 22 minutes

1 tbsp olive oil
1 pound ground beef
Salt and pepper, to taste
1 tbsp garlic, minced
¼ cup onions, diced
½ cup carrots, diced
½ cup potatoes, shredded
Soy sauce
20 lumpia wrappers
1 egg, whisked

Prepare a pan with olive oil and ground meat. Stir fry for a few minutes, then add salt and pepper. Stir sauté garlic, onions, carrots, potatoes, and soy sauce. Stir fry until cooked, then set aside. Preheat Air Fryer at 390ºF. While the Air Fryer is heating up, lay out your lumpia wrappers and add a tablespoon of the stuffing near one corner. Roll up halfway up, fold the corners, then seal with the whisked egg. Place the lumpia in one layer into the Air Fryer, then cook for 12 minutes at 390ºF.

RECIPE 66: BEEF MEATBALLS

Serve: 4 | Total Time: 85 minutes

1 lb. ground beef
1/4 cup carrots, finely chopped.
1/2 cup onions, finely chopped.
1/2 cup breadcrumbs
1 egg
2 tbsp. chives, chopped.
2 tbsp. garlic, minced.
2 tbsp. fresh parsley, chopped.
1 tbsp. soy sauce
1 tsp. paprika

In a large bowl, mix in the ground beef, onions, carrots and garlic. Add in the paprika, soy sauce, parsley and chives. Add the egg with the breadcrumbs and knead well to combine. Form meatballs of your desired size and chill for an hour. Preheat the Air Fryer to temperature of 350 degrees F. Arrange the meatballs in the Air Fryer Basket. Prepare the meatballs as directed. Serve and enjoy!

RECIPE 67: BEEF ROLL-UP

Serve: 4 | Total Time: 15 minutes

2 lbs beef flank steak
Salt and pepper to taste
¾ cup baby spinach, fresh
3 oz red bell peppers, roasted
6 slices provolone cheese
3 tbsp Pesto

Open the steak and spread the pesto evenly over the meat. Layer the cheese, roasted red peppers and spinach ¾ of the way down the meat. Roll up and secure with toothpicks. Season with sea salt and pepper. Preheat Air Fryer to 400°Fahrenheit. Place the roll-ups in the fry basket and into the Air Fryer and cook it for 14-minutes. Halfway through the cooking time, rotate the meat. When cook time is completed, allow the meat to rest for 10-minutes before cutting and serving.

RECIPE 68: BEEF ROLLS

Serve: 4 | Total Time: 24 minutes

2 lbs beef steak, opened and flattened with a meat tenderizer
Salt and black pepper to the taste
3 oz red bell pepper, roasted and chopped
6 slices provolone cheese
3 tbsp pesto

Arrange flattened beef steak on a cutting board, spread pesto all over, add cheese in a single layer, add bell peppers, salt and pepper to the taste. Roll your steak, secure with toothpicks, season again with salt and pepper, place roll in your Air Fryer's basket and cook at 400 degrees F for 14 minutes, rotating roll halfway. Leave aside to cool down, cut into 2-inch smaller rolls, arrange on a platter and serve them as an appetizer. Enjoy!

RECIPE 69: BEEF STRIP WITH SNOW PEA AND MUSHROOMS

Serve: 2 | Total Time: 30 minutes

2 beef steaks (cut into strips)
2 tbsp. soy sauce
7 oz. snow pea
1 medium yellow onion (cut into rings)
1 tbsp. olive oil
8 oz. white mushroom (cut into halves)
Salt and black pepper to taste

Preheat the Air Fryer to 3500F. Pour the olive oil and soy sauce, into a bowl then whisk. Toss in the beef strip to coat. In a separate bowl, mix the mushroom, snow pea, onions, salt, and pepper. Transfer the contents in the bowl to a pan and fit it into the Air Fryer. Set the timer for about 16 minutes and start cooking. Turn up the Air Fryer's temperature to 4000F, add the beef strip, and cook for another 6 minutes. Serve.

RECIPE 70: BEETS CHIPS

Serve: 4 | Total Time: 22 minutes

4 beets, washed

2 tsp coconut oil
1/4 tsp salt

Preheat the Air Fryer toaster oven to 175 ° C. Place one basket on the Air Fryer toaster oven. Peel the beets into thin strips with a vegetable peeler. Put in a large bowl. Spray coconut oil on the beet strips and stir to cover. Season with salt; throw it again. Spread the beets in a layer on 2 baking sheets so that they do not overlap. Place one baking sheet on the top basket. Bake the beets in the preheated oven for 6 minutes, change the racks and continue cooking until the beets are crispy, another 6 minutes. Cool the chips before serving until they are cold enough.

RECIPE 71: BLACK BEANS AND QUINOA

Serve: 4 | Total Time: 50 minutes

1/3 cup of hot sauce
1 cup of cooked quinoa
1 tsp oil
1 onion
1 tsp garlic powder
1 tsp pepper
1 potato
½ tsp cumin
½ tsp oregano
½ cup of potatoes
1 green pepper
1 red pepper
6 oz of cooked black beans

Preheat the Air Fryer to 390F. Cut potatoes in the pieces. Mix with oil and cook in the Air Fryer for 20 minutes. Then chop pepper and onion and put in the bowl. Add beans and mix together. After that add cooked quinoa, pepper, salt, cumin, oregano, chopped potatoes and mix everything well. Cook for 10 minutes more at the same temperature. Then cover with sauce and cook for 5 minutes. Serve hot with tortillas.

RECIPE 72: BLACK COD WITH GRAPES, PECANS, FENNEL AND KALE

Serve: 2 | Total Time: 15 minutes

2 fillets black cod (8-ounces)
3 cups kale, minced
2 tsp white balsamic vinegar
½ cup pecans
1 cup grapes, halved
1 small bulb fennel, cut into inch-thick slices
4 tbsp extra-virgin olive oil
Salt and black pepper to taste

Preheat your Air Fryer to 400°Fahrenheit. Use salt and pepper to season your fish fillets. Drizzle with 1 teaspoon of olive oil. Place the fish inside of Air Fryer with the skin side down and cook for 10-minutes. Take the fish out and cover loosely with aluminum foil. Combine fennel, pecans, and grapes. Pour 2 tablespoons of olive oil and season with salt and pepper. Add to the Air Fryer basket. Cook for an additional 5-minutes. In a bowl combine minced kale and cooked grapes, fennel and pecans. Cover ingredients with balsamic vinegar and remaining 1 tablespoon of olive oil. Toss gently. Serve fish with sauce and enjoy!

RECIPE 73: BOW TIE PASTA CHIPS

Serve: 2 | Total Time: 35 minutes

2 cups whole wheat bow tie pasta
1 tbsp olive oil
1 tbsp nutritional yeast
1 1/2 tsp Italian Seasoning mix
1/2 tsp salt

Cook and boil the pasta for ½ of the cooking time, as mentioned on the package. Once cooked, drain this pasta and mix with the olive oil, nutritional yeast, Italian seasoning, and salt in a suitable. Spread about half of the pasta in the Air Fryer's Basket. Air fry it for 5 minutes at 390 F. Shake the fryer basket and cook for another 5 minutes. Cook the remaining pasta in the same manner as the first batch. And serve.

RECIPE 74: BRAISED LAMB SHANKS

Serve: 4 | Total Time: 30 minutes

4 lamb shanks
1 ½ tsp salt
½ tsp black pepper
4 garlic cloves, crushed
2 tbsp olive oil
4 to 6 sprigs fresh rosemary
3 cups beef broth, divided
2 tbsp balsamic vinegar

Place the sham shanks in a baking pan. Whisk rest of the ingredients in a bowl and pour over the shanks. Place these shanks in the Air Fryer basket. Press "Power Button" of Air Fry Oven and turn the dial to select the "Air Fry" mode. Press the Time button and again turn the dial to set the cooking time to 20 minutes. To adjust the temperature to 360 degrees F, press the Temp button and move the dial. Place the Air frying basket in the oven and shut the lid after it has been warmed. Slice and serve warm.

RECIPE 75: BREADED ARTICHOKE HEARTS

Serve: 2 | Total Time: 25 minutes

1 can artichoke hearts in water, drained
1 egg
¼ cup bread crumbs
¼ tsp salt
¼ tsp hot paprika
½ lemon
¼ cup garlic aioli

Preheat Air Fryer to 380°F. In a bowl, whisk the egg and 1 tbsp water. Mix together the bread crumbs, salt, and hot paprika in a separate bowl. Dip the artichoke hearts into the egg mixture, then coat in the bread crumb mixture. Put the artichoke hearts in a single layer in the frying basket. Air Fry for 15 minutes. Pour fresh lemon juice over the artichokes and serve. Serve with garlic aioli.

RECIPE 76: BREADED FLOUNDER

Serve: 3 | Total Time: 27 minutes

1 egg
1 cup dry breadcrumbs
1/4 cup vegetable oil
3 (6-oz.) flounder fillets
1 lemon, sliced

In a bowl, beat the egg In another bowl, attach the breadcrumbs and oil and merge until crumbly mixture is formed. Dip flounder fillets into the beaten egg and then, coat with the breadcrumb mixture. Choose "Power Button" of Air Fry Oven and turn the dial to select the "Air Fry" mode. Choose the Time button and again turn the dial to set the cooking time to 12 minutes. Now press the Temp button and rotate the dial to set the temperature at 356 degrees F. Press "Start/Pause" button to start. When the unit beeps to show that it is preheated, open the lid. Arrange the flounder fillets in greased "Air Fry Basket" and insert in the oven. Season with the lemon slices and serve hot.

RECIPE 77: BREADED MUSHROOMS

Serve: 4 | Total Time: 55 minutes

1 lb. small Button mushrooms, cleaned
2 cups breadcrumbs
2 eggs, beaten
Salt and pepper to taste
2 cups Parmigiano Reggiano cheese, grated

Prepare an Air Fryer by preheating it to 360 degrees. Pour the breadcrumbs in a bowl, add salt and pepper and mix well. Pour the cheese in a separate bowl and set aside. Dip each mushroom in the eggs, then in the crumbs, and then in the cheese. Slide out the fryer basket and add 6 to 10 mushrooms. Cook them for 20 minutes, in batches, if needed. Serve with cheese dip.

RECIPE 78: BREADED PARMESAN PERCH

Serve: 5 | Total Time: 15 minutes

¼ cup grated Parmesan
½ tsp salt
¼ tsp paprika
1 tbsp chopped dill
1 tsp dried thyme
2 tsp Dijon mustard
2 tbsp bread crumbs
4 ocean perch fillets
1 lemon, quartered
2 tbsp chopped cilantro

Preheat Air Fryer to 400°F. Combine salt, paprika, pepper, dill, mustard, thyme, Parmesan, and bread crumbs in a wide bowl. Coat all sides of the fillets in the breading, then transfer to the greased frying basket. Air Fry for 8 minutes until outside is golden and the inside is cooked through. Garnish with lemon wedges and sprinkle with cilantro. Serve and enjoy!

RECIPE 79: BREADED SHRIMP WITH LEMON

Serve: 3 | Total Time: 29 minutes

½ cup plain flour
2 egg whites
1 cup breadcrumbs
1-pound large shrimp, peeled and deveined
Salt and ground black pepper, as required
¼ tsp lemon zest
¼ tsp cayenne pepper
¼ tsp red pepper flakes, crushed
2 tbsp vegetable oil

Preheat the Air Fryer to 400 o F and grease an Air Fryer basket. Mix flour, salt, and black pepper in a shallow bowl. In another dish, combine the breadcrumbs, lime zest, and spices. Coat each shrimp with the flour, dip into egg whites and finally, dredge in the breadcrumbs. Drizzle the shrimp evenly with olive oil and arrange half of the coated shrimps into the Air Fryer basket. Cook for about 7 minutes and dish out the coated shrimps onto serving plates. Repeat with the remaining mixture and serve hot.

RECIPE 80: BREAKFAST BEEF CHILI

Serve: 4 | Total Time: 10 minutes

8 oz ground beef
½ yellow onion, diced
1 tsp tomato puree
6 oz cheddar cheese, shredded
1 tsp parsley, dried
1 tsp cilantro, dried
1 tsp oregano, dried
1 tbsp dill weed
1 tsp mustard
1 tbsp butter

Combine ground beef with diced onion in a bowl. Sprinkle the mixture with tomato puree, cilantro, parsley, oregano and dried dill. Then add the butter and mustard and mix well. Preheat your Air Fryer to 380°Fahrenheit. Add ground beef mixture to Air Fryer basket tray and cook the chili for 9-minutes. After about 6-minutes of cooking stir the chili. When the chili is cooked, sprinkle the top with shredded cheddar cheese and stir carefully. Transfer chili mixture into serving bowls. Serve warm.

RECIPE 81: BREAKFAST BUNS

Serve: 4 | Total Time: 60 minutes

2 tsp. baking powder
1 cup, Greek- yogurt, nonfat, plain
¾ tsp. cinnamon
1 egg white/whole egg beaten
1 cup, flour, all purpose, unbleached, whole/ gluten free
2 tbsp. raw sugar
½ tsp. kosher salt
3 tbsp. raisins
Icing (reserve half)
1 tsp. water/milk
1/4 powdered sugar

Prepare the icing by whisking together the milk and powdered sugar. Pour the smooth mixture into a Ziploc bag. Set the Air Fryer

at 325 degrees Fahrenheit to preheat. Cook the iced rolls in the Air Fryer for eleven to twelve minutes. Let cool. Trim off the tip of the icing bag. Pipe the icing onto the rolls' surfaces in your desired pattern. (Reserve the remaining icing for another recipe.)

RECIPE 82: BREAKFAST CHERRY AND ALMOND BARS

Serve: 8 | Total Time: 17 minutes

2 cups old-fashioned oats
½ cup quinoa, cooked
½ cup chia seeds
½ cup prunes, pureed
¼ tsp salt
2 tsp liquid Stevia
¾ cup almond butter
½ cup dried cherries, chopped
½ cup almonds, sliced

Preheat your Air Fryer to 375°Fahrenheit. In a large mixing bowl, add quinoa, chia seeds, oats, cherries, almonds. In a saucepan over medium heat melt almond butter, liquid Stevia and coconut oil for 2-minutes and stir to combine. Add salt and prunes and mix well. Pour into baking dish that will fit inside of your Air Fryer and cook for 15-minutes. Allow to cool for an hour once cook time is completed, then slice the bars and serve.

RECIPE 83: BREAKFAST CHICKEN HASH

Serve: 3 | Total Time: 14 minutes

6-ounces of cauliflower, chopped
7-ounce chicken fillet
1 tbsp water
1 green pepper, chopped
½ yellow onion, diced
1 tsp ground black pepper
3 tbsp butter
1 tbsp cream

Chop the cauliflower and place into the blender and blend it carefully until you get cauliflower rice. Chop the chicken fillet into

small pieces. Sprinkle the chicken fillet with ground black pepper and stir. Preheat your Air Fryer to 380°Fahrenheit. Dice the yellow onion and chop the green pepper. In a large mixing bowl, combine ingredients, then add mixture to fryer basket. Then cook and serve chicken hash warm!

RECIPE 84: BREAKFAST COCONUT PORRIDGE

Serve: 4 | Total Time: 7 minutes

1 cup coconut milk
3 tbsp blackberries
2 tbsp walnuts
1 tsp butter
1 tsp ground cinnamon
5 tbsp chia seeds
3 tbsp coconut flakes
¼ tsp salt

Pour the coconut milk into the Air Fryer basket tray. Add the coconut, salt, chia seeds, ground cinnamon, and butter. Ground up the walnuts and add them to the Air Fryer basket tray. Sprinkle the mixture with salt. Mash the blackberries with a fork and add them also to the Air Fryer basket tray. Cook the porridge at 375°Fahrenheit for 7-minutes. After cooking, remove the Air Fryer basket and let it rest for 5 minutes. Stir porridge with a wooden spoon and serve warm.

RECIPE 85: BREAKFAST COD NUGGETS

Serve: 4 | Total Time: 10 minutes

1 lb. of cod

For breading:
2 eggs, beaten
2 tbsp olive oil
1 cup almond flour
¾ cup breadcrumbs
1 tsp dried parsley
Pinch of sea salt
½ tsp black pepper

Preheat the Air Fryer to 390°Fahrenheit. Cut the cod into strips about 1-inch by 2-inches in length. Blend breadcrumbs, olive oil, salt, parsley and pepper in a food processor. In three separate bowls add breadcrumbs, eggs, and flour. Place each piece of fish into flour, then the eggs and lastly the breadcrumbs. Add pieces of cod to Air Fryer basket and cook for 10-minutes. Serve warm.

RECIPE 86: BREAKFAST GRANOLA

Serve: 6 | Total Time: 10 minutes

1 ½ cups rolled oats
½ cup pecans, chopped
½ cup raisins, divided
2 tbsp. butter, melted
3 tbsp. honey
Salt to taste

Put oats, pecans, sunflower seeds and half of the raisins in a bowl. Mix well. Add butter and honey and blend well. Cover your Air Fryer basket with foil. Preheat your Air Fryer to temperature of 350 degrees F. Cook mixture for three minutes. Cook for two more minutes or until golden, after stirring. Pour in a serving tray. Garnish with the other half of the raisins, let cool, and serve.

RECIPE 87: BREAKFAST LIVER PATE

Serve: 7 | Total Time: 10 minutes

1 lb. chicken liver
1 tsp salt
½ tsp cilantro, dried
1 yellow onion, diced
1 tsp ground black pepper
1 cup water
4 tbsp butter

Chop the chicken liver roughly and place it in the Air Fryer basket tray. Add water to Air Fryer basket tray and add diced onion. Preheat your Air Fryer to 360°Fahrenheit and cook chicken liver for 10-minutes. When it is finished cooking, drain the chicken liver. Transfer the chicken liver to blender, add butter, ground black pepper and dried cilantro and

blend. Once you get a pate texture, transfer to liver pate bowl and serve immediately or keep in the fridge for later.

RECIPE 88: BREAKFAST MEATLOAF SLICES

Serve: 6 | Total Time: 20 minutes

8 oz ground pork
7 oz ground beef
1 tsp olive oil
1 tsp butter
1 tbsp oregano, dried
1 tsp cayenne pepper
1 tsp salt
1 tbsp chives
1 tbsp almond flour
1 egg
1 onion, diced

Beat egg in a bowl. Add the ground beef and ground pork. Add the chives, almond flour, cayenne pepper, salt, dried oregano, and butter. Add diced onion to ground beef mixture. Use hands to shape a meatloaf mixture. Preheat the Air Fryer to 350°Fahrenheit. Place the meatloaf in the Air Fryer basket after spraying the interior with olive oil. Cook the meatloaf for 20-minutes. When the meatloaf has cooked, allow it to chill for a bit. Slice and serve it.

RECIPE 89: BREAKFAST MUSHROOM CAKES

Serve: 8 | Total Time: 28 minutes

35 oz mushrooms, chopped
1 small yellow onion, chopped
Salt and black pepper to the taste
¼ tsp nutmeg, ground
2 tbsp olive oil
1 tbsp breadcrumbs
14 oz coconut milk

Heat up a pan with half of the oil over medium-high heat, add onion and mushrooms, stir and cook for 3 minutes. Add coconut milk. salt, pepper and nutmeg, stir, take off heat and leave aside for 2 hours. In a bowl, mix the rest of the oil with breadcrumbs and stir well. Take 1

tablespoon mushroom filling, roll in breadcrumbs and put them in your Air Fryer's basket. Repeat with the rest of the mushroom mix and cook cakes at 400 degrees F for 8 minutes. Divide mushroom cakes between plates and serve them for breakfast. Enjoy!

RECIPE 90: BREAKFAST POTATOES

Serve: 4 | Total Time: 35 minutes

2 russet potatoes
1 red bell pepper
1 white onion
Cooking spray
Salt and pepper to taste

Cut the potatoes into 1-inch small cubes. Put them in the basket, spray with cooking spray, and sprinkle with a little salt and pepper. Cook the potatoes at 400 °F for 10 minutes, shaking once at the halfway point. While the potatoes cook, dice up the peppers and onions into small cubes. Mix in the onions and peppers with the potatoes. Season with salt and pepper. Cook at 400 °F for another 15 minutes, shaking a few times and checking to ensure that the potatoes aren't being overcooked.

RECIPE 91: BREAKFAST SAUSAGE CASSEROLE

Serve: 8 | Total Time: 25 minutes

1/4 cup diced white onion
1 diced green bell pepper
1 lb ground sausage
8 whole eggs, beaten
½ cup shredded Colby jack cheese
½ tsp garlic salt
1 tsp fennel seed
Cooking spray

Sauté sausage ground in a skillet greased with cooking spray, until brown. Stir in bell pepper, and onion then sauté until soft. Grease an 8 ½ inches pan with cooking spray and spread the sautéed sausage mixture in it. Beat eggs with garlic salt in a bowl and pour over the sausage layer: drizzle fennel seeds and jack cheese on top. Place the prepared pan in the Air Fryer and cook for 15 minutes at 390 F. Once done, remove the casserole from the Air Fryer. Slice and serve.

RECIPE 92: BREAKFAST TUNA AND BACON

Serve: 4 | Total Time: 10 minutes

6-ounces bacon, sliced
1 tsp butter
4-ounces parmesan cheese, shredded
1 tsp cream
6-ounces tuna
½ tsp ground black pepper
¼ tsp turmeric
¼ tsp sea salt

Place bacon inside of four ramekins. Add a small amount of butter in each ramekin. Mix the sea salt, turmeric, and ground black pepper. Combine chopped tuna with spice mix. Place some tuna mix into each ramekin on top of bacon. Add the cream and shredded cheese on top of tuna mix. Preheat your Air Fryer to 360°Fahrenheit. Put the tuna boards into the Air Fryer basket and cook for 10-minutes. When the tuna boards are done cooking, they will have a sweet, crunchy taste with a light brown color to them. Serve hot!

RECIPE 93: BROCCOLI CASSEROLE

Serve: 4 | Total Time: 29 minutes

4 cups steamed broccoli florets (about 1 large head), chopped
1/4 cup peeled diced yellow onion
1/2 cup diced white mushrooms
1 large egg
2 tbsp sour cream
1/4 cup mayonnaise
1tsp salt
1/2 tsp freshly ground black pepper
1 cup coarsely crushed Cheddar cheese crisps

In a large bowl, combine broccoli, onion, mushrooms, egg, sour cream, mayonnaise, salt, and

pepper. Spoon mixture into a round cake barrel. Preheat Air Fryer at temperature of 350°F for 3 minutes. Cook casserole 14 minutes. Remove barrel from Air Fryer and let rest 10 minutes. Evenly distribute crushed Cheddar Cheese crisps over the top of casserole and serve warm.

RECIPE 94: BROCCOLI CHEESE QUICHE

Serve: 4 | Total Time: 50 minutes

1 large broccoli
3 large carrots
1 large tomato
3 ½ oz cheddar cheese grated
¼ oz feta cheese
½ cup milk
1 tsp parsley
1 tsp thyme
2 eggs, large
Salt and black pepper, to taste

Cut the broccoli into small florets. Set a cooking pot filled with water over medium-high heat and place the steamer basket over it. Place broccoli and carrots in the steamer and cook for only 20 minutes, then remove them from the steamer—beat eggs with milk and seasonings in a bowl. Add broccoli and carrots to the egg mixture then mix well. Layer the cheese on top of the mixture in the baking pan. Place the prepared pan in the Air Fryer basket and return the fryer basket to the Air Fryer. Cook for 20 minutes at 325 F. Serve warm.

RECIPE 95: BROCCOLI HASH

Serve: 2 | Total Time: 38 minutes

10 oz. mushrooms
1 broccoli head
1 garlic clove
1 tbsp. balsamic vinegar
1 yellow onion
1 tbsp. olive oil
Salt and black pepper
1 tbsp. dried basil
1 avocado
A pinch of red pepper flakes

Mix in mushrooms with onion, garlic, broccoli and avocado in a bowl. Mix in oil, salt, pepper, vinegar and basil and beat properly. Get this over veggies. Toss to coat, leave for 30 minutes. Put into Air Fryer's basket and then cook at 350 F for 8 minutes, Share in plates. Serve with pepper flakes over.

RECIPE 96: BROCCOLI PESTO WITH QUINOA

Serve: 4 | Total Time: 30 minutes

1 cup of quinoa
2 cups of water
5 cups of broccoli
1 tbsp basil
½ tsp salt
½ tsp pepper
¼ cup of cream
2 tbsp lemon juice
¼ cup of oil
2/3 cup of almonds
4 garlic cloves
1 cup of cheese, grated

Cook the quinoa in 2 glasses of water until it is tender. When it is ready, place it in the bowl. Then add broccoli and blend the products well. After that, put salt, pepper, chopped basil, almonds, cloves of garlic and blend the components well. Sprinkle the Air Fryer with oil. Then preheat it to 350F. Cook for 10 minutes. Then shake everything, add cream, lemon juice and cheese. Cook for 5 minutes more. Enjoy with the meal.

RECIPE 97: BROCCOLI STUFFED PEPPERS

Serve: 2 | Total Time: 50 minutes

4 eggs
1/2 cup cheddar cheese, grated
2 bell peppers cut in half and remove seeds
1/2 tsp garlic powder
1 tsp dried thyme
1/4 cup feta cheese, crumbled
1/2 cup broccoli, cooked
1/4 tsp pepper

1/2 tsp salt

Preheat the Air Fryer to 325 F. Stuff feta and broccoli into the bell peppers halved. Beat egg in a bowl with seasoning and pour egg mixture into the pepper halved over feta and broccoli. Place bell pepper halved into the Air Fryer basket and cook for 35-40 minutes. Top with grated cheddar cheese and cook until cheese melted. Serve and enjoy.

RECIPE 98: BROCCOLI WITH CHEESE SAUCE

Serve: 4 | Total Time: 30 minutes

6 cups broccoli florets
Cooking spray
10 tbsp low-fat evaporated milk
1 1/2 oz queso fresco, crumbled
4 tsp Amarillo paste
6 lower-sodium saltine crackers

Place half of the broccoli florets in the Air Fryer Basket, spray them with cooking spray and cook them for 8 minutes at 375 F until crispy. Cook the remaining broccoli florets in the same way. Meanwhile, add evaporated milk, Amarillo paste, saltines, and queso fresco in a blender. Press the pulse button to blend for 45 seconds until smooth. Pour this sauce in a microwave-safe bowl and heat for 30 seconds in the microwave. Pour this sauce on top of the roasted broccoli. Serve.

RECIPE 99: BROWN SUGAR GLAZED SALMON

Serve: 3 | Total Time: 27 minutes

3 salmon filets
1 tbsp brown sugar
2 tbsp coconut oil, melted
A pinch of salt and pepper

Preheat the Airfryer to 360 degrees F. Combine the coconut oil with the brown sugar and salt and pepper in a medium sized bowl. Place the salmon fillets in the bowl. Cover with the glaze. Pour the mixture over the salmon with a spoon taking care not to cut up the salmon in the process. Put the glazed salmon in the Airfryer. Cook for about 15 minutes, checking progress from 12 minutes on. Serve with your choice of vegetable fries and salad.

RECIPE 100: BRUSSELS SPROUT SALAD WITH PANCETTA

Serve: 4 | Total Time: 50 minutes

2/3 pound Brussels sprouts
1 tbsp olive oil
salt and ground black pepper, to taste
2ounces baby arugula
1 shallot, thinly sliced
4 ounces pancetta, chopped

Lemon Vinaigrette:
2 tbsp extra virgin olive oil
2 tbsp fresh lemon juice
1 tbsp honey
1 tsp Dijon mustard

Start by preheating your Air Fryer to temperature of 380 degrees F. Add the Brussels sprouts to the cooking basket. Brush with olive oil and cook for 15 minutes. Let it cool to room temperature about 15 minutes. Toss the Brussels sprouts with the salt, black pepper, baby arugula, and shallot. Mix all ingredients for the dressing. Then, dress your salad, garnish with pancetta, and serve well chilled. Bon appétit!

RECIPE 101: BUFFALO CAULIFLOWER

Serve: 4 | Total Time: 15 minutes

2 cups Cauliflower Florets
1 cup Panko Breadcrumbs
1 tsp Sea Salt
¼ cup Vegan Butter, melted
¼ cup Vegan Buffalo Sauce

Melt the vegan butter in a bowl. Add buffalo sauce into the butter and stir. Hold the stem and dip each floret into the buffalo mixture, making sure most floret is coated with sauce. Shake off the excess. Mix sea salt with breadcrumbs and coat the dipped floret evenly with it. Place the floret into the Air Fryer and cook for 10 minutes at 350°F. After 5 minutes, shake the florets, making sure they are evenly cooked. Once done, serve and enjoy.

RECIPE 102: BUFFALO CHICKEN STRIPS

Serve: 3 | Total Time: 25 minutes

1 egg
¼ cup flour
¾ cup breadcrumbs
Salt and pepper, to taste
12 oz. chicken breast strips
Buffalo sauce

Place the egg, flour, and breadcrumbs into separate bowls for dredging. You may add the salt and pepper to the breadcrumbs bowl. Then, dip a piece of chicken into the flour bowl, then the egg bowl, and finally the breadcrumbs basin. Cooking spray the bottom of the Air Fryer and drop the chicken pieces inside. Mist the strips with some more cooking spray, then fry at 375°F (≈190°C) for 10 minutes. Flip and cook for 3-5 minutes until flesh is no longer pink. Remove the strips and place in a mixing bowl, adding the buffalo sauce. Mix until well-coated, then serve.

RECIPE 103: BUFFALO RANCH CHICKPEAS

Serve: 2 | Total Time: 45 minutes

1 (15 oz) can chickpeas, drained and rinsed
2 tbsp Buffalo wing sauce
1 tbsp dry ranch dressing mix

Ensure that your Air Fryer is preheated to 350 F. After lining your baking sheet with paper towels, spread the chickpeas over the lined paper towels. Cover the chickpeas with another layer of paper towels, and press gently to drain any excess moisture. Pour the wing sauce over the chickpeas. Stir the mixture to combine. Add ranch dressing powder and mix well to combine. Arrange the Air Fryer in an even layer in the Air Fryer basket. Allow cooking for 8 minutes. Stop, shake, and cook for an extra 5 minutes, shake again, and cook for 5 minutes more, and shake again for the last time, before cooking for the final 2 minutes. Set aside the cooked chickpeas for about 5 minutes to allow cooling. Serve immediately.

RECIPE 104: BUTTERMILK CHICKEN

Serve: 4 | Total Time: 18 minutes

2 lbs. chicken thighs
2 tsp black pepper
1 tsp salt
1 tbsp garlic powder
1 tsp cayenne pepper
1 tbsp baking powder
2 cups almond flour
2 cups buttermilk
1 tbsp paprika

Rinse the chicken thighs then pat dry. Add black pepper, paprika, and salt in a bowl. Toss the chicken pieces in paprika mixture. Pour buttermilk over chicken until coated. Place in the fridge for about 6-hours. Preheat your Air Fryer to 355°Fahrenheit. Use a different bowl to mix flour, baking powder, salt, garlic powder and black pepper. Coat chicken thighs in seasoned flour. Remove any excess flour then place on a plate. Arrange the chicken in one layer on fryer basket and place basket inside Air Fryer and cook for 8-minutes. Pull out the tray and turn chicken pieces over and cook for an additional 10-minutes.

RECIPE 105: CABBAGE AND SWEET POTATOES

Serve: 2 | Total Time: 23 minutes

1/8 cup carrots, diced.
1/4 cup celery, chopped.
1 cup sweet potatoes, diced.
1/4 cup onions, finely chopped.
1/4 head red cabbage, chopped.
4 rashers bacon, chopped.
1 tbsp. fresh parsley, finely chopped.
1 tbsp. garlic, minced.
1 tbsp. button mushrooms, minced.
½ tsp. ground allspice
½ tsp. garlic powder

Preheat the Air Fryer to temperature of 350 degrees F. Place the bacon in the Air Fryer Baking Pan and place the Air Fryer Baking Pan in the Air Fryer Basket. Cook for 10 minutes or until the bacon is crispy. Add the onions, red cabbage, sweet potatoes, minced garlic, carrots, celery and mushrooms. Mix well with the garlic powder and ground allspice. Cook for another 8 minutes. Remove from the Air Fryer and top with the fresh parsley. Serve and enjoy!

RECIPE 106: CAJUN CHEESE STICKS

Serve: 4 | Total Time: 20 minutes

1/2 cup all-purpose flour
2 eggs
1/2 cup parmesan cheese, grated
1 tablespoon Cajun seasonings
8 cheese sticks, kid-friendly

To begin, set up your breading station. Place the all-purpose flour in a dish. In a separate dish, whisk the eggs. Finally, mix the parmesan cheese and Cajun seasoning in a third dish. Start by dredging the cheese sticks in the flour; then, dip them into the egg. Press the cheese sticks into the parmesan mixture, coating evenly. Place the breaded cheese sticks in the lightly greased Air Fryer basket. Cook with settings at 380 degrees F for 6 minutes. Serve with ketchup and enjoy!

RECIPE 107: CAJUN CHICKEN KEBABS

Serve: 4 | Total Time: 30 minutes

3 tbsp lemon juice
2 tsp olive oil
2 tbsp chopped parsley
½ tsp dried oregano
½ Cajun seasoning
1 lb chicken breasts, cubed
1 cup cherry tomatoes
1 zucchini, cubed

Preheat Air Fryer to 400°F. Combine the lemon juice, olive oil, parsley, oregano, and Cajun seasoning in a bowl. Toss in the chicken and stir, making sure all pieces are coated. Allow to marinate for 10 minutes. Take 8 bamboo skewers and poke the chicken, tomatoes, and zucchini, alternating the pieces. Use a brush to put more marinade on them, then lay them in the Air Fryer. Air Fry the kebabs for 15 minutes, turning once, or until the chicken is cooked through, with no pink showing. Get rid of the leftover marinade. Serve and enjoy!

RECIPE 108: CAJUN CHICKEN LIVERS

Serve: 2 | Total Time: 45 minutes

1 lb chicken livers, rinsed, connective tissue discarded
1 cup whole milk
½ cup cornmeal
3/4 cup flour
1 tsp salt and black pepper
1 tsp Cajun seasoning
2 eggs
1 ½ cups bread crumbs
1 tbsp olive oil
2 tbsp chopped parsley

Pat chicken livers dry with paper towels, then transfer them to a small bowl and pour in the milk and black pepper. Let sit covered in the fridge for 2 hours. Preheat Air Fryer at 375ºF. In a bowl, combine cornmeal, flour, salt, and Cajun seasoning. In another bowl, beat the eggs, and in a third bowl, add bread crumbs. Dip chicken livers first in the cornmeal mixture, then in the egg, and finally in the bread crumbs. Place chicken livers in the greased frying basket, brush the tops lightly with olive oil, and Air Fry for 16 minutes, turning once. Serve right away sprinkled with parsley.

RECIPE 109: CAJUN FLOUNDER FILLETS

Serve: 2 | Total Time: 5 minutes

2 4-ounce skinless flounder fillet(s)
2 tsp Peanut oil
1 tsp Purchased or homemade Cajun dried seasoning blend

Preheat the Air Fryer to 400°F. Oil the fillet(s) by drizzling on the peanut oil, then gently rubbing in the oil with your clean, dry fingers. Sprinkle the seasoning blend evenly over both sides of the fillet(s). When the machine is at temperature, set the fillet(s) in the basket. If working with more than one fillet, they should not touch, although they may be quite close together, depending on the basket's size. Air-fry undisturbed for 5 minutes, or until lightly browned and cooked through. Use a nonstick-safe spatula to transfer the fillets to a serving platter or plate(s). Serve at once.

RECIPE 110: CARAMEL APPLE CRISPS

Serve: 2 | Total Time: 25 minutes

1/4 cup caster sugar
4 apples; peeled, cored and sliced thinly
1/4 cup caramel discs, melted.
2 tsp. ground cinnamon

Preheat the Air Fryer to temperature of 350 degrees F. Place the apples in the Air Fryer Basket and spray lightly with cooking spray. Cook for about at least 15 minutes or until the apples are crisp. Shake the Air Fryer Basket halfway through the cooking time to allow the apples to cook evenly. In a bowl, combine sugar and cinnamon. Remove the apples from the Air Fryer and coat evenly with the cinnamon and

sugar mixture. Drizzle over with the melted caramel. Serve and enjoy!

RECIPE 111: CARIBBEAN JERK COD FILLETS

Serve: 2 | Total Time: 20 minutes

¼ cup chopped cooked shrimp
¼ cup diced mango
1 tomato, diced
2 tbsp diced red onion
1 tbsp chopped parsley
¼ tsp ginger powder
2 tsp lime juice
Salt and pepper to taste
2 (6-oz) cod fillets
2 tsp Jerk seasoning

In a bowl, combine the shrimp, mango, tomato, red onion, parsley, ginger powder, lime juice, salt, and black pepper. Let chill the salsa in the fridge until ready to use. Preheat Air Fryer to 350°F. Sprinkle cod fillets with Jerk seasoning. Place them in the greased frying basket and Air Fry for 10 minutes or until the cod is opaque and flakes easily with a fork. Divide between 2 medium plates. Serve topped with the Caribbean salsa.

RECIPE 112: CAULIFLOWER BUFFALO BITES

Serve: 3 | Total Time: 25 minutes

1 large head cauliflower, cut into florets
1 tbsp olive oil
2 tsp garlic powder
½ cup Buffalo Style sauce or other hot sauce
1 tbsp melted butter
¼ tsp salt
¼ tsp ground pepper

Cut cauliflower into bite-sized florets. Place cauliflower florets into large plastic bag add olive oil, garlic powder, salt, and pepper. Close bag and toss ingredients and make sure all florets coated. Preheat the Air Fryer to 400°F. Place coated florets to the cooking

basket and cook for 15 minutes, turning once during cooking. Remove cauliflower from the fryer. Add the spicy sauce to the melted butter. Toss florets and cover all of them with this mixture. Return to the Air Fryer for another 5 minutes of cooking. Serve warm with any sauce you prefer, for example, blue cheese dip or sour cream.

RECIPE 113: CAULIFLOWER BURGER

Serve: 4 | Total Time: 35 minutes

3 large eggs
3 cups cauliflower florets
½ cup almond flour
3 tbsp coconut flour
1 tsp coconut oil, melted
½ tsp garlic powder
½ tsp turmeric
½ tsp parsley
Salt and black pepper to taste
Cooking oil spray

Preheat your Air Fryer machine to 375 F. Add cauliflower to a food processor and chop it finely. Toss cauliflower rice with coconut flour, turmeric, parsley, almond flour garlic powder, and parsley in a large bowl. Whisk together the eggs and coconut oil in a mixing bowl. Pour this egg mixture over the cauliflower rice. Mix well and use ¼ cup of this mixture to form a 4-burger patty. Place the prepared patties in the Air Fryer's Basket. Top the patties with some oil. Cook for about 30 minutes at 375 F. Serve warm over lettuce leaves.

RECIPE 114: CAULIFLOWER HASH

Serve: 6 | Total Time: 25 minutes

1-pound cauliflower
2 eggs
1 tsp salt
½ tsp ground paprika
4-ounce turkey fillet, chopped

Wash the cauliflower, chop, and set aside. In a different bowl, crack the eggs and whisk well. Add the salt and ground paprika; stir. Place the chopped turkey in the Air Fryer basket and cook it for 4 minutes at 365° F, stirring halfway through. After this, add the chopped cauliflower and stir the mixture. Cook the turkey/cauliflower mixture for 6 minutes more at 370° F, stirring it halfway through. Then pour in the whisked egg mixture and stir it carefully. Cook the cauliflower hash for 5 minutes more at 365° F. When the cauliflower hash is done, let it cool and transfer to serving bowls. Serve; enjoy.

RECIPE 115: CAULIFLOWER PATTIES

Serve: 2 | Total Time: 40 minutes

2 cup cauliflower florets, grated
1 chopped green onion
1 tsp minced garlic
2 tbsp ranch seasoning mix
1 cup cilantro
1/2 tsp chili powder
1/4 tsp cumin
2 tbsp xanthan gum
1/4 cup ground flaxseed
1/4 cup sunflower seeds
1/4 tsp Kosher Salt and pepper
Dipping sauce of choice

Let your oven preheat at 400 F. Grease its basket with cooking oil. Toss all the vegetables in the food processor and grind them. Add flaxseed, sunflower seeds, all the seasoning, xanthan gum, and cilantro. Mix well until it forms a thick patties batter. Make 1 ½ inch thick patties out of it. Place 4 patties in the Air Fryer's Basket then return the basket to the Air Fryer. Cook them for 20 minutes while flipping them halfway through. Cook the remaining patties using the same steps. Serve.

RECIPE 116: CAULIFLOWER WITH LIME JUICE

Serve: 4 | Total Time: 17 minutes

2 cups chopped cauliflower florets
2 tbsp coconut oil, melted
2 tsp chili powder
1/2 tsp garlic powder

1 medium lime
2 tbsp chopped cilantro

In a bowl, merge cauliflower with coconut oil. Sprinkle with chili powder and garlic powder. Set seasoned cauliflower into the Air Fryer basket. Set the temperature to 350F (180C). Cauliflower will be juicy and begin to turn golden at the edges. Set into serving bowl. Divide the lime into quarters and squeeze juice over cauliflower. Garnish with cilantro.

RECIPE 117: CHEESE AND BACON FILLED SWEET POTATOES

Serve: 4 | Total Time: 40 minutes

12 ounces sweet potatoes
1 tsp melted butter
¼ cup shredded Monterey Jack cheese
¼ cup buttermilk
2 slices bacon, cooked and crumbled
1 tbsp chopped scallions
Salt to taste

Close crisping lid. Preheat your cooker by choosing Air Fry at 390 F for 5 minutes. Mix the sweet potatoes with the melted butter until evenly coated. Add to the Cook & Crisp basket. Close the lid, choose Air Fry, set the temperature to 345 F, and set the time to 30 minutes. Press Start. After 15 minutes, open the lid, pull out the basket and shake the potatoes. At the 15-minute mark, check the potatoes to see if they're crisped to your liking. In a bowl, mix cheese, buttermilk, bacon, and scallions, season with salt and set aside. Get the potatoes from the basket and halve the potatoes lengthwise. Top with the bacon-cheese filling and serve.

RECIPE 118: CHEESE AND EGG BREAKFAST SANDWICH

Serve: 1 | Total Time: 9 minutes

1 egg
2 slices cheddar or Swiss cheese

A bit of butter
1 roll either English muffin or Kaiser Bun, halved

Both sides of the cut buns should be brushed with butter. In an oven-safe dish, whisk together the eggs. Place the cheese, egg dish, and rolls in the Air Fryer to cook until the cheese has melted. Make sure the greased sides of the roll are facing up while baking them in the oven. Adjust the Air Fryer to 390 °F. Cook for 6 minutes on medium heat. Using two pieces of bread, sandwich the egg and cheese together. Serve warm..

RECIPE 119: CHEESE CAULIFLOWER MASH

Serve: 6 | Total Time: 25 minutes

1 (12-ounce / 340-g) steamer bag cauliflower florets, cooked according to package instructions
2 tbsp salted butter, softened
2 ounces (57 g) cream cheese, softened
1/2 cup shredded sharp Cheddar cheese
1/4 cup pickled jalapeños
1/2 tsp salt
1/4 tsp ground black pepper

Set cooked cauliflower into a food processor with remaining ingredients. Pulse twenty times until cauliflower is smooth and all ingredients are combined. Spoon mash into an ungreased 6-inch round nonstick baking dish. Place dish into Air Fryer basket. Adjust the temperature to 380F (193C) and set the timer for 15 minutes. When done, the top will be golden. Serve warm.

RECIPE 120: CHEESE CRUSTED BRUSSELS SPROUTS

Serve: 4 | Total Time: 20 minutes

1 lb. Brussels sprouts, halved
1 tbsp. paprika
2 tbsp. Grana Padano cheese, grated.
3 tbsp. breadcrumbs

2 tbsp. sage, chopped.
2 tbsp. canola oil

Preheat your Air Fryer to temperature of 400 degrees F. Line the Air Fryer basket with parchment paper. Take a bowl and, mix breadcrumbs and paprika with Grana Padano cheese. Drizzle the Brussels sprouts with the canola oil and pour in the breadcrumb/cheese mixture; toss to coat. Place in the Air Fryer basket and cook for 15 minutes, shaking it every 4-5 minutes. Serve sprinkled with chopped sage.

RECIPE 121: CHEESE STICKS

Serve: 4 | Total Time: 15 minutes

6 cups broccoli florets
1 tbsp olive oil
1/4 tsp salt
2 tbsp sesame seeds
2 tbsp rice vinegar
2 tbsp coconut aminos
2 tbsp sesame oil
1/2 tsp Swerve
1/4 tsp red pepper flakes (optional)
Preheat the Air Fryer to 400F (205C). In a bowl, merge the broccoli with the olive oil and salt until thoroughly coated. Placing the broccoli in the Air Fryer Pausing halfway through the cooking time to shake the basket, air fry for 10 minutes. Meanwhile, in the same large bowl, whisk together the sesame seeds, vinegar, coconut aminos, sesame oil, Serve, and red pepper flakes (if using). Transfer the broccoli to the bowl and toss until thoroughly coated with the seasonings. Serve warm or at room temperature.

RECIPE 122: CHEESY BACON POCKETS

Serve: 5 | Total Time: 20 minutes

1 box puff pastry sheets
5 eggs
½ cup sausage crumbles, cooked
Cooking spray
½ cup bacon, cooked
½ cup shredded cheddar cheese

Grease a regular skillet with cooking spray and set it over medium heat. Crack eggs in the skillet and stir as you cook them to make scrambled eggs. Add bacon, sausage and cheese, mix well and remove the skillet from the heat. Spread half of the pastry sheets on the working surface and divide the egg cheese filling at the center of each sheet. Use the remaining sheets to cover all the fillings and pinch the edges to the pastry to sheets to seal the pockets. Place the bacon pockets in the Air Fryer Basket and return the fryer basket to the Air Fryer. Cook for 10 minutes at 370 F until golden brown. Serve warm.

RECIPE 123: CHEESY BELL PEPPER EGGS

Serve: 4 | Total Time: 25 minutes

4 medium green bell peppers
ounces (85 g) cooked ham, chopped
1/4 medium onion, peeled and chopped
8 large eggs
1 cup mild Cheddar cheese

Cut the tops off each bell pepper. Remove the seeds and the white membranes with a small knife. Place ham and onion into each pepper. Crack 2 eggs into each pepper. Top with 1/4 cup cheese per pepper. Place into the Air Fryer basket. Adjust the temperature to 390F (199C) and air fry for 15 minutes. When fully cooked, peppers will be tender and eggs will be firm. Serve immediately.

RECIPE 124: CHEESY BOMBS IN BACON

Serve: 8 | Total Time: 20 minutes

8 Bacon Slices, cut in half
16 oz Mozzarella Cheese, cut into 8 pieces
3 tbsp Butter, melted

Wrap each cheese string with a slice of bacon and secure the ends

with toothpicks. Set aside. Grease the crisp basket with the melted butter and add in the bombs. Close the crisping lid, select Air Fry mode, and set the temperature to 370 F and set the time to 10 minutes. At the 5-minute mark, turn the bombs. When ready, remove to a paper-lined plate to drain the excess oil. Serve on a platter with toothpicks.

RECIPE 125: CHEESY CAULIFLOWER HASH BROWNS

Serve: 4 | Total Time: 22 minutes

1 1/2 (12-ounce) steamer bag cauliflower
1 large egg
1 cup shredded sharp Cheddar cheese

Microwave bag as directed on box. After cooling, compress cauliflower in a cheesecloth or a dish towel to remove extra liquid. Pulse cauliflower with a fork and add egg and cheese. Divide a piece of parchment to fit your Air Fryer basket. Set 1/4 of the mixture and form it into a hash brown patty shape. Place it onto the parchment and into the Air Fryer basket, working in batches if necessary. Set the oven to 400°F and the timer for 12 minutes. Flip the hash browns halfway through the cooking time. When completely cooked, they will be golden brown. Serve immediately.

RECIPE 126: CHEESY FINGERLING POTATOES

Serve: 4 | Total Time: 31 minutes

1 lb fingerling potatoes, cut into wedges
1 tsp olive oil
½ tsp salt
1 tsp black pepper ground
1 ½ tsp dry garlic powder
Cheese sauce
Raw cashews
1 tsp turmeric
1 tsp paprika
2 tbsp nutritional yeast

1 tsp lemon juice
2 tbsp water
Preheat your Air Fryer machine to 400 F. Wash and cut the potatoes in half, lengthwise. Place the fingerling potatoes wedges in a bowl and add oil, salt, pepper, and garlic powder Toss well and transfer the potatoes to the Air Fryer's Basket. Cook for 16 minutes and stir well when halfway through. Blend all the ingredients for cheese sauce in a blender Place the potatoes in the Air Fryer's Basket. Pour over the cheese sauce. Cook for 2 minutes in the fryer. Serve warm.

RECIPE 127: CHEESY FRIED BROCCOLI

Serve: 4 | Total Time: 35 minutes

2 pounds broccoli, cut into florets
2 tbsp olive oil
1/3 cup Kalamata olives, halved
½ tsp ground black pepper
2 tsp lemon zest, grated
4-6 slices Parmesan cheese
A pinch of salt

Cook broccoli florets into salted water. Remove from the water drain well and toss with olive oil, salt, and pepper. Preheat the Air Fryer to 370-390°F. Place oiled broccoli into the Fryer and cook for 15 minutes, shaking couple times during frying. When the timer goes off, remove cooked broccoli and transfer to the serving bowl. Toss with halved olives, lemon zest, and Parmesan slices and serve.

RECIPE 128: CHEESY GARLIC BREAD

Serve: 2 | Total Time: 20 minutes

2 dinner rolls
½ cup grated Parmesan cheese
2 tbsp butter, melted
2 tbsp garlic and herb seasoning, or more to taste

Into each roll, cut a crisscross that almost reaches the base, while leaving the bottom crusts untouched. Fill all the holes with Parmesan cheese. Use melted butter to paint the tops of the rolls, and sprinkle garlic seasoning also. Ensure that your Air Fryer is preheated to 350 F. Transfer the rolls in the Air Fryer basket, and allow to cook for 5 minutes, or until you have the cheese melted.

.

RECIPE 129: CHEESY ROASTED SWEET POTATOES

Serve: 4 | Total Time: 25 minutes

2 large sweet potatoes, peeled and sliced
1 tsp olive oil
1 tbsp white balsamic vinegar
1 tsp dried thyme
¼ cup grated Parmesan cheese

In a big bowl, shower the sweet potato slices with the olive oil and toss. Sprinkle with the balsamic vinegar and thyme and toss again. Sprinkle the potatoes with the Parmesan cheese and toss to coat. Roast the slices, in batches, in the Air Fryer basket for 18 to 23 minutes, tossing the sweet potato slices in the basket once during cooking, until tender. Repeat with the remaining sweet potato slices. Serve immediately.

RECIPE 130: CHEESY SPINACH MACARONI

Serve: 2 | Total Time: 20 minutes

6 ounces elbow pasta, cooked.
1/4 cup grated gruyere cheese
1 cup baby spinach leaves
1/4 cup grated cheddar cheese
1/4 cup grated mozzarella cheese
1/4 cup whole milk
1/4 cup cream
½ tbsp. unsalted butter, melted.
salt and pepper, to taste

Preheat the Air Fryer to temperature of 350 degrees F. Place the pasta in the Air Fryer Baking Pan or another casserole dish that can fit snugly in the Air Fryer Basket. Add the butter, milk, cream, mozzarella cheese, gruyere cheese and cheddar cheese and season with salt and pepper. Stir in the baby spinach leaves. Place the Air Fryer Baking Pan in the Air Fryer Basket and cook for 15 minutes. Serve and enjoy!

RECIPE 131: CHICKEN AND PEPPER FAJITAS

Serve: 4 | Total Time: 40 minutes

1 pound (454 g) chicken legs, boneless, skinless, cut into pieces
2 tbsp canola oil
1 red bell pepper, sliced
1 yellow bell pepper, sliced
1 jalapeño pepper, sliced
1 onion, sliced
½ tsp onion powder
½ tsp garlic powder
salt and black pepper, to taste
Pat the chicken dry with paper towels. Toss the chicken legs with 1 tablespoon of the canola oil. Cook the chicken at 380°F (193°C) for 15 minutes, shaking the basket halfway through the cooking time. Add the remaining ingredients to the Air Fryer basket and turn the heat to 400°F (204°C). Let it cook for 15 minutes more or until cooked through. Bon appétit!

RECIPE 132: CHICKEN AND VEGETABLE FRIED RICE

Serve: 4 | Total Time: 25 minutes

2 tbsp vegetable oil
½ cup of green onions, chopped
1 cup of celery, chopped
½ cup carrot, thinly sliced
2 cups rice, boiled
1 pound cooked chicken meat
1 cup green peas, boiled
4 egg whites, whisked
2 tsp ginger, grated
½ tsp garlic
Salt, to taste
Pinch of black pepper
4 tbsp lemon juice
2 tbsp soya sauce
Place the garlic and ginger into the Air Fryer and add oil along with onions. Set the timer to 2 minutes and cook. Then beat the eggs and

set aside. Add celery, carrots, chicken meat, peas, salt, pepper, lemon juice and soy sauce in an Air Fryer and cook for 7 minutes to 10 minutes. Then open the fryer and add eggs and rice. Set timer to 10 minutes. Once it's cooked, serve.

RECIPE 133: CHICKEN AVOCADO BURGERS

Serve: 2 | Total Time: 15 minutes

14 oz avocado, peeled
14 oz chicken, minced
1 tbsp mexican seasoning

Slice the peeled avocado and cut three slices into small cubes. Keep the rest aside as whole slices. Transfer the minced chicken into a mixing bowl, and add the chunks of avocado alongside the Mexican seasoning. After mixing the contents of the bowl above thoroughly, form the mixture into chicken burger patty shapes. Transfer the burger into the Air Fryer and allow to cook for 12 minutes at 360 F for 12 minutes. To get that ideal Mexican meal, serve the burger alongside potato wedges.

RECIPE 134: CHICKEN BITES

Serve: 4 | Total Time: 15 minutes

¼ cup blue cheese salad dressing
1 lb. chicken breast, skinless and boneless
½ tsp salt
1 tbsp olive oil
½ cup sour cream
1 cup breadcrumbs
¼ cup blue cheese, crumbled
½ tsp pepper

Mix salad dressing, blue cheese, and sour cream. Stir and set aside. In another bowl, mix olive oil, salt, pepper, and breadcrumbs. Cut chicken breasts into 2-inch pieces and roll in breadcrumbs mixture. Preheat Air Fryer to 380°Fahrenheit. Transfer the chicken bites to the frying basket.

Cook for 15-minutes. Serve with sauce and enjoy!

RECIPE 135: CHICKEN BREASTS WRAPPED IN BACON

Serve: 4 | Total Time: 35 minutes

¼ cup mayonnaise
¼ cup sour cream
3 tbsp ketchup
1 tbsp yellow mustard
1 tbsp light brown sugar
1 lb chicken tenders
1 tsp dried parsley
8 bacon slices

Preheat the Air Fryer to 370°F. Combine the mayonnaise, sour cream, ketchup, mustard, and brown sugar in a bowl and mix well, then set aside. Sprinkle the chicken with the parsley and wrap each one in a slice of bacon. Put the wrapped chicken in the frying basket in a single layer and Air Fry for 18-20 minutes, flipping once until the bacon is crisp. Serve with sauce.

RECIPE 136: CHICKEN BURGERS WITH BLUE CHEESE SAUCE

Serve: 4 | Total Time: 40 minutes

¼ cup crumbled blue cheese
¼ cup sour cream
2 tbsp mayonnaise
1 tbsp red hot sauce
Salt to taste
3 tbsp buffalo wing sauce
1 lb ground chicken
2 tbsp grated carrot
2 tbsp diced celery
1 egg white

Whisk the blue cheese, sour cream, mayonnaise, red hot sauce, salt, and 1 tbsp of buffalo sauce in a bowl. Let sit covered in the fridge until ready to use. Preheat Air Fryer at 350°F. In another bowl, combine the remaining ingredients. Form mixture into 4 patties, making a slight indentation in the middle of each. Place patties in the greased frying basket and Air Fry for 13 minutes until you reach your

desired doneness, flipping once. Serve with the blue cheese sauce.

RECIPE 137: CHICKEN CHEESE DINNER ROLLS

Serve: 4 | Total Time: 22 minutes

1 lb (454 g) ground chicken
½ cup crushed tortilla chips
2 oz (57 g) Cheddar cheese, grated
1 tsp dried parsley flakes
1 tsp cayenne pepper
½ tsp paprika
salt and ground black pepper, to taste
4 dinner rolls

Mix the chicken, tortilla chips, cheese, and spices until everything is well combined. Now, roll the mixture into four patties. Cook the burgers at 380ºF (193ºC) for about 17 minutes or until cooked through; make sure to turn them over halfway through the cooking time. Serve your burgers in dinner rolls. Bon appétit!

RECIPE 138: CHICKEN CHEESE TORTILLA

Serve: 4 | Total Time: 20 minutes

1 egg, whisked
½ cup grated Parmesan cheese
½ cup crushed tortilla chips
½ tsp onion powder
½ tsp garlic powder
1 tsp red chili powder
1½ pounds (680 g) chicken breasts, boneless, skinless, cut into strips

Whisk the egg in a shallow bowl. In a separate bowl, whisk the Parmesan cheese, tortilla chips, onion powder, garlic powder, and red chili powder. Dip the chicken pieces into the egg mixture. Then, roll the chicken pieces over the bread crumb mixture. Cook the chicken at 380ºF (193ºC) for 12 minutes, turning them over halfway through the cooking time. Bon appétit!

RECIPE 139: CHICKEN CILANTRO WITH BEETS

Serve: 2 | Total Time: 16 minutes

1 chicken breast, cubed.
1/4 cup fresh cilantro, chopped.
1/4 cup red bell peppers, diced.
1/4 cup radish, sliced.
1/4 cup goat cheese
1 large beet, thinly sliced.
salt and pepper, to taste

Preheat the Air Fryer to temperature o350 degrees F. Place the chicken cubes in the Air Fryer Baking Pan and season with salt and pepper. Place the Air Fryer Baking Pan in the Air Fryer Basket and cook for 8 minutes. Add the bell peppers, beets and radish to the Air Fryer Baking Pan and cook for 3 more minutes or until the chicken is cooked through. Top with the goat cheese and fresh cilantro. Serve and enjoy!

RECIPE 140: CHICKEN CORDON BLEU PATTIES

Serve: 4 | Total Time: 30 minutes

1/3 cup grated Fontina cheese
3 tbsp milk
1/3 cup bread crumbs
1 egg, beaten
½ tsp dried parsley
Salt and pepper to taste
1 ¼ lb ground chicken
¼ cup finely chopped ham

Preheat Air Fryer to 350°F. Mix milk, breadcrumbs, egg, parsley, salt and pepper in a bowl. Using your hands, add the chicken and gently mix until just combined. Divide into 8 portions and shape into thin patties. Place on waxed paper. On 4 of the patties, top with ham and Fontina cheese, then place another patty on top of that. Gently pinch the edges together so that none of the ham or cheese is peeking out. Arrange the burgers in the greased frying basket and Air Fry until cooked through, for 14-16 minutes. Serve and enjoy!

RECIPE 141: CHICKEN DRUMSTICKS

Serve: 8 | Total Time: 30 minutes

8 chicken drumsticks
2 tbsp olive oil
1 tsp salt
1 tsp pepper
1 tsp garlic powder
1 tsp paprika
1/2 tsp cumin
Mix olive oil with salt, black pepper, garlic powder, paprika, and cumin in a bowl. Rub this mixture liberally over all the drumsticks. Place these drumsticks in the Air Fryer basket. Turn the dial to select the "Air Fry" mode. Hit the Time button and again use the dial to set the cooking time to 20 minutes. Now push the Temp button and rotate the dial to set the temperature at 375 degrees F. Once preheated, place the Air Fryer basket inside the oven. Flip the drumsticks when cooked halfway through. Resume air frying for another rest of the 10 minutes. Serve warm.

RECIPE 142: CHICKEN FILLED MUSHROOM BITES

Serve: 12 | Total Time: 30 minutes

12 large fresh mushrooms, stems removed

Stuffing:
1 cup chicken meat, cubed
1 (8 oz.) package cream cheese, softened
½ lb. imitation crabmeat, flaked
2 cups butter
2 garlic cloves, peeled and minced
Black pepper and salt to taste
Garlic powder to taste
Crushed red pepper to taste

Melt and heat butter in a skillet over medium heat. Add chicken and sauté for 5 minutes. Add in all the remaining ingredients for the stuffing. Cook for 5 minutes then turn off the heat. Allow the mixture to cool. Stuff each mushroom with a tbsp of this mixture. In the Air Fryer basket, place the mushrooms. Spray some oil on top and cook for 10 minutes at 375 F. Serve warm.

RECIPE 143: CHICKEN FILLET WITH BRIE AND HAM

Serve: 4 | Total Time: 30 minutes

2 large chicken fillets
Freshly ground pepper
4 small slices Brie cheese
1 tbsp chives, chopped
4 slices cured ham
4 tablespoons olive oil

Preheat the Air Fryer to 360 F. Cut the chicken fillets into four equal pieces and slit them horizontally to ½ inch from the edge. After the chicken fillets have been opened, season them with salt and pepper. Place a slice of Brie and some chives on top of each piece of brie. Close the chicken fillets and firmly wrap a piece of ham around them to make a ring around them. Cook the packed fillets in the Air Fryer after coating them with olive oil on a thin layer. Cook for 15 minutes until brown and ready. Enjoy!

RECIPE 144: CHICKEN FILLETS WITH CORIANDER

Serve: 4 | Total Time: 17 minutes

1 pound (454 g) chicken fillets
1 egg
1 tbsp olive oil
1 cup crushed crackers
1 tbsp minced fresh coriander
1 tbsp minced fresh parsley
salt and black pepper, to taste
¼ tsp ground cumin
¼ tsp mustard seeds
1 tsp celery seeds

Dry the chicken fillets. Whisk the egg in a shallow bowl. Mix the remaining ingredients in a separate shallow bowl. Dip the chicken fillets into the egg mixture. Then, roll the chicken fillets over the bread crumb mixture. Cook the chicken at 380°F (193°C) for 12 minutes, turning them over halfway through the cooking time. Bon appétit!

RECIPE 145: CHICKEN HAWAIIAN ROLLS

Serve: 3 | Total Time: 22 minutes

¾ pound (340 g) ground chicken
1 tsp minced garlic
1 small onion, minced
2 tbsp minced fresh parsley
2 tbsp minced fresh cilantro
½ tsp mustard seeds
½ tsp ground cumin
½ tsp paprika
salt and black pepper, to taste
2 tbsp olive oil
6 Hawaiian rolls

Mix all ingredients, except for the burger buns, until everything is well combined. Shape the mixture into six patties. Cook the burgers at 380°F (193°C) for about 17 minutes or until cooked through; make sure to turn them over halfway through the cooking time. Serve your burgers over Hawaiian rolls and garnish with toppings of choice. Bon appétit!

RECIPE 146: CHICKEN KEBABS

Serve: 3 | Total Time: 15 minutes

1 lb. chicken breasts, diced
1 small zucchini, cut into rings
3 medium-sized bell peppers, sliced
2 medium tomatoes, sliced
6 large mushrooms, cut in halves
¼ cup sesame seeds
½ cup soy sauce
5 tbsp honey
1 tbsp olive oil
Salt and pepper to taste
Wooden skewers

Cut the chicken breasts into cubes and transfer to mixing bowl. Add salt and pepper. Add 1 tablespoon of olive oil and stir to blend. Add soy sauce and honey and sprinkle with sesame seeds. Set aside for 30-minutes. Alternately add chicken pieces and vegetables to wooden skewers. Preheat your Air

Fryer to 340°Fahrenheit. Place the chicken kebabs in fryer basket. Cook for 15-minutes.

RECIPE 147: CHICKEN LEGS WITH PINEAPPLE

Serve: 4 | Total Time: 40 minutes

1 pound (454 g) chicken legs, boneless
salt and black pepper, to taste
2 tbsp tamari sauce
1 tbsp hot sauce
1 cup peeled and diced pineapple
1 tbsp roughly chopped fresh cilantro

Pat the chicken dry with paper towels. Toss the chicken legs with the salt, black pepper, tamari sauce, and hot sauce. Cook the chicken at 380°F (193°C) for 30 minutes, turning them over halfway through the cooking time. Top the chicken with the pineapple and continue to cook for 5 minutes more. Serve warm, garnished with the fresh cilantro. Bon appétit!

RECIPE 148: CHICKEN MEATBALLS

Serve: 2 | Total Time: 20 minutes

½ lb chicken breast
1 tbsp of garlic
1 tbsp of onion
½ chicken broth
1 tbsp of oatmeal, whole wheat flour or of your choice

Place all of the ingredients in a food processor and beat well until well mixed and ground. If you don't have a food processor, ask the butcher to grind it and then add the other ingredients, mixing well. Make balls and place them in the Air Fryer basket. Program the Air Fryer for 15 minutes at 400°F. Half the time shake the basket so that the meatballs loosen and fry evenly.

RECIPE 149: CHICKEN POTATOES AND CHICKPEA

Serve: 2 | Total Time: 25 minutes

2 chicken breast fillets, cubed.
1 cup potatoes, diced.
1 cup canned chickpeas
1 tsp. dried sage
1 tsp. garlic powder
salt and pepper, to taste

Preheat the Air Fryer to temperature of 350 degrees F. Place the chicken cubes in the Air Fryer Baking Pan and season with the garlic powder, sage, salt & pepper. Add the chickpeas and potatoes to the Air Fryer Baking Pan. Season with pepper and spray with cooking spray. Place the Air Fryer Baking Pan in the Air Fryer Basket and cook for 15 minutes or until the chicken is cooked through. Serve and enjoy!

RECIPE 150: CHICKEN SCOTCH EGGS

Serve: 4 | Total Time: 25 minutes

1 lb ground chicken
2 tsp Dijon mustard
2 tsp grated yellow onion
1 tbsp chopped chives
1 tbsp chopped parsley
⅛ tsp ground nutmeg
1 lemon, zested
Salt and pepper to taste
4 hard-boiled eggs, peeled
1 egg, beaten
1 cup bread crumbs
2 tsp olive oil

Preheat Air Fryer to 350°F. In a bowl, mix the ground chicken, mustard, onion, chives, parsley, nutmeg, salt, lemon zest and pepper. Shape into 4 oval balls and form the balls evenly around the boiled eggs. Submerge them in the beaten egg and dip in the crumbs. Brush with olive oil. Place the scotch eggs in the frying basket and Air Fry for 14 minutes, flipping once. Serve hot.

RECIPE 151: CHICKEN TENDERS WITH BASIL-STRAWBERRY GLAZE

Serve: 2 | Total Time: 15 minutes

1 lb chicken tenderloins
¼ cup strawberry preserves
3 tbsp chopped basil
1 tsp orange juice
½ tsp orange zest
Salt and pepper to taste

Combine all ingredients, except for 1 tbsp of basil, in a bowl. Marinade in the fridge covered for 30 minutes. Preheat Air Fryer to 350ºF. Place the chicken tenders in the frying basket and Air Fry for 4-6 minutes. Shake gently the basket and turn over the chicken. Cook for 5 more minutes. Top with the remaining basil to serve.

RECIPE 152: CHICKEN THIGHS WITH LEMON GARLIC

Serve: 4 | Total Time: 35 minutes

4 skin-on, bone-in chicken thighs
4 lemon wedges
¼ cup lemon juice
2 cloves garlic, minced
2 tbsp olive oil
1 tsp Dijon mustard
¼ tsp salt
⅛ tsp ground black pepper

Mix the lemon juice, Dijon mustard, olive oil, garlic, salt, and pepper in a bowl. Refrigerate to marinate for an hour. Put the chicken thighs into a zip lock bag and pour the marinade all over the chicken and zip the bag. Refrigerate for at least 2 hours. Take the chicken out from the bag. Pat dry with paper towels. Arrange them in the Air Fryer basket. Put the air fry lid on and cook in batches in the preheated instant pot at 350ºF for 15 to 18 minutes or until cooked through. Transfer the chicken thighs to a platter. Squeeze the lemon wedges over before serving.

RECIPE 153: CHICKEN WITH SAUCE, VEGETABLES AND RICE

Serve: 4 | Total Time: 16 minutes

1 lb. chicken breasts, skinless and boneless

½ lb. button mushrooms, sliced
1 medium-sized onion, chopped
1 tbsp olive oil
2 cups cooked rice
1 jar (10-ounces) Alfredo sauce
Salt and pepper to taste
½ tsp thyme, dried

Cut the chicken breasts into 1-inch cubes. Mix chicken, onion, and mushrooms in a large bowl. Season with salt and dried thyme and mix well. Preheat your Air Fryer to 370˚Fahrenheit and sprinkle basket with olive oil. Transfer chicken and vegetables to fryer and cook for 12-minutes and stir occasionally. Stir in the Alfredo sauce. Cook for another 4-minutes. Serve with cooked rice.

RECIPE 154: CHILI AVOCADO CHIMICHURRI APPETIZER

Serve: 4 | Total Time: 35 minutes

4 zero carb bread slices
1/4 cup + 2 tbsp. olive oil
2 tbsp red wine vinegar
1 lemon, juiced
Salt and black pepper to taste
2 garlic cloves, minced
1/2 tsp red chili flakes
1/2 tsp dried oregano
1/2 cup chopped fresh parsley
2 avocados, cubed

Cut bread slices in half, brush both sides with 2 tbsp. of the olive oil, and arrange on a baking sheet. Place under the broiler and toast for 1-2 minutes per side. In a bowl, mix 1/4 cup olive oil, vinegar, lemon juice, salt, pepper, garlic, red chili flakes, oregano, and parsley. Fold in avocado. Spoon the mixture onto the bread and serve.

RECIPE 155: CHILI CON CARNE

Serve: 3 | Total Time: 40 minutes

300 g minced meat (mixed)
150 g kidney beans
1 onion
500 g tomato pieces
250 g chili beans

A small can of corn
Chili powder
1 clove of garlic
salt and pepper
Some dark chocolate

Put the chopped garlic, salt, pepper, chopped onions and the minced meat in the Air Fryer. Fry for a good 8 minutes at 100 degrees in the Air Fryer and after this time add the corn, beans and tomatoes. Also cook the chili powder for 30 minutes. If necessary, add water so that the chili does not get too dry. After the cooking time, add the chocolate and let it melt with the dish in the Air Fryer for a few more minutes. Good Appetite.

RECIPE 156: CHILI CHEESE TOASTS

Serve: 4 | Total Time: 15 minutes

1 tsp garlic powder
1 tsp red chili flakes
6 pieces sandwich bread
4 tbsp butter
1 cup grated cheddar cheese
2 little fresh red chilies, deseeded and minced
½ tsp salt
1 tbsp sliced fresh parsley

Preheat the oven in Broil mode at 375 °F for 2 to 3 minutes. Place each bread slice on a clean, flat surface. Divide the cheddar cheese on top and followed with the remaining ingredients. Lay 3 pieces of the bread on the cooking tray, slide the tray onto the middle rack of the oven, and close the oven. Set the timer for 3 to 4 minutes and press Start. Cook till the cheese melts and is golden brown on top. Remove the first batch when ready and prepare the other three bread pieces. Slice them into triangle halves and serve immediately.

RECIPE 157: CHILI HASH BROWNS

Serve: 3 | Total Time: 50 minutes

1 lb. potatoes, peeled and shredded
1 egg, beaten
1 tbsp. olive oil
1 tsp. garlic powder
1 tsp. chili flakes
1 tsp. onion powder
Salt and pepper to taste
Cooking spray

Melt olive oil in a skillet. 10 minutes sauté potatoes Move to a bowl. Add the egg, pepper, salt, chili flakes, onion powder, and garlic powder when they cool. In a flat plate, spread the mixture and pat firmly with your fingers. Refrigerate for 20 minutes. Preheat your Air Fryer to temperature of 350 degrees F. Remove from the fridge and divide into equal sizes. Grease the fryer basket with cooking spray and add in the patties. Cook at 350 degrees F for 15 minutes; flip and cook for 6 more minutes. Serve with sunshine eggs.

RECIPE 158: CHIMICHURRI SKIRT STEAK

Serve: 2 | Total Time: 10 minutes

1 lb. skirt steak

Chimichurri:
1 cup parsley, finely chopped
2 tsp smoked paprika
1 tsp cayenne pepper
1 tbsp ground cumin
1 tsp crushed red pepper
3 garlic cloves, finely chopped
2 tbsp oregano, finely chopped
¼ cup mint, finely chopped
3 tbsp red wine vinegar
¾ cup olive oil
¼ tsp black pepper
Salt to taste

Mix the ingredients for the chimichurri in a mixing bowl. Cut the steak into 2 (8-ounce) portions and put into a re-sealable bag, along with ¼ cup of chimichurri. Place in the fridge for 24-hours. Remove from the fridge 30-minutes before cooking. Preheat your Air Fryer to 390°Fahrenheit. Pat the steak dry with paper towel. Add the steak to cooking basket

and cook for 10-minutes for medium-rare. Serve with 2 tablespoons chimichurri garnish.

RECIPE 159: CHINESE STYLE BEEF AND BROCCOLI

Serve: 4 | Total Time: 12 minutes

3 cups oyster sauce
2 tsp sesame oil
1 tsp cornstarch
1/3 cup sherry
1 tsp soy sauce
1 tsp liquid Stevia
¾ lb. steak, cut into strips
1 lb. broccoli, cut into pieces
1 tbsp olive oil
1 clove garlic, minced
1 slice of ginger, fresh

For the marinade, in a bowl, pour in the oyster sauce, sesame oil, cornstarch, sherry, soy sauce and Stevia. Mix well. Place your steak strips into the sauce and leave to marinate for about 1-hour. Remove from the marinade and place in the wire basket of Air Fryer, along with broccoli, topped with garlic, ginger and olive oil. Cook for 12-minutes at 390°Fahrenheit.

RECIPE 160: CHIPOTLE CHICKEN DRUMSTICKS

Serve: 4 | Total Time: 40 minutes

1 can chipotle chilies packed in adobo sauce
2 tbsp grated Mexican cheese
6 chicken drumsticks
1 egg, beaten
½ cup bread crumbs
1 tbsp corn flakes
Salt and pepper to taste

Preheat Air Fryer to 350°F. Place the chilies in the sauce in your blender and pulse until a fine paste is formed. Transfer to a bowl and add the beaten egg. Combine thoroughly. Mix the breadcrumbs, Mexican cheese, corn flakes, salt, and pepper in a separate bowl, and set aside. Coat the chicken drumsticks with the crumb mixture, then dip into the bowl

with wet ingredients, then dip again into the dry ingredients. Arrange the chicken drumsticks on the greased frying basket in a single flat layer. Air Fry for 14-16 minutes, turning each chicken drumstick over once. Serve warm.

RECIPE 161: CHORIZO AND BEEF BURGER

Serve: 4 | Total Time: 25 minutes

3/4 pound 80/20 ground beef
1/4 pound Mexican-style ground chorizo
1/4 cup chopped onion
5 slices pickled jalapeños, chopped
2 tsp chili powder
1 tsp minced garlic
1/4 tsp cumin

In a large bowl, mix all ingredients. Form the ingredients into four burger patties. Place burger patties into the Air Fryer basket, working in batches if necessary. Adjust the temperature to 375F and set the timer for 15 minutes. Turn over the patties halfway through the cooking time. Serve warm.

RECIPE 162: CILANTRO AND FETA BEEF MEATBALLS

Serve: 5 | Total Time: 20 minutes

1 lb. ground beef
1/4 cup feta cheese, crumbled.
1/2 cup fresh cilantro, chopped.
1/2 cup breadcrumbs
1 tbsp. garlic, minced.
1 tsp. paprika
salt and pepper, to taste

Preheat the Air Fryer to temperature of 400 degrees F. Mix together the ground beef, minced garlic, fresh cilantro, paprika and feta cheese. Season with salt and pepper. Add the breadcrumbs. Divide the beef mixture into 10 balls and smoothen them wet palms. Arrange the meatballs into the Air Fryer Basket and use the Air Fryer Double Layer Rack if needed. Simmer for 10 minutes with meatballs. Serve and enjoy!

RECIPE 163: CLASSIC CHICKEN WINGS

Serve: 4 | Total Time: 50 minutes

2 lbs. Chicken wings
For sauce:
1/4 tsp tabasco
1/4 tsp Worcestershire sauce
6 tbsp. butter, melted
12 oz. hot sauce
Spray Air Fryer basket with cooking spray. Cook for 25 minutes at 380°F in the Air Fryer basket. Shake every 5 minutes. After 25 minutes turn the temperature to 400 f and cook for 10-15 minutes more. Meanwhile, in a large bowl, mix all sauce ingredients. Add cooked chicken wings in a sauce bowl and toss well to coat. Serve and enjoy.

RECIPE 164: CLASSIC BEEF MEATBALLS

Serve: 4 | Total Time: 30 minutes

3 tbsp buttermilk
1/3 cup bread crumbs
1 tbsp ketchup
1 egg
½ tsp dried marjoram
Salt and pepper to taste
1 lb ground beef
20 Swiss cheese cubes

Preheat Air Fryer to 390°F. Mix buttermilk, crumbs, ketchup, egg, marjoram, salt, and pepper in a bowl. Using your hands, mix in ground beef until just combined. Shape into 20 meatballs. Take one meatball and shape it around a Swiss cheese cube. Repeat this for the remaining meatballs. Lightly spray the meatballs with oil and place into the frying basket. Bake the meatballs for 10-13 minutes, turning once until they are cooked through. Serve and enjoy!

RECIPE 165: COCONUT CRUSTED CHICKEN TENDERS

Serve: 8 | Total Time: 15 minutes

3 Eggs

1 lb. Chicken tenders
1 cup Cornstarch
2 cups. Sweetened shredded coconut
1 tsp. Cayenne pepper

Set the Air Fryer temperature at 360° Fahrenheit. Prepare three dishes. Add cornstarch, cayenne, and other ingredients to the first. In the second bowl, add the eggs. Lastly, add the coconut to the third dish. Dredge the chicken through the cornstarch, egg, and coconut. Lightly spritz the fryer basket with a cooking oil spray as needed. Set the timer for 8 minutes and air-fry until it's golden brown before serving.

RECIPE 166: COCONUT-CUSTARD PIE

Serve: 4 | Total Time: 20 minutes

1 cup milk
¼ cup plus 2 tablespoons sugar
¼ cup biscuit baking mix
1 tsp vanilla
2 eggs
2 tbsp melted butter
cooking spray
½ cup shredded, sweetened coconut

Place all ingredients except coconut in a medium bowl. 3 minutes with a hand mixer on high speed. Let sit for 5minutes. Preheat Air Fryer to 330°F. Spray a 6-inch round or 6 x 6-inch square baking pan with cooking spray and place pan in Air Fryer basket. Pour filling into pan and sprinkle coconut over top. Cook pie at 330°F for 20 minutes or until center sets.

RECIPE 167: COD FILLETS AND PEAS

Serve: 4 | Total Time: 20 minutes

4 cod fillets
2 tbsp freshly chopped parsley
2 cups peas
4 tbsp wine
½ tsp oregano, dried

½ tsp sweet paprika
2 garlic cloves, minced
Salt and pepper to the taste

Place garlic with parsley, salt, pepper, oregano, paprika and wine in your food processor and blend until smooth. Prepare the heat of the Air Fryer to 360 F. Rub fish fillets with half of this mix, place in your Air Fryer and cook for 10 minutes. Meanwhile, put peas in a pot, add water to cover, add salt, bring to a boil over medium high heat, and cook for 10 minutes. When cooked, drain and divide among plates. Add fish, spread the rest of the herb dressing all over and serve.

RECIPE 168: COD FILLETS WITH HONEY GLAZED GREENS

Serve: 4 | Total Time: 30 minutes

4 cod fillets
10 spears asparagus
2 mandarins; segmented
8 ounces fresh green beans; trimmed
1 tsp. rice wine vinegar
1 tbsp. soy sauce
1 tbsp. Dijon mustard
4 tbsp. honey
salt and pepper, to taste

Toss the asparagus and green beans in a bowl with the honey, soy sauce, mustard and rice wine vinegar and set aside. Preheat the Air Fryer to temperature of 350 degrees F. Season the cod fillets with the salt and pepper. Place the cod fillets into the Air Fryer and spray with a little cooking spray. Cook for 10 minutes. Flip the fish and add the vegetables to the Air Fryer Basket. Cook for 10 more minutes. Remove from Air Fryer and mix in the mandarin segments. Serve and enjoy!

RECIPE 169: COLESLAW STUFFED WONTONS

Serve: 6 | Total Time: 35 minutes

1 package won ton wrappers

1 package coleslaw mix
2 tbsp soy sauce
2 tbsp butter

Firstly, melt the butter and stir in the coleslaw until fully combined. Sauté it for 5 minutes then add soy sauce. Adjust seasoning with black pepper and salt, then turn off the heat. Spread the wonton wrapper over a sheet of wax paper. Add a tbsp of coleslaw to the center of each wrap. Wet the edges of all the wonton wrappers and fold them into a triangle to seal the filling. Set the wontons in the Air Fryer basket. Let your Air Fryer preheat at 375 F. Return the basket to its fryer then cook for 10 minutes approximately. Flip the wontons and cook for another 4 minutes. Serve warm.

RECIPE 170: CORN-CRUSTED CHICKEN TENDERS

Serve: 4 | Total Time: 50 minutes

2 chicken breasts, cut into strips
Salt and black pepper to taste
2 eggs
1 cup ground cornmeal

Preheat Air Fryer to 390 °F. In a bowl, mix ground cornmeal, salt, and black pepper. In another bowl, beat the eggs; season with salt and pepper. The chicken should be dipped into the eggs and then coated in cornmeal. Spray the prepared sticks with cooking spray and place them in the Air Fryer basket in a single layer. Air Fry for 6 minutes, slide the basket out, and flip the sticks; cook for 6-8 more minutes until golden brown.

RECIPE 171: CORNFLAKE CHICKEN NUGGETS

Serve: 4 | Total Time: 25 minutes

1 egg white
1 tbsp lemon juice
½ tsp dried basil
½ tsp ground paprika
1 lb chicken breast fingers
½ cup ground cornflakes

2 slices bread, crumbled

Preheat Air Fryer to 400°F. Whisk the egg white, lemon juice, basil, and paprika, then add the chicken and stir. Combine the cornflakes and breadcrumbs on a plate, then put the chicken fingers in the mix to coat. Put the nuggets in the frying basket and Air Fry for 10-13 minutes, turning halfway through, until golden, crisp and cooked through. Serve hot!

RECIPE 172: CORNFLAKES TOAST STICKS

Serve: 4 | Total Time: 26 minutes

2 eggs
½ cup milk
⅛ tsp salt
½ tsp pure vanilla extract
¾ cup crushed cornflakes
6 slices sandwich bread, each slice cut into 4 strips
Maple syrup, for dipping
Cooking spray

Prepare the Air Fryer to a temperature of 390ºF (199ºC). Firstly, beat together the eggs, milk, salt, and vanilla. Put crushed cornflakes on a plate or in a shallow dish. Dip bread strips in egg mixture, shake off excess, and roll in cornflake crumbs. Spray both sides of bread strips with oil. Put bread strips in Air Fryer basket in a single layer. Air fry it for about 6 minutes or until golden brown. Repeat steps 5 and 6 to air fry remaining French toast sticks. Serve with maple syrup.

RECIPE 173: CORNMEAL COATED CATFISH

Serve: 4 | Total Time: 29 minutes

2 tbsp cornmeal
2 tsp Cajun seasoning
½ tsp paprika
½ tsp garlic powder
Salt
2 catfish fillets
1 tbsp olive oil

Mix together the cornmeal, Cajun seasoning, paprika, garlic powder, and salt. Add the catfish fillets and coat with the mixture. Coat each fillet with oil. Press the "Power" button on the Air Fry Oven and choose "Air Fry" mode. Press the Time button again and flip the dial to 14 minutes. Press the Temp button and crank the dial to 400°F. To begin, press "Start/Pause". When the machine beeps, open the lid. Arrange the catfish fillets in greased "Air Fry Basket" and insert in the oven. After 10 minutes of cooking, flip the fillets and spray with the cooking spray.

RECIPE 174: COWBOY RIB EYE STEAK

Serve: 2 | Total Time: 20 minutes

¼ cup barbecue sauce
1 clove garlic, minced
⅛ tsp chili pepper
¼ tsp sweet paprika
¼ tsp cumin
1 rib-eye steak

Preheat Air Fryer to 400°F. In a bowl, whisk the barbecue sauce, garlic, chili pepper, paprika, and cumin. Divide in half and brush the steak with half of the sauce. Add steak to the lightly greased frying basket and Air Fry for 10 minutes until you reach your desired doneness, turning once and brushing with the remaining sauce. Let rest for 5 minutes onto a cutting board before slicing. Serve warm.

RECIPE 175: CRAB CAKES

Serve: 8 | Total Time: 22 minutes

2 pounds crab meat, cooked
½ cup mayonnaise
1 cup saltine crackers, crushed
2 eggs
Juice of 1 lemon
1 tsp seafood seasoning of choice

Combine the mayonnaise and egg in a mixing dish and stir until completely combined. Add the lemon juice, seafood seasoning, then add the crab meat and crushed crackers. Mix everything well, but be sure not to overcook. Let it rest for 20-30 minutes in the refrigerator. Take a bit of the mixture and form into patties. Spray the basket with oil spray, then cook the patties in batches for 10-12 minutes at 350°F (≈177°C). Serve.

RECIPE 176: CRAB WONTONS

Serve: 12 | Total Time: 20 minutes

1 cup crab meat
8 oz cream cheese
2 tsp Worcestershire sauce
½ tsp light soy sauce
1 tbsp minced garlic
48 wonton wrappers

1 teaspoon cream cheese, smeared in the center of each wonton wrapper Wipe the wonton wrappers' edges with water. Secure the edges by bringing all four corners together in the middle. Using cooking spray, coat the bottom of the fryer basket. Place as many as your Air Fryer can accommodate without overcrowding it. Coat the wontons' tops with frying spray. Cook for 7-10 minutes in an Air Fryer at 390°F (198°C), turning halfway through. Warm the dish before serving.

RECIPE 177: CRANBERRY NUTMEG SCONES

Serve: 4 | Total Time: 20 minutes

2 cups of flour
¼ cup brown sugar
1 tbsp baking powder
¼ tsp ground nutmeg
¼ tsp salt
¼ cup butter, chilled and diced
1 cup fresh cranberry
⅓ cup sugar
1 tbsp orange zest
¾ cup half and half cream
1 egg

Whisk flour with baking powder, salt, nutmeg, and both the sugars in a bowl. Stir in egg and cream, mix well to form a smooth dough. Fold in cranberries along with the orange zest. Knead this dough well on a work surface. Make 3-inch circles out of the dough. Place the scones in the Air Fryer's Basket and spray them cooking oil. Return the fryer basket to the Air Fryer and cook for 10 minutes at 365 F. Once done, allow them to cool. Enjoy.

RECIPE 178: CRASHED BONES WITH CHIPS AND HAM

Serve: 4 | Total Time: 25 minutes

600 g potatoes
Salt
1 tbsp olive oil
100 g Iberian Ham
4 eggs

Cut the elongated French fries, rinse through plenty of water and dry well with paper towels. Spray with oil and adjust the Air Fryer to 392 °F for a few minutes. Put all the potatoes in the Air Fryer and set the timer for 25 minutes at 392 °F. When we see that they are starting to brown, put paper under the potatoes and lay the eggs. Put in the Air Fryer again for 5 more minutes. Finally, add Iberian ham flakes. If you want to go faster while the potatoes are fried in the Air Fryer, you can prepare the grilled eggs in a small pan and then mix with the potatoes and ham on the plate. Serve.

RECIPE 179: CREAM POTATO

Serve: 2 | Total Time: 35 minutes

3 medium potatoes, scrubbed
½ tsp kosher salt
1 tbsp Italian seasoning
1/3 cup cream
½ tsp ground black pepper

Slice the potatoes. Preheat the Air Fryer to 365 F. Make the layer from the sliced potato in the Air

Fryer basket. Sprinkle the potato layer with the kosher salt and ground black pepper. After this, make the second layer of the potato and sprinkle it with Italian seasoning. Make the last layer of the sliced potato and pour the cream. Cook the scallop potato for 20 minutes. When the scalloped potato is cooked – let it chill till the room temperature. Enjoy!

RECIPE 180: CREAMY CHICKEN SALAD

Serve: 4 | Total Time: 17 minutes

1 pound (454 g) chicken breasts, skinless and boneless
¼ cup mayonnaise
¼ cup sour cream
1 tbsp lemon juice
salt and black pepper, to taste
½ cup chopped celery

Pat the chicken dry with paper towels. Place the chicken in a lightly oiled Air Fryer basket. Cook the chicken breasts at 380ºF (193ºC) for 12 minutes, turning them over halfway through the cooking time. Shred the chicken breasts using two forks; transfer it to a salad bowl and add in the remaining ingredients. Toss to combine and serve chilled. Bon appétit!

RECIPE 181: CREAMY PESTO SPAGHETTI SQUASH

Serve: 4 | Total Time: 30 minutes

2 tsp olive oil
1(11/2-pound) spaghetti squash, halved and seeded
1/2 tsp salt, divided
1/2 cup pesto
1/2 cup ricotta cheese
2 tbsp chopped fresh basil leaves

Preheat Air Fryer at 375F for 3 minutes. Rub olive oil over both halves of spaghetti squash. Season with half of salt. Place both halves, flat sides down, in ungreased Air Fryer basket. Cook 25 minutes. Transfer squash to a cutting board and let cool for 5 minutes until easy to handle. Once cooled, use a fork to gently pull the strands out of squash and place into a medium bowl. Toss squash noodles with pesto, ricotta cheese, and remaining salt. Garnish with basil leaves. Serve warm.

RECIPE 182: CREOLE CHICKEN DRUMETTES

Serve: 4 | Total Time: 50 minutes

1 lb chicken drumettes
½ cup flour
½ cup heavy cream
½ cup sour cream
½ cup bread crumbs
1 tbsp Creole seasoning
2 tbsp melted butter

Preheat Air Fryer to 370°F. Combine chicken drumettes and flour in a bowl. Shake away excess flour and set aside. Mix the heavy cream and sour cream in a bowl. In another bowl, combine bread crumbs and Creole seasoning. Dip floured drumettes in cream mixture, then dredge them in crumbs. Place the chicken drumettes in the greased frying basket and Air Fry for 20 minutes, tossing once and brushing with melted butter. Let rest for a few minutes on a plate and serve.

RECIPE 183: CREOLE TURKEY WITH PEPPERS

Serve: 4 | Total Time: 65 minutes

2 pounds turkey thighs, skinless and boneless
1 red onion, sliced
2 bell peppers, deveined and sliced
1 habanero pepper, deveined and minced
1 carrot, sliced
1 tbsp Creole seasoning mix
1 tbsp fish sauce
2 cups chicken broth

Preheat your Air Fryer to temperature of 360 degrees F. Now, spritz the bottom and sides of the casserole dish with a nonstick

cooking spray. Arrange the turkey thighs in the casserole dish. Add the onion, pepper, and carrot. Sprinkle with Creole seasoning. Afterward, add the fish sauce and chicken broth. Cook in the preheated Air Fryer for 30 minutes. Serve warm and enjoy!

RECIPE 184: CRISPY AIR FRIED PICKLES

Serve: 4 | Total Time: 30 minutes

14 dill pickles, sliced
¼ cup all-purpose flour
1/8 tsp baking powder
a pinch of salt
2 tbsp cornstarch + 3 tbsp water
6 tbsp panko bread crumbs
½ tsp paprika
oil for spraying

Dry the pickles using a paper towel then set aside. In a bowl, mix together the all-purpose flour, baking powder and salt. Add the cornstarch and water slurry. Whisk until well combined. Combine the panko bread crumbs and paprika in a shallow dish or platter. Mix until combined. Dredge the pickles in the flour batter first then on to the panko. Place on a plate and spray all pickles with oil. Put inside a preheated Air Fryer and cook at 400F for 15 minutes or until golden brown.

RECIPE 185: CRISPY AND CRUNCHY BABY CORN

Serve: 4 | Total Time: 10 minutes

1 cup almond flour
1 tsp garlic powder
¼ tsp chili powder
4 baby corns, boiled
Salt to taste
½ tsp carom seeds
Pinch of baking soda

In a bowl, add flour, chili powder, garlic powder, baking soda, carom seed, and salt. Mix well. Pour a little water into the batter to make a nice batter. Dip boiled baby corn into the batter to coat. Preheat

your Air Fryer to 350°Fahrenheit. Line the Air Fryer basket with foil and place the baby corns on foil. Cook baby corns for 10-minutes.

RECIPE 186: CRISPY BANANA BITES

Serve: 6 | Total Time: 15 minutes

1 large banana, sliced
6 wonton wrappers
½ cup peanut butter
1-2 tsp vegetable oil

Add-Ins
Chocolate chips
Raisins
M&M's
Ground cinnamon

Spread the wonton wrappers out on a work surface. Place a banana slice and a tsp of peanut butter at the center of each wonton wrapper. Add any of the add ins of your choice, to the filling and avoid over filling. Wet the edges and bring them together. Pinch them together to seal the stuffing. Place the wrappers in the Air Fryer's Basket and spray them with cooking oil. Return the fryer basket to the Air Fryer and cook for 6 minutes at 380 F. Enjoy with ice cream and cinnamon sugar.

RECIPE 187: CRISPY BREAKFAST PIES

Serve: 4 | Total Time: 35 minutes

8 oz frozen dough sheet
4 eggs
1/3 cup ham, cooked & crushed
1/3 cup bacon, cooked chopped
1/3 cup cheese, shredded

Preheat your Air Fryer to 380 F. Unroll the dough on a work surface. Unroll the paper to make a 13x9-inch rectangle. Separate into 4 equal rectangles (6 1/2x4 1/2 inches). Place rectangles of dough on a cookie sheet. Make a 1/2-inch rimmed border around each rectangle by bringing the edges toward the center. 1 egg should be carefully broken in the middle of each dough rectangle. Each pie should be topped with ham, bacon, and cheese. Cook for 15-20 minutes in the Air Fryer, until the edges of the crescent dough are golden brown and the egg whites and yolks are cooked. Serve and enjoy a delicious and nutritious breakfast.

RECIPE 188: CRISPY BREAKFAST AVOCADO FRIES

Serve: 2 | Total Time: 8 minutes

2 eggs, beaten
2 large avocados, peeled, pitted, cut into 8 slices each
¼ tsp pepper
½ tsp cayenne pepper
Salt to taste
Juice of ½ a lemon
½ cup of whole wheat flour
1 cup whole wheat breadcrumbs
Greek yogurt to serve

Add flour, salt, pepper and cayenne pepper to bowl and mix. Add bread crumbs into another bowl. Beat eggs in a third bowl. First, dredge the avocado slices in the flour mixture. Next, dip them into the egg mixture and finally dredge them in the breadcrumbs. Place avocado fries into the Air Fryer basket. Preheat the Air Fryer to 390°Fahrenheit. Place the Air Fryer basket into the Air Fryer and cook for 6-minutes. When cook time is completed, transfer the avocado fries onto a serving platter. Sprinkle with lemon juice and serve with Greek yogurt.

RECIPE 189: CRISPY BREAKFAST TACO WRAPS

Serve: 4 | Total Time: 30 minutes

1 tbsp water
4 pieces commercial vegan nuggets, chopped
1 small yellow onion, diced
1 small red bell pepper, chopped
2 cobs grilled corn kernels
4 large tortillas mixed greens for garnish

Preheat the Air Fryer to 400F. In a skillet heated over medium heat, water sauté the vegan nuggets together with the onions, bell peppers, and corn kernels. Set aside. Place filling inside the corn tortillas. Fold the tortillas and place inside the Air Fryer and cook for 15 minutes until the tortilla wraps are crispy. Serve with mix greens on top.

RECIPE 190: CRISPY BRUSSELS SPROUTS

Serve: 2 | Total Time: 25 minutes

1 pound Brussels sprouts, cut into bite-sized pieces
1 tbsp olive oil
1 tbsp balsamic vinegar
A pinch of kosher salt to taste
Freshly ground black pepper to taste

In a large mixing bowl place Brussels sprouts Drizzle oil and balsamic vinegar over Brussels sprouts. Season with salt & pepper to taste. Toss to combine the Brussels sprouts well to completely coat with the mixture. Preheat the Air Fryer for 370 F. Transfer coated Brussels sprouts to the Air Fryer basket and cook for about 8-10 minutes, shaking couple times during cooking. Cook until golden brown, crispy and cooked. When you're finished, move the dish to a serving platter and serve it.

RECIPE 191: CRISPY CHEESE STICKS

Serve: 4 | Total Time: 5 minutes

1 (16-ounce) package mozzarella cheese
½ tsp salt
1 tsp garlic powder
1 tsp onion powder
1 tsp cayenne pepper
1 cup breadcrumbs
1 cup almond flour
2 eggs, beaten

Cut the mozzarella cheese into 3 (1/2 inch) sticks. Add beaten eggs in small bowl. In a bowl, add flour. In another small bowl, combine breadcrumbs, cayenne pepper, onion powder, garlic powder, and salt. Dip cheese sticks into beaten egg, then dip into flour, then return to egg, and coat with breadcrumbs. Place coated cheese in the fridge for 20-minutes. Preheat your Air Fryer to 400°Fahrenheit. Spray Air Fryer basket with cooking spray. Place the coated cheese sticks into Air Fryer and cook for 5-minutes. Serve hot!

RECIPE 192: CRISPY CHICKEN NUGGETS

Serve: 4 | Total Time: 25 minutes

1 lb. chicken breast, boneless, skinless, cubed
2 tbsp. panko breadcrumbs
2 tbsp. grated Parmesan cheese
2 tbsp. olive oil
5 tbsp. plain breadcrumbs
Salt and black pepper to taste

Preheat your Air Fryer to temperature of 380 degrees F. and grease. Season the chicken with pepper and salt. Take a bowl and, pour olive oil. In a separate bowl, add crumb and Parmesan cheese. Place the chicken pieces in the oil to coat, then dip into breadcrumb mixture and transfer to the Air Fryer. Work in batches if needed. Lightly spray chicken with cooking spray. Cook for 10 minutes, flipping once halfway through.

RECIPE 193: CRISPY CHICKEN SKINS

Serve: 2 | Total Time: 25 minutes

9 ounces chicken skins
2 tsp. garlic powder
2 tsp. onion powder
1 tsp. paprika
salt and pepper, to taste

Preheat the Air Fryer to temperature of 400 degrees F. Wash the chicken skins and pat dry with paper towels. Rub the garlic, onion, and paprika into the chicken skins. Place the skins, fat sides down, into the Air Fryer Basket. Cook for 15 minutes, and flip the skins over halfway through the cooking time. Season with salt and pepper to taste. Serve and enjoy!

RECIPE 194: CRISPY CHICKEN STRIPS

Serve: 4 | Total Time: 15 minutes
1 cup breadcrumbs
2 lbs. chicken breast, skinless, boneless
½ cup almond flour
1 tsp sea salt
¼ tsp black pepper
6 tbsp skimmed milk
3 large eggs
2 tbsp olive oil

In a bowl, mix breadcrumbs and olive oil. Mix well and set aside. Whisk the eggs and milk in a different bowl, adding salt and pepper. In a third bowl, add the flour. Cut the chicken breast into strips about 1-inch long. Dip the strips into flour, then egg mixture, and finally into breadcrumbs. Preheat your Air Fryer to 380°Fahrenheit. Cook the coated chicken strips for 15-minutes. Shake a couple of times during cook time.

RECIPE 195: CRISPY COCONUT TILAPIA

Serve: 4 | Total Time: 20 minutes

4 medium tilapia fillets
1/2 tsp salt
Freshly ground black pepper to taste
½ cup coconut milk
1 tsp ginger, grated
½ cup cilantro, chopped
2 garlic cloves, minced
½ tsp garam masala
2 tbsp olive oil
½ jalapeno, chopped

Add coconut milk with salt, pepper, cilantro, ginger, garlic, jalapeno and garam masala in the food processor, and pulse well. Cover the fish fillets with the olive oil, spread coconut mix all over, rub well. Preheat the Air Fryer to 380 F. Transfer fish to the fryer and cook for about 10 minutes, until ready and crisp. Serve and enjoy.

RECIPE 196: CRISPY CRABSTICK CRACKERS

Serve: 3 | Total Time: 25 minutes
1 packet Crabstick Filament, thawed
Cooking Spray

Ensure that your Air Fryer is set at 360 F. After detaching the plastic wrapper on each crabstick filament, peel and unroll them. Finally, separate them into little pieces, ½-inch wide is good for thicker crackers. Before transferring them into the frying basket, spray them with some cooking spray. Transfer the crab sticks in batches into the Air Fryer. Air fry each batch for 8-10 minutes. In the 4th minute, remove the tray and stir the crabstick crackers with your kitchen tongs. When air frying is completed, withdraw and allow to cool before storing them in an airtight container.

RECIPE 197: CRISPY FRIED PORK CHOPS THE SOUTHERN WAY

Serve: 4 | Total Time: 40 minutes

1/2 cup all-purpose flour
1/2 cup low-fat buttermilk
1/2 tsp black pepper
11/2 tsp Tabasco sauce
1 tsp paprika
4 bone-in pork chops

Place the buttermilk and hot sauce in a Ziploc bag and add the pork chops. Allow to marinate for at least an hour in the fridge. In a bowl, combine the flour, paprika, and black pepper. Remove pork from the Ziploc bag and dredge in the flour mixture. Preheat the Air Fryer to 390F. Spray the pork chops with oil. Set in the device and cook for 25 minutes.

RECIPE 198: CRISPY LAMB

Serve: 4 | Total Time: 30 minutes

1 tbsp bread crumbs
2 tbsp macadamia nuts, toasted and crushed
1 tsp olive oil
1 garlic clove, minced
28 oz rack of lamb
Salt and black pepper to the taste
1 egg,
1 tbsp rosemary, chopped

In a bowl, mix oil with garlic and stir well. Season lamb with salt, pepper and brush with the oil. In another bowl, mix nuts with breadcrumbs and rosemary. Put the egg in a separate bowl and whisk well. Dip lamb in egg, then in macadamia mix, place them in your Air Fryer's basket, cook at 360 degrees F and cook for 25 minutes, increase heat to 400 degrees F and cook for 5 minutes more. Divide among plates and serve right away. Enjoy!

RECIPE 199: CRISPY MUSTARD PORK TENDERLOIN

Serve: 4 | Total Time: 26 minutes

3 tbsp low-sodium grainy mustard
2 tsp olive oil
¼ tsp dry mustard powder
1 (1-pound) pork tenderloin, silver skin and excess fat trimmed and discarded
2 slices low-sodium whole-wheat bread, crumbled
¼ cup ground walnuts
2 tbsp cornstarch

Mix mustard, olive oil, and mustard powder in a small basin. Spread this mixture over the pork. On a plate, mix the bread crumbs, walnuts, and cornstarch. Dip the mustard-coated pork into the crumb mixture to coat. Air-fry the pork for 12 to 16 minutes, or until it registers at least 145°F on a meat thermometer. Slice to serve.

RECIPE 200: CRISPY NACHOS PRAWNS

Serve: 6 | Total Time: 25 minutes

18 large prawns, peeled and deveined
1 egg, beaten
1 (10 oz) bag nacho-cheese flavored corn chips, finely crushed

Rinse the prawns and dry by patting them. Whisk the egg in a small bowl. Transfer the crushed chips in a separate bowl. Dip a prawn in the whisked egg and the crushed chips respectively. Transfer the coated prawn into a plate and do the same for the remaining prawns. Ensure that your Air Fryer is preheated to 350 F. Transfer the coated prawns into the Air Fryer and allow to cook for 8 minutes. Opaque prawns mean they are well cooked. Withdraw from the Air Fryer and serve.

RECIPE 201: CRISPY ONION RINGS

Serve: 2 | Total Time: 10 minutes

1 tsp baking powder
¾ cup breadcrumbs
1 cup milk
1 egg, beaten
1 large onion, sliced
1 tsp salt
1 ¼ cup almond flour

Preheat the Air Fryer for 5-minutes. Combine the baking powder, flour, and salt in a small bowl. Use a different bowl to whisk the egg and milk in. Place the breadcrumbs in another bowl. Coat onion slices with flour, dip in egg mixture and coat with breadcrumbs. Place coated onion rings into Air Fryer basket and cooked at 350°Fahrenheit for 10-minutes. Serve and enjoy!

RECIPE 202: CRISPY PAPRIKA FISH FILLETS

Serve: 4 | Total Time: 20 minutes

1/2 cup seasoned bread crumbs

1 tbsp balsamic vinegar
1/2 tsp seasoned salt
1 tsp paprika
1/2 tsp ground black pepper
1 tsp celery seed
2 fish fillets, halved
1 egg, beaten

Add the breadcrumbs, vinegar, salt, paprika, ground black pepper, and celery seeds to your food processor. Process for about 30 seconds. Coat the fillets with the beaten egg, then the breadcrumbs. Cook at 350 degrees F for about 15 minutes.

RECIPE 203: CRISPY PARMESAN CRUSTED PORK CHOPS

Serve: 4 | Total Time: 30 minutes

½ tsp salt
½ tsp onion powder
4 thick pork chops, center-cut boneless
¼ tsp pepper
1 tsp smoked paprika
¼ tsp chili powder
1 cup pork rind crumbs
2 large eggs, beaten
3 tbsp Parmesan cheese, grated
Preheat your Air Fryer to temperature of 400 degrees F. Season pork chops with salt and pepper. Take a bowl and mix in pork rind crumbs, Parmesan cheese, seasoning. Place beaten eggs in another bowl. Dip each pork chop into the egg mix, then in crumb mix. Transfer to an Air Fryer and cook for 20 minutes. Serve and enjoy!

RECIPE 204: CRISPY POPCORN CHICKEN

Serve: 12 | Total Time: 10 minutes

1 chicken breast, boneless
Salt and pepper to taste
1 cup breadcrumbs
2 tsp mix spice
¼ cup almond flour
1 egg, beaten

Add the chicken to your food processor and process it until it is

minced. In a bowl, add the beaten egg. In another bowl, add the flour. Blend the breadcrumbs, spice, pepper, and salt in a third shallow dish and toss to combine. Make small chicken balls from minced chicken. Roll chicken balls in flour, then dip into egg, then coat with breadcrumbs. Place coated chicken balls into Air Fryer and air fry at 350°Fahrenheit for 10-minutes. Serve hot!

RECIPE 205: CRISPY PORK BELLY

Serve: 2 | Total Time: 65 minutes

½ lb. whole pork belly; with skin
1/4 cup onions, sliced.
1/4 cup fresh rosemary, chopped.
3 garlic cloves; smashed
2 tsp. garlic powder
2 tsp. onion powder
1 tsp. paprika

Preheat the Air Fryer to temperature of 400 degrees F. Remove excess water from the pork belly with paper towels. Mix together the prepared garlic powder, the onion powder, paprika and fresh rosemary and rub the mixture evenly on the pork belly. Line with pork belly with the garlic and onion slices. Roll the belly into a log and secure it with kitchen yarn. Place the log in the Air Fryer and cook for 30 minutes. Flip over the log and cook for 25 minutes more or until the skin is crispy. Serve and enjoy!

RECIPE 206: CRISPY PORK DUMPLINGS

Serve: 8 | Total Time: 20 minutes

5 lb. Ground pork
1 tbsp. Olive oil
5 tsp. each Black pepper and salt
Half of 1 pkg. Dumpling wrappers

Set the Air Fryer temperature setting at 390 Fahrenheit. Mix the fixings. Prepare each dumpling using two tsp of the pork mixture. Seal the edges with a portion of water to make the triangle form.

Lightly spritz the Air Fryer basket using a cooking oil spray as needed. Add the dumplings to air-fry for eight minutes. Serve when they're ready.

RECIPE 207: CRISPY SHRIMP

Serve: 8 | Total Time: 8 minutes

4 egg whites
1 cup almond flour
2 lbs. shrimp, peeled and deveined
½ tsp cayenne pepper
2 tbsp olive oil
1 cup breadcrumbs
Salt and black pepper to taste

In a dish mix flour, pepper, and salt. In a small bowl, whisk egg whites. In another bowl, mix breadcrumbs, cayenne pepper, and salt. Preheat your Air Fryer to 400°Fahrenheit. Coat the shrimp with flour mixture, dip in egg white, then finally coat with breadcrumbs. Place shrimp in Air Fryer basket and drizzle with olive oil and cook in batches for 8-minutes each.

RECIPE 208: CRISPY SHRIMP SCAMPI

Serve: 6 | Total Time: 20 minutes

4 tbsp butter
1 tbsp lemon juice
1 tbsp minced garlic
2 tsp red pepper flakes
1 tbsp chopped chive
1 tbsp minced basil leaves
2 tbsp chicken stock
1 lb defrosted shrimp

Melt butter in a 6-inch hot pan. Add garlic and red pepper flakes to sauté for 2 minutes approximately. Transfer the pan to the Air Fryer. Add all the remaining scampi ingredients to the pan. Cook for 5 minutes with occasional stirring. Thoroughly mix well and remove the hot pan from the fryer. Let the shrimp rest for 1 minute. Thoroughly mix gently and garnish with basil. Serve warm.

RECIPE 209: CRISPY SOUTHWESTERN HAM EGG CUPS

Serve: 2 | Total Time: 17 minutes

4 (1-ounce) slices deli ham
4 large eggs
2 tbsp full-fat sour cream
1/4 cup diced green bell pepper
2 tbsp diced red bell pepper
2 tbsp diced white onion
1/2 cup shredded medium Cheddar cheese
Four baking cups each with one ham slice. Mix eggs and sour cream in a big basin. Mix in green, red, and onion. Into the ham-lined baking cups. Add Cheddar. Put cups in frying basket. Adjust the temperature to 320F and set the timer for 12 minutes or until the tops are browned. Serve warm.

RECIPE 210: CRISPY SWEET-AND-SOUR COD FILLETS

Serve: 2 | Total Time: 15 minutes

1 ½ cups Plain panko bread crumbs
2 tbsp Regular or low-fat mayonnaise
¼ cup Sweet pickle relish
3 4- to 5-ounce skinless cod fillets

Preheat the Air Fryer to 400°F. Pour the bread crumbs into a shallow soup plate or a small pie plate. Mix the mayonnaise and relish in a small bowl until well combined. Smear this mixture all over the cod fillets. Set them in the crumbs and turn until evenly coated on all sides, even on the ends. Set the coated cod fillets in the basket with as much air space between them as possible. They should not touch. Air-fry undisturbed for 12 minutes, or until browned and crisp. Use a nonstick-safe spatula to transfer the cod pieces to a wire rack. Cool for only a minute or two before serving hot.

RECIPE 211: CRISPY TOFU BITES

Serve: 4 | Total Time: 20 minutes

1 pound Extra firm unflavored tofu
Vegetable oil spray

Wrap the piece of tofu in a triple layer of paper towels. Place it on a wooden cutting board and set a large pot on top of it to press out excess moisture. Set aside for 10 minutes. Preheat the Air Fryer to 400°F. Remove the pot and unwrap the tofu. Cut it into 1-inch cubes. Place these in a bowl and coat them generously with vegetable oil spray. Toss gently, then spray generously again before tossing, until all are glistening. Gently pour the tofu pieces into the basket, spread them into as close to one layer as possible, and air-fry for 20 minutes, using kitchen tongs to gently rearrange the pieces at the 7- and 14-minute marks, until light brown and crisp. Gently pour the tofu pieces onto a wire rack. Cool for 5 minutes before serving warm.

RECIPE 212: CRUMBED FISH FILLETS WITH TARRAGON

Serve: 4 | Total Time: 45 minutes

2 eggs, beaten
1/2 tsp tarragon
4 fish fillets, halved
2 tbsp dry white wine
1/3 cup parmesan cheese, grated
tsp seasoned salt
1/3 tsp mixed peppercorns
1/2 tsp fennel seed
Add the parmesan cheese, salt, peppercorns, fennel seeds, and tarragon to your food processor; blitz for about 20 seconds. Drizzle fish fillets with dry white wine. Dump the egg into a shallow dish. Now, coat the fish fillets with the beaten egg on all sides; then, coat them with the seasoned cracker mix. Air-fry at 345 degrees f for about 17 minutes.

RECIPE 213: CRUNCHY CANADIAN BACON

Serve: 4 | Total Time: 10 minutes

10-ounces Canadian bacon, sliced
1 tsp cream

½ tsp salt
¼ tsp ground black pepper
½ tsp ground coriander
½ tsp ground thyme

In a mixing bowl combine the thyme, coriander, black pepper, and salt. Sprinkle this spice mix on top of the bacon slices on each side. Preheat your Air Fryer to 360°Fahrenheit. Place prepared bacon inside the Air Fryer and cook it for 5-minutes. After this turn, the sliced bacon over and cook for an additional 5-minutes more. Remove cooked bacon from Air Fryer, sprinkle with cream, and serve immediately.

RECIPE 214: CRUNCHY CHICKEN STRIPS

Serve: 4 | Total Time: 40 minutes

1 chicken breast, sliced into strips
1 tbsp grated Parmesan cheese
1 cup breadcrumbs
1 tbsp chicken seasoning
2 eggs, beaten
Salt and pepper to taste

Preheat Air Fryer to 350°F. Mix the breadcrumbs, Parmesan cheese, chicken seasoning, salt, and pepper in a mixing bowl. Coat the chicken with the crumb mixture, then dip in the beaten eggs. Finally, coat again with the dry ingredients. Arrange the coated chicken pieces on the greased frying basket and Air Fry for 15 minutes. Turn over halfway through cooking and cook for another 15 minutes. Serve immediately.

RECIPE 215: CRUNCHY FISH TACO

Serve: 6 | Total Time: 20 minutes

12 ounces cod filet
1 cup breadcrumbs
4-6 flour tortillas
4 tbsp tempura butter
½ cup salsa
½ cup guacamole
2 tbsp freshly chopped cilantro
½ tsp salt
¼ tsp black pepper

Lemon wedges for garnish

Cut cod fillets lengthwise into 2-inch pieces and season with salt and pepper from all sides. Place tempura butter to a bowl and dip each cod piece into it. Then dip filets into breadcrumbs. Preheat the Air Fryer for about 340 degrees F and cook the fish sticks for 10 to 13 minutes, flipping once. Meanwhile, spread guacamole on each tortilla. Place cod stick to a tortilla and top with chopped cilantro and salsa. Squeeze lemon juice, fold and serve.

RECIPE 216: CRUNCHY GOLDEN NUGGETS

Serve: 4 | Total Time: 15 minutes

2 chicken breasts, cut into nuggets
4 tbsp sour cream
½ cup bread crumbs
½ tbsp garlic powder

From the Cupboard:
½ tsp cayenne pepper
Salt and ground black pepper, to taste

Preheat the Air Fryer to temperature of 360°F (182°C). Cooking spray the Air Fryer basket. Put the sour cream in a large bowl. Combine the bread crumbs, cayenne pepper, garlic powder, salt, and black pepper on a large plate. Dredge the chicken nuggets in the bowl of sour cream, shake the excess off, then roll the nuggets through the bread crumbs mixture to coat well. Cook for 10 minutes in the Air Fryer basket until golden brown and crispy. Flip the nuggets halfway through the cooking time. Remove the nuggets from the basket and serve warm.

RECIPE 217: CRUSTED TILAPIA COCONUT FLAVOR

Serve: 4 | Total Time: 20 minutes

4 (4 ounces filets) tilapia fillets
3/4 cup unsweetened flaked coconut

1/2 cup coconut flour
1 tsp. sea salt
3 eggs, beaten

Mix coconut flour, unsweetened flaked, coconut, and sea salt together. Crack an egg into a bowl. Then sink the fillets into the cracked egg and then into the coconut mixture. Grease the Air Fryer pan with oil. Put the fish in the pan and spray with olive oil. Place the pan into the Air Fryer and set to cook at 400 F for 4 minutes. Check and flip the fish after 4 minutes and continue cooking for another 4 minutes. Serve and enjoy

RECIPE 218: CURRIED CAULIFLOWER FLORETS

Serve: 4 | Total Time: 10 minutes

1/4 cup sultanas or golden raisins
¼ tsp salt
1 tbsp curry powder
1 head cauliflower, broken into small florets
¼ cup pine nuts
½ cup olive oil

In a cup of boiling water, soak your sultanas to plump. Preheat your Air Fryer to 350°Fahrenheit. Add oil and pine nuts to Air Fryer and toast for a minute or so. In a bowl toss the cauliflower and curry powder as well as salt, then add the mix to Air Fryer mixing well. Cook for 10-minutes. Drain the sultanas, toss with cauliflower, and serve.

RECIPE 219: CURRIED CHICKEN LEGS

Serve: 4 | Total Time: 40 minutes

¾ cup Greek yogurt
1 tbsp tomato paste
2 tsp curry powder
½ tbsp oregano
1 tsp salt
1 ½ lb chicken legs
2 tbsp chopped fresh mint

Combine yogurt, tomato paste, curry powder, oregano and salt in a bowl. Divide the mixture in half. Cover one half and store it in the fridge. Into the other half, toss in the chicken until coated and marinate covered in the fridge for 30 minutes up to overnight. Preheat Air Fryer to 370ºF. Shake excess marinade from chicken. Place chicken legs in the greased frying basket and Air Fry for 18 minutes, flipping once and brushing with yogurt mixture. Serve topped with mint.

RECIPE 220: DELICATE STEAK WITH GARLIC

Serve: 3 | Total Time: 40 minutes

1 pound halibut steak
2/3 cup soy sauce
¼ cup sugar
½ cup Japanese cooking wine
2 tbsp lime juice
1 garlic clove, crushed
¼ cup orange juice
¼ tsp ground ginger
¼ tsp crushed red pepper flakes
½ tsp salt

Mix all ingredients in a saucepan and make a fine marinade. Bring to a boil over high heat. Divide in halves. One half of the marinade put with the halibut in releasable bag and set aside in the refrigerator for 30 minutes. Set the Air Fryer's heat to 390 degrees Fahrenheit and cook the marinated steak for 10 to 12 minutes. The other half of the marinade serves with cooked steak.

RECIPE 221: DESSERT FRIES

Serve: 4 | Total Time: 25 minutes

2 medium sweet potatoes peeled
½ tbsp of coconut oil.
1 tbsp arrowroot starch
2 tsp melted butter
1/4 cup coconut Sugar
2 tbsp cinnamon
Powdered Sugar for dusting
Dipping Sauces
Dessert Hummus

Honey or Vanilla Greek Yogurt

Slice the peeled sweet potatoes into long ½ thick strips. Toss these slices with arrowroot starch and ½ tbsp coconut oil in a large bowl. Spread the slices in the Air Fryer's Basket and return the basket to the fryer. Cook them for 18 minutes at 370 F by pressing the Start button. Toss them well once cooked half way through. Whisk sugar with cinnamon in a small bowl. Toss the fried potatoes with 2 tsp butter and drizzle cinnamon on top. Serve with dipping sauces.

RECIPE 222: DIJON LIME CHICKEN

Serve: 6 | Total Time: 20 minutes

8 chicken drumsticks
1 lime, juiced
1 lime zest
1 tsp salt
1 tbsp light mayonnaise
½ tsp black pepper
2 garlic cloves, minced
3 tbsp Dijon mustard
1 tsp dried parsley
1 tsp olive oil

Preheat the Air Fryer to 370 F. Get rid of the skin of the chicken. Season the chicken with salt and black pepper. In a large bowl mix Dijon mustard with lime juice. Stir in lime zest, minced garlic and parsley. Mix to combine. Cover the chicken with the lime mixture. Set aside for 10-20 minutes. Sprinkle the Air Fryer with olive oil and add chicken drumsticks. Cook for 5 minutes on each side until cooker and crispy. Serve with mayonnaise.

RECIPE 223: DIJON MUSTARD BREADED CHICKEN

Serve: 4 | Total Time: 20 minutes

3 tbsp Dijon mustard
⅓ cup seasoned bread crumbs
1 cup panko breadcrumbs
Salt and pepper
1 lb skinless chicken cutlets
Cooking spray

Add mustard to one gallon-sized plastic bag and the bread crumbs, panko, salt, and pepper to another bag. Set aside. Dip 1-2 chicken pieces at a time into the mustard and lightly coat all sides. Remove the chicken from the mustard bag and place into the bag of bread crumbs. Seal and shake to coat with the crumb mixture. Gently press the crumbs into the chicken to ensure they are completely coated. Preheat the Air Fryer as per manufacturer directions. Lightly spray both sides of the coated chicken with the cooking spray, then add to the fryer. Cook at 360°F, and depending on thickness of cutlets cook them for 6-10 minutes until golden brown.

RECIPE 224: DILL MASHED POTATO

Serve: 2 | Total Time: 25 minutes

2 potatoes
2 tbsp fresh dill, chopped
1 tsp butter
½ tsp salt
¼ cup half and half

Preheat the Air Fryer to 390 F. Rinse the potatoes thoroughly and place them in the Air Fryer. Cook the potatoes for 15 minutes. After this, remove the potatoes from the Air Fryer. Peel the potatoes. Mash the potatoes with the help of the fork well. Then add chopped fresh dill and salt. Stir it gently and add butter and half and half. Take the hand blender and blend the mixture well. When the mashed potato is cooked – serve it immediately. Enjoy!

RECIPE 225: DILLY RED SNAPPER

Serve: 4 | Total Time: 40 minutes

Salt and pepper to taste
½ tsp ground cumin
¼ tsp cayenne
¼ teaspoon paprika
1 (1½-lb) whole red snapper
2 tbsp butter
2 garlic cloves, minced

¼ cup dill
4 lemon wedges

Preheat Air Fryer to 360°F. Combine salt, pepper, cumin, paprika and cayenne in a bowl. Brush the fish with butter, then rub with the seasoning mix. Stuff the minced garlic and dill inside the cavity of the fish. Put the snapper into the basket of the Air Fryer and Roast for 20 minutes. Flip the snapper over and Roast for 15 more minutes. Serve with lemon wedges and enjoy!

RECIPE 226: DUCK WITH MISO PASTE

Serve: 5 | Total Time: 35 minutes

2 pounds (907 g) duck breasts
1 tbsp butter, melted
2 tbsp pomegranate molasses
2 tbsp miso paste
1 tsp minced garlic
1 tsp peeled and minced ginger
1 tsp five-spice powder

Towel-dry the duck breasts. Toss the duck breast with the remaining ingredients. Cook the duck breasts at 330°F (166ºC) for 15 minutes, turning them over halfway through the cooking time. Turn the heat to 350ºF (177ºC); continue to cook for about 15 minutes or until cooked through. Allow it to rest for 10 minutes before cutting. Bon appétit!

RECIPE 227: EGGPLANT FRIES

Serve: 4 | Total Time: 15 minutes

2 large eggplants, thinly sliced
Salt, to taste
1 tsp red chilies
½ tsp coriander
1/ tsp baking powder
½ tsp dry pomegranate seeds
1 cup chickpea flour
½ cup water

Combine water, chickpea flour, baking powder, salt, coriander, red chili and dry pomegranate seeds in a bowl. Mix well to make a paste.

If the mixture is sticky, add additional water. Then dump all the eggplants into the mixture and mix to coat well. Place the eggplant into the Air Fryer basket and let it cook at 390 degrees until brown on top. Serve.

RECIPE 228: EGGPLANT PARMESAN

Serve: 4 | Total Time: 50 minutes

1 large eggplant,
1/2 cup whole wheat bread crumbs
3 tbsp finely grated parmesan cheese
Salt, to taste
1 tsp Italian seasoning mix
3 tbsp whole wheat flour
1 free-range egg
1 tbsp water
Olive oil spray
1 cup marinara sauce
1/4 cup grated mozzarella cheese
Fresh parsley or basil to garnish

Set your Air Fryer to 360F. Merge the flour, egg and water in a large bowl. Add the breadcrumbs, parmesan, Italian seasoning and salt in a shallow bowl. Mix properly to combine. Put the eggplant into the egg mixture, drip off any excess, place into the breadcrumbs and coat evenly. Cook in the Air Fryer until perfectly cooked.

RECIPE 229: EGGPLANTS SATAY

Serve: 1 | Total Time: 25 minutes

2 large eggplants, center cored
1/3 cup cornstarch+1/4 cups water
4 tbsp Olive Oil
Pinch of sea salt
1 cup tomatoes
½ cup chopped mint leaves
1 tsp ginger garlic paste
1 large onion, chopped

Preheat the Air Fryer to temperature of 392 degrees F. Wash and cut the top of the eggplant. Center core the eggplants. Now, in a skillet, sauté the onion in oil along with ginger

and garlic paste. Then add in the tomatoes and mint leaves. Season it with salt. Mix cornstarch in water and add to the skillet. Let the mixture cook for 2 minutes. Then turn off the heat. Now fill the cavity of the eggplants with the prepared mixture. Place eggplant into the Air Fryer. Cook for 16 minutes. Then serve.

RECIPE 230: EGGS IN ZUCCHINI NESTS

Serve: 4 | Total Time: 7 minutes

4 tsp butter
½ tsp paprika
½ tsp black pepper
¼ tsp sea salt
4-oz cheddar cheese, shredded
4 eggs
8-oz zucchini, grated

Grate the zucchini and place the butter in ramekins. Add the grated zucchini in ramekins in the shape of nests. Sprinkle the zucchini nests with salt, pepper, and paprika. Beat the eggs and pour over zucchini nests. Top egg mixture with shredded cheddar cheese. Preheat the Air Fryer basket and cook the dish for 7-minutes. When the zucchini nests are cooked, chill them for 3-minutes and serve them in the ramekins.

RECIPE 231: FENNEL AND CHICKEN RATATOUILLE

Serve: 4 | Total Time: 30 minutes

1 lb boneless, skinless chicken thighs, cubed
2 tbsp grated Parmesan cheese
1 eggplant, cubed
1 zucchini, cubed
1 bell pepper, diced
1 fennel bulb, sliced
1 tsp salt
1 tsp Italian seasoning
2 tbsp olive oil
1 (14-oz) can diced tomatoes
1 tsp pasta sauce
2 tbsp basil leaves

Preheat Air Fryer to 400°F. Mix the chicken, eggplant, zucchini, bell pepper, fennel, salt, Italian seasoning, and oil in a bowl. Place the chicken mixture in the frying basket and Air Fry for 7 minutes. Transfer it to a cake pan. Mix in tomatoes along with juices and pasta sauce. Air Fry for 8 minutes. Scatter with Parmesan and basil. Serve.

RECIPE 232: FENNEL WITH SHIRATAKI NOODLES

Serve: 3 | Total Time: 65 minutes

1 fennel bulb, quartered
Salt and white pepper, to taste
1 clove garlic, finely chopped
1 green onion, thinly sliced
1 cup Chinese cabbage, shredded
2 tbsp rice wine vinegar
2 tbsp sesame oil
1 tsp ginger, freshly grated
1 tbsp soy sauce
1 1/3 cups Shirataki noodles, boiled

Start by preheating your Air Fryer to temperature of 370 degrees F. Now, cook the fennel bulb in the lightly greased cooking basket for 15 minutes, shaking the basket once or twice. Let it cool completely and toss with the remaining ingredients. Serve well chilled.

RECIPE 233: FETA AND MUSHROOM FRITTATA

Serve: 4 | Total Time: 30 minutes

1 red onion, thinly sliced
4 cups button mushrooms, thinly sliced
Salt to taste
6 tbsp feta cheese, crumbled
6 medium eggs
Non-stick cooking spray
2 tbsp olive oil

Sauté onion and mushrooms in olive oil till soft. Remove the vegetables from pan and drain on a paper towel-lined plate. In a mixing bowl, whisk eggs and salt.

Coat all sides of baking dish with cooking spray. Preheat your Air Fryer to 325°Fahrenheit. Pour the beaten eggs into prepared baking dish and scatter the sautéed vegetables and crumble feta on top. Bake in the Air Fryer for 30-minutes. Allow to cool slightly and serve!

RECIPE 234: FETA ORZO AND LAMB CHOPS

Serve: 4 | Total Time: 35 minutes

1 tbsp. lemon juice, fresh
4 garlic cloves, chopped finely
8 lamb loin chops, 1/4 pound, fat-trimmed
½ tsp. salt
2 tbsp. sundried tomatoes, oil-packed, drained' chopped finely
1 cup, orzo/rosamarina pasta, uncooked
1 tsp. oregano leaves, dried
½ tbsp. pepper
1/3 feta cheese, basil-tomato, crumbled

Preheat Air Fryer at 375 degrees Fahrenheit. Follow package direction in cooking pasta without adding oil and salt. Drain and keep warm. Combine salt (1/4 teaspoon), pepper, garlic, and oregano. Rub mixture all over lamb chops. Cook lamb chops in Air Fryer for 30 minutes, turning halfway. Toss pasta with tomatoes, oil, cheese, lemon juice, and remaining pepper (1/4 teaspoon) and salt (1/4 teaspoon). Serve with the lamb chops.

RECIPE 235: FIGS WITH HONEY AND MASCARPONE

Serve: 4 | Total Time: 12 minutes

8 figs
1/3 cup butter
2 tbsp honey
150ml mascarpone
1 tsp almonds, to serve
A Few tsp Rosewater, as per needed

Preheat your Air Fryer to temperature of 390 degrees F.
Make a cut on the top of each fig and squeeze slightly to open them.
Place them on a heatproof dish and place butter on each of the figs.
Drizzle a generous amount of honey over the top
Then place in the Air Fryer basket and cook for 6 minutes.
Stir rosewater into the mascarpone.
Place a dollop of mascarpone on each caramelized fig and top it off with almonds.
Serve and enjoy.

RECIPE 236: FIJIAN COCONUT FISH

Serve: 2 | Total Time: 35 minutes

1 cup coconut milk
2 tbsp lime juice
2 tbsp shoyu sauce
Salt and white pepper, to taste
1 tsp turmeric powder
1/2 tsp ginger powder
1/2 Thai bird's eye chili, seeded and finely chopped
1-pound tilapia
2 tbsp olive oil

In a mixing bowl, thoroughly combine the coconut milk with the lime juice, shoyu sauce, salt, pepper, turmeric, ginger, and chili pepper. Add tilapia and let it marinate for 1 hour. Olive oil the Air Fryer basket. Discard the marinade and place the tilapia fillets in the Air Fryer basket. Cook the tilapia in the preheated Air Fryer at 400 degrees f for 6 minutes; turn them over and cook for 6 minutes more. Work in batches. Serve with some extra lime wedges if desired.

RECIPE 237: FILLED MUSHROOMS WITH CRAB AND CHEESE

Serve: 6 | Total Time: 30 minutes

16 oz baby bella mushrooms, stems removed
½ cup lump crabmeat, shells discarded
2 oz feta cheese, crumbled

1 tsp prepared horseradish
1 tsp lemon juice
Salt and pepper to taste
2 tbsp bread crumbs
2 tbsp butter, melted
¼ cup chopped dill

Preheat Air Fryer to 350°F. Combine the feta, crabmeat, horseradish, lemon juice, salt, and pepper in a bowl. Evenly stuff the crab mixture into mushroom caps, scatter bread crumbs over and drizzle with melted butter over the crumbs. Place the stuffed mushrooms in the frying basket. Bake for 10 minutes. Scatter with dill to serve.

RECIPE 238: FISH AND CAULIFLOWER CAKES

Serve: 4 | Total Time: 15 minutes

1/2-pound cauliflower florets
1/2 tsp English mustard
2 tbsp butter, room temperature
1/2 tbsp cilantro, minced
2 tbsp sour cream
2 ½ cups cooked white fish
Salt and freshly cracked black pepper, to savor

Boil the cauliflower until tender. Then, purée the cauliflower in your blender. Transfer to a mixing dish. Now, stir in the fish, cilantro, salt, and black pepper. Add the sour cream, English mustard, and butter; mix until everything's well incorporated. Using your hands, shape them into patties. Refrigerate the patties for 2 hours. Cook for 13 minutes at 395 degrees f. Serve with some extra English mustard.

RECIPE 239: FISH FILLETS WITH PARMESAN CHEESE

Serve: 4 | Total Time: 17 minutes

1 cup Parmesan cheese, grated
1 egg whisked
1 tsp garlic powder
1/2 tsp shallot powder
4 white fish fillets

Preheat the Air Fryer to 370F (188C). In a shallow dish, put the Parmesan cheese. Mix the whisked egg, garlic powder, and shallot powder in a bowl, and stir to combine. On a clean surface, season the fillets generously with salt and pepper. Dredge the fillets into the egg mixture, and then roll over the cheese until thickly coated. Assemble the fillets in the Air Fryer basket and air fry until golden brown, about 10 to 12 minutes. Let the fish fillets cool for 5 minutes before serving.

RECIPE 240: FISH TORTILLAS WITH COLESLAW

Serve: 4 | Total Time: 30 minutes

1 tbsp olive oil
1 lb cod fillets
3 tbsp lemon juice
2 cups chopped red cabbage
½ cup salsa
1/3 cup sour cream
6 taco shells, warm
1 avocado, chopped

Preheat Air Fryer to 400°F. Brush oil on the cod and sprinkle with some lemon juice. Place in the frying basket and Air Fry until the fish flakes with a fork, 9-12 minutes. Meanwhile, mix together the remaining lemon juice, red cabbage, salsa, and sour cream in a medium bowl. Put the cooked fish in a bowl, breaking it into large pieces. Then add the cabbage mixture, avocados, and warmed tortilla shells ready for assembly. Enjoy!

RECIPE 241: FIVE SPICE CREAM CHEESE CHICKEN

Serve: 4 | Total Time: 35 minutes

1 pound chicken thighs, boneless
¼ tsp garlic powder
¼ cup milk or almond milk
¼ tsp mustard, ground
½ tsp adobo seasoning
½ tsp cayenne pepper
¼ tsp paprika, smoked
½ tsp salt

1 tbsp olive oil, extra virgin
1 tbsp butter
¼ cup cream cheese
2 tbsp heavy cream

Except for the chicken thighs, put all of the ingredients in a pan. Mix thoroughly to desired consistency. Add the thighs to the pan, coating slightly with the mixture. Cook in Air Fryer for 20 minutes at 356°F (180°C). If chicken is still raw, cook for another 5 minutes at 392°F (200°C). Serve.

RECIPE 242: FIVE SPICE DUCK BREAST

Serve: 3 | Total Time: 35 minutes

1 pound (454 g) duck breast
1 tbsp Hoisin sauce
1 tbsp five-spice powder
Sea salt and black pepper, to taste
¼ tsp ground cinnamon

Towel-dry the duck breasts. Toss the duck breast with the remaining ingredients. Cook the duck breast at 330ºF (166ºC) for 15 minutes, turning them over halfway through the cooking time. Turn the heat to 350ºF (177ºC); continue to cook for about 15 minutes or until cooked through. Wait 10 minutes before cutting or serving. Bon appétit!

RECIPE 243: FLUFFY POTATO CAKES

Serve: 3 | Total Time: 55 minutes

3 medium-sized potatoes, peeled
1 small-sized red onion, minced
1 small-sized garlic, minced
1 serrano pepper, seeded and minced
1 tbsp flax seeds, ground
2 tbsp oat flour
1 tsp smoked paprika
Sea salt and ground pepper, to taste
2 tbsp olive oil
2 tbsp fresh parsley leaves, chopped

Place your potatoes in the Air Fryer cooking basket; cook the potatoes at 400 degrees F for about 40 minutes, shaking the basket occasionally to promote even cooking. Mash your potatoes with a fork or potato masher. Mix together the remaining ingredients and make equal patties. Cook the potato cakes at 390 degrees F for about 10 minutes, flipping them halfway through the cooking time. Garnish with fresh herbs, if desired. Bon appétit!

RECIPE 244: FRENCH TOAST SOLDIERS

Serve: 2 | Total Time: 22 minutes

4 slices whole meal bread
2 large eggs
¼ cup whole milk
¼ cup brown sugar
1 tbsp honey
1 tsp cinnamon
A pinch of nutmeg
A pinch of icing sugar

Chop up the bread into soldiers, or fingers. Each slice yields 4 soldiers. Then, place the rest of the ingredients apart from the icing sugar into a mixing bowl. Mix well. Dip each soldier into the mixture until well-coated and place into the Air Fryer. Cook at 320°F (160°C) for 10 minutes until toasted. Halfway through cooking, flip each soldier over. Serve with a sprinkle of icing sugar.

RECIPE 245: FRENCH TOAST STICKS

Serve: 12 | Total Time: 15 minutes

1 tsp ground cinnamon
1 tsp vanilla extract
1 tbsp butter, melted
2 large eggs, beaten
3 oz milk
4 slices day-old bread, cut into thirds
1 tsp confectioners sugar, or to taste

Combine the cinnamon, vanilla extract, butter, eggs, and milk in a mixing bowl. After lining the Air Fryer basket with parchment paper, dip each bread piece into the milk mixture and place in the basket. Ensure that there are spaces between them, and divide into batches if there is the need to. Ensure that your Air Fryer is preheated to 360 F, then place in the basket containing the bread. Allow to cook for 6 minutes, and change to the other side, and cook for an extra 3 minutes. Sprinkle each stick with confectioner's sugar. Serve.

RECIPE 246: FRIDAY NIGHT CHEESEBURGERS

Serve: 4 | Total Time: 20 minutes

1 lb ground beef
1 tsp Worcestershire sauce
1 tbsp allspice
Salt and pepper to taste
4 cheddar cheese slices
4 buns

Preheat Air Fryer to 360°F. Combine beef, Worcestershire sauce, allspice, salt and pepper in a large bowl. Form 4 equal patties. Place the burgers in the greased frying basket and Air Fry for 8 minutes. Flip and cook for another 3-4 minutes. Top each burger with cheddar cheese and cook for another minute so the cheese melts. Transfer to a bun and serve.

RECIPE 247: FRIED BANANAS

Serve: 2 | Total Time: 12 minutes

2 large bananas
½ cup plain flour
2 eggs, whisked
¾ cup breadcrumbs
½ cup cinnamon sugar
1 tbsp olive oil
A pinch of salt

Take 4 bowls and place separately: flour with salt, whisked eggs, breadcrumbs, and cinnamon sugar. Peel bananas and cut them into thirds. Evenly cover bananas with the flour, then with eggs, and finally with breadcrumbs. Preheat the Air Fryer to 360°F. Sprinkle covered bananas with olive oil and put into the Air Fryer. Cook for 4-5 minutes, and then make a shake to move bananas. Cook for another 4-5 minutes. Remove the bananas and through then directly into the cinnamon sugar. Get them cool for a minute and eat!

RECIPE 248: FRIED CATFISH WITH FISH FRY

Serve: 4 | Total Time: 18 minutes

4 catfish fillets rinsed and patted dry
1/4 cup seasoned fish fry
1 tbsp chopped parsley
1 tbsp olive oil
Warm the Air Fryer to 400F (205C). Put the fillets and seasoned fish fry in a Ziploc bag. Cover the bag and shake well until the fish is nicely coated. Brush both sides of each piece of fish with olive oil. Put the fillets in the Air Fryer basket. Cook in the preheated Air Fryer for 13 minutes. Flip the fillets once during cooking or until the fish is cooked through. Remove from the basket and garnish with chopped parsley.

RECIPE 249: FRIED CHEESECAKE BITES

Serve: 8 | Total Time: 50 minutes

8 oz. cream cheese, at room temp
1/2 cup + 2 tbsp Erythritol
4 tbsp cream, divided
1/2 tsp vanilla extract
1/2 cup almond flour

Add the cream cheese, 1/2 cup Erythritol, vanilla and 2 tbsp of the heavy cream in a large bowl. Stir to combine. Whisk with a wooden spoon until smooth. Scoop out the batter and place in a lined baking sheet. Place in the freezer for 30 minutes. Warm-up your Air Fryer to 350F. Merge the almond flour with the rest of the Erythritol in a bowl and stir together. In another bowl add the remaining cream. Dip the batter into the cream, and then roll up in the almond flour. Cook for 2-3 minutes in the Air Fryer. Serve and enjoy.

RECIPE 250: FRIED CHICKEN THIGHS AND LEGS

Serve: 4 | Total Time: 20 minutes

3 chicken legs, bone-in, with skin
3 chicken thighs, bone-in, with skin
1 cup buttermilk
2 tbsp extra-virgin olive oil
1 tsp ground cumin
1 tsp onion powder
1 tsp garlic powder
Salt and pepper to taste
2 cups almond flour

Wash and dry chicken and transfer to large bowl. Pour in buttermilk and set aside in the fridge for 2-hours. In another bowl, mix flour and all seasonings. Dip the chicken into flour mixture, then into buttermilk, and again into flour. Preheat your Air Fryer to 360°Fahrenheit and place the chicken legs and thighs into the fryer basket. Sprinkle with olive oil and cook for 20-minutes, turning chicken halfway through cook time.

RECIPE 251: FRIED COD AND SPRING ONION

Serve: 4 | Total Time: 20 minutes

7 oz cod fillet, washed and dried
Spring onion, white and green parts, chopped
A dash of sesame oil
5 tbsp light soy sauce
1 tsp dark soy sauce
3 tbsp olive oil
5 slices of ginger
1 cup of water
Salt and pepper to taste

Season the cod fillet with a dash of sesame oil, salt, and pepper. Preheat your Air Fryer to 356°Fahrenheit. Cook the cod fillet in Air Fryer for 12-minutes. For the seasoning sauce, boil water in a pan on the stovetop, along with both light and dark soy sauce and stir. In another small saucepan, heat the oil and add the ginger and white part of the spring onion. Fry until the ginger browns, then remove the ginger and onions. Top the cod fillet with shredded green onion. Pour the oil over the fillet and add the seasoning sauce on top.

RECIPE 252: FRIED HASSELBACK POTATOES

Serve: 4 | Total Time: 40 minutes

4 medium Yukon Gold potatoes
3 tbsp melted butter
1 tbsp olive oil
3 cloves garlic, crushed
½ tsp ground paprika
Salt and black pepper ground, to taste
1 tbsp chopped fresh parsley

Preheat your Air Fryer Machine to 350 F. Slice each potato from top to make 1/4-inch slices, without cutting its 1/2-inch bottom, keeping the potato's bottom intact. Mix butter, with olive oil, garlic, and paprika in a small bowl. Brush the garlic mixture on top of each potato and add the mixture into the slits. Season them with salt and black pepper. Place the seasoned potatoes in the Air Fryer's Basket and cook them for 15 minutes. Brushing the potatoes again with butter mixture. Cook the potatoes for 15 minutes more. Garnish with parsley. Serve warm.

RECIPE 253: FRIED HOT PRAWNS WITH COCKTAIL SAUCE

Serve: 4 | Total Time: 20 minutes

1 tsp chili powder
1 tsp chili flakes
½ tsp freshly ground black pepper
½ tsp sea salt
8-12 fresh king prawns

For sauce:

1 tbsp cider or wine vinegar
1 tbsp ketchup
3 tbsp mayonnaise

Ensure that your Air Fryer is set to 360 F. Get a clean bowl and combine the spices in it. Coat the prawns by tossing them in the spices mixture. Transfer the spicy prawns into the Air Fryer basket and place the basket in the Air Fryer. Allow the prawns to cook for 6 to 8 minutes (how long depends on the size of the prawns). Get another clean bowl and make a mixture of the sauce ingredients. Serve the prawns while hot alongside the cocktail sauce.

RECIPE 254: FRIED MEATBALLS IN TOMATO SAUCE

Serve: 2 | Total Time: 20 minutes

1 small onion
1 egg, beaten
11 oz minced beef
1 tbsp fresh thyme leaves, chopped
1 tbsp fresh parsley, chopped
3 tbsp bread crumbs
¾ cup tomato sauce
Salt and ground black pepper to taste

Ensure that your Air Fryer is preheated to 390F. Chop your onion into fine pieces and transfer it, alongside all other ingredients, into a clean mixing bowl. Mix thoroughly and form 10-12 balls. Separate the balls into two batches and transfer each batch into the Air Fryer basket. Fry each batch for 7 minutes. Transfer the meatballs into an oven dish, put the tomato sauce and place the oven dish into the Air Fryer basket. Then set the temperature to 320 F and allow to cook for 5 minutes. This will warm everything through before you finally serve.

RECIPE 255: GARLIC CHICKEN KEBAB

Serve: 2 | Total Time: 10 minutes

1 lb. chicken fillet, cut into small pieces
1 tbsp garlic, minced
½ cup plain yogurt
1 tbsp olive oil
Juice of one lime
1 tsp turmeric powder
1 tsp red chili powder
1 tsp black pepper
1 tbsp chicken masala

Mix the yogurt and spices in a bowl. Add the oil and squeeze half a lime into it and stir. Coat the chicken pieces with mixture one at a time. Marinate the chicken pieces in the fridge for 2 hours. Preheat your Air Fryer to 356°Fahrenheit. Place the grill pan into the Air Fryer and put the chicken pieces into it. Cook chicken for 10-minutes.

RECIPE 256: GARLIC LEMON COD FILLET

Serve: 4 | Total Time: 50 minutes

8 lemon slices
5 cloves garlic, sliced.
4 cod fillets
1/4 cup low sodium soy sauce
2-tbsp. lemon juice
1/4-tsp. ground ginger
1/4-tsp. ground red pepper

Place the soy sauce, lemon juice, garlic, ground red pepper and ground ginger in a large zip lock bag. Place the cod fillets in the zip lock bag and marinate well with the seasonings. Chill for at least 30 minutes. Preheat the Air Fryer to temperature of 350 degrees F. Drip off the excess seasoning from the fillets and arrange the fillets in the Air Fryer Basket. Use the Air Fryer Double Layer Rack if needed. Top each fillet with lemon slices and cook for 8 minutes or until the fish is cooked through. Serve and enjoy!

RECIPE 257: GARLIC MOZZARELLA STICKS

Serve: 4 | Total Time: 60 minutes

1 tbsp Italian seasoning

1 cup Parmesan cheese
8 string cheeses, diced
2 eggs, beaten
1 clove garlic, minced

Start by combining your parmesan, garlic, and Italian seasoning in a bowl. Dip your cheese into the egg, and mix well. Roll it into your cheese crumbles, and then press the crumbs into the cheese. Place them in the fridge for an hour, and then preheat your Air Fryer to 375 °F. Spray your Air Fryer down with oil, and then arrange the cheese strings into the basket. Cook for eight to nine minutes at 365 °F. Allow them to cool for at least five minutes before serving.

RECIPE 258: GARLIC MUSSELS

Serve: 2 | Total Time: 13 minutes

1-lb. fresh mussels, cleaned.
1/2 cup white wine
5 cloves garlic, minced.
1 tbsp. fresh cilantro, chopped.
1 tbsp. olive oil
1 tbsp. onions, sliced.
½ tsp. paprika
salt and pepper, to taste

Preheat the Air Fryer to temperature of 350 degrees F. Mix the mussels, olive oil, garlic, onions and paprika in the Air Fryer Baking Pan. Add salt, pepper, and white wine to taste. Place the Air Fryer Baking Pan in the Air Fryer Basket and cook for 5 minutes. Add the cilantro and cook for 3 more minutes. Serve and enjoy!

RECIPE 259: GARLIC SALMON BALLS

Serve: 2 | Total Time: 15 minutes

6 oz of tinned salmon
1 large egg
3 tbsp olive oil
5 tbsp wheat germ
½ tsp garlic powder
1 tsp dill, fresh, chopped
4 tbsp spring onion, diced
4 tbsp celery, diced

Preheat your Air Fryer to 370°Fahrenheit. Combine the salmon, egg, celery, onion, dill, and garlic in a large mixing bowl. Shape the mixture into golf ball size balls and roll them in the wheat germ. In a small pan, warm olive oil over medium-low heat. Add the salmon balls and slowly flatten them. Transfer them to your Air Fryer and cook for 10-minutes.

RECIPE 260: GARLICKY ROSEMARY LAMB CHOPS

Serve: 4 | Total Time: 22 minutes

4 lamb chops
2 sp olive oil
1 tsp fresh rosemary
2 garlic cloves, minced
2 tsp garlic puree
Salt & black pepper

Place the 4 lamb chops in the Air Fryer basket. Rub them with olive oil, rosemary, garlic, garlic puree, salt, and black pepper. Press "Power Button" of Air Fry Oven and turn the dial to select the "Air Fry" mode. Press the Time button and again turn the dial to set the cooking time to 12 minutes. To adjust the temperature to 350 degrees F, press the Temp button and move the dial. Place the Air frying basket in the oven and shut the lid after it has been warmed. Flip the chops when cooked halfway through then resume cooking. Serve warm.

RECIPE 261: GARLICKY SEA BASS WITH ROOT VEGGIES

Serve: 4 | Total Time: 25 minutes

1 carrot, diced
1 parsnip, diced
½ rutabaga, diced
½ turnip, diced
¼ cup olive oil
Celery salt to taste
4 sea bass fillets
½ tsp onion powder
2 garlic cloves, minced
1 lemon, sliced

Preheat Air Fryer to 380°F. Coat the carrot, parsnip, turnip and rutabaga with olive oil and salt in a small bowl. Lightly season the sea bass with and onion powder, then place into the frying basket. Spread the garlic over the top of the fillets, then cover with lemon slices. Pour the prepared vegetables into the basket around and on top of the fish. Roast for 15 minutes. Serve and enjoy!

RECIPE 262: GERMAN-STYLE PORK PATTIES

Serve: 6 | Total Time: 35 minutes

1 lb ground pork
¼ cup diced fresh pear
1 tbsp minced sage leaves
1 garlic clove, minced
2 tbsp chopped chives
Salt and pepper to taste
Preheat the Air Fryer to 375°F. Combine the pork, pear, sage, chives, garlic, salt, and pepper in a bowl and mix gently but thoroughly with your hands, then make 8 patties about ½ inch thick. Lay the patties in the frying basket in a single layer and Air Fry for 15-20 minutes, flipping once halfway through. Remove and drain on paper towels, then serve. Serve and enjoy!

RECIPE 263: GINGER PORK CHOPS

Serve: 5 | Total Time: 45 minutes

2 tbsp. of ground ginger
1 lb. of pork chop
1 cup of soy sauce
1 tsp. of parsley
1 tsp. of ground black pepper
1 cup of water
1 tbsp. of freshly-squeezed lemon juice
1 tsp. of garlic powder

Combine the soy sauce and water in a mixing bowl. Add fresh lemon juice and mix. Sprinkle the mixture with ground ginger, parsley, ground black pepper, and garlic powder. Add freshly squeezed lemon juice and stir well. Cut the pork chop roughly using a sharp object. Put the pork on the soy sauce mixture and allow it to sit for about 15 minutes. Set pressure cooker to Sauté mode. Place the amalgamation into the cooker and close its lid. Cook the dish for about 35 minutes. When cooked, open pressure cooker lid and serve the ginger pork chops while hot.

RECIPE 264: GINGERED BACON WRAPPED SCALLOPS

Serve: 6 | Total Time: 25 minutes

¼ cup tamarind sauce
1 tbsp dark brown sugar
1 ½ tsp minced fresh ginger
6 very large "dry" sea scallops
6 slices bacon, cut in half crosswise

Insert the dripping pan at the bottom of the Air Fryer and preheat in Air Fry mode at 350 F for 2 to 3 minutes. In a medium bowl, mix the tamarind sauce, brown sugar, ginger, and scallops. Allow marinating for 15 minutes and then, wrap each scallop with two bacon slices. Secure with toothpicks. Arrange the wrapped scallops on the cooking tray. Put the cooking tray onto the middle rack of the Air Fryer and close the lid. Set the timer for 15 minutes and push the Start button. Cook until the bacon is golden brown and crispy whole turning the food halfway the Cooking Time. Plate it and serve warm.

RECIPE 265: GLAZED CHICKEN THIGHS

Serve: 4 | Total Time: 25 minutes

1 lb boneless, skinless chicken thighs
¼ cup balsamic vinegar
3 tbsp honey
2 tbsp brown sugar
1 tsp whole-grain mustard
¼ cup soy sauce
3 garlic cloves, minced
Salt and pepper to taste
½ tsp smoked paprika

2 tbsp chopped shallots
Preheat Air Fryer to 375°F. Whisk vinegar, honey, sugar, soy sauce, mustard, garlic, salt, pepper, and paprika in a small bowl. Arrange the chicken in the frying basket and brush the top of each with some of the vinegar mixture. Air Fry for 7 minutes, then flip the chicken. Brush the tops with the rest of the vinegar mixture and Air Fry for another 5 to 8 minutes. Allow resting for 5 minutes before slicing. Serve warm sprinkled with shallots.

RECIPE 266: GOLDEN BREADED TURKEY SCHNITZEL

Serve: 3 | Total Time: 29 minutes

1½ pounds (680 g) turkey thighs, skinless, boneless
1 egg, beaten
½ cup all-purpose flour
½ cup seasoned bread crumbs
½ tsp crushed red pepper flakes
salt and black pepper, to taste
1 tbsp olive oil

Flatten the turkey thighs with a mallet. Whisk the egg in a shallow bowl. Place the flour in a second bowl. Then, in a third shallow bowl, place the bread crumbs, red pepper, salt, and black pepper. Dip the turkey first in the flour, then, in the beaten egg, and roll them in the bread crumb mixture. Place the breaded turkey thighs in the Air Fryer basket. Mist your schnitzel with the olive oil and transfer them to the basket. Cook the schnitzel at 380°F (193°C) for 22 minutes, turning them over halfway through the cooking time. Bon appétit!

RECIPE 267: GREEK CHICKEN WINGS

Serve: 4 | Total Time: 30 minutes

8 whole chicken wings
½ lemon, juiced
½ tsp garlic powder
1 tsp shallot powder
½ tsp Greek seasoning
Salt and pepper to taste

¼ cup buttermilk
½ cup all-purpose flour

Preheat Air Fryer to 400°F. Put the wings in a resealable bag along with lemon juice, garlic, shallot, Greek seasoning, salt and pepper. Seal the bag and shake to coat. Set up bowls large enough to fit the wings. In one bowl, pour the buttermilk. In the other, add flour. Using tongs, dip the wings into the buttermilk, then dredge in flour. Transfer the wings in the greased frying basket, spraying lightly with cooking oil. Air Fry for 25 minutes, shaking twice, until golden and cooked through. Allow to cool slightly, and serve.

RECIPE 268: GREEK EGGPLANT ROUNDS

Serve: 4 | Total Time: 20 minutes

2 tsp olive oil
1long, narrow eggplant, sliced into rounds
1/2 tsp salt
1/2 cup no-sugar-added marinara sauce
1/2 cup feta cheese crumbles
8 kalamata olives, pitted and halved
2 tbsp chopped fresh dill

Preheat Air Fryer at 350F for 3 minutes. Rub olive oil over both sides of eggplant circles. Lay out slices on a large plate and season evenly with salt. Top evenly with marinara sauce, feta crumbles, and olives. Place half of eggplant pizzas in ungreased Air Fryer basket. Cook 5 minutes. Transfer back to plate. Repeat cooking with remaining pizzas. Garnish with chopped dill and serve warm.

RECIPE 269: GREEK STREET TACOS

Serve: 8 | Total Time: 5 minutes

8 small flour tortillas (4-inch diameter)
8 tbsp hummus
4 tbsp crumbled feta cheese

4 tbsp chopped kalamata or other olives (optional)
olive oil for misting

Place 1 tablespoon of hummus or tapenade in the center of each tortilla. Top with 1 teaspoon of feta crumbles and 1 teaspoon of chopped olives, if using. Using your finger or a small spoon, moisten the edges of the tortilla all around with water. Fold tortilla over to make a half-moon shape. Press center gently. Then press the edges firmly to seal in the filling. Mist both sides with olive oil. Place in Air Fryer basket very close but try not to overlap. Cook at 390°F for 3minutes, just until lightly browned and crispy.

RECIPE 270: GREEK-STYLE DEVILED EGGS

Serve: 2 | Total Time: 15 minutes

3 eggs
1 tbsp chives, chopped
1 tbsp parsley, chopped
2 tbsp Kalamata olives, pitted and chopped
1 tbsp Greek-style yogurt
1 tsp habanero pepper, seeded and chopped
Sea salt and red pepper flakes

Set the wire rack in the Air Fryer basket and lower the eggs onto the rack. Cook the eggs at 260 degrees F for 15 minutes. Transfer the eggs to an ice-cold water bath to stop cooking. Skin the eggs under cold running water; slice them into halves, separating the whites and yolks. Press the egg yolks with the remaining ingredients and mix to combine. Spoon the yolk mixture into the egg whites and serve well chilled. Enjoy!

RECIPE 271: GREEK STYLES MINI BURGER PIES

Serve: 6 | Total Time: 55 minutes

Burger mixture:
1 onion, large, chopped

½ cup, Red bell peppers, roasted, diced
1 pound, ground lamb, 80% lean
¼ tsp. red pepper flakes
2 oz. feta cheese, crumbled

Baking mixture:
½ cup, milk
½ cup biscuit mix, classic
2 eggs

Preheat the Air Fryer at temperature of 350 degrees Fahrenheit. Grease 12 muffin cups using cooking spray. Cook the onion and beef in a skillet heated on medium-high. Once beef is browned and cooked through, drain and let cool for five minutes. Stir together with feta cheese, roasted red peppers, and red pepper flakes. Whisk the baking mixture ingredients together. Fill each muffin cup with baking mixture (1 tablespoon). Air-fry for twenty-five to thirty minutes. Let cool before serving.

RECIPE 272: GREEK VEGGIE WITH THYME

Serve: 4 | Total Time: 30 minutes

A handful cherry tomatoes, halved
Salt and black pepper to the taste
1 parsnip, roughly chopped
1 zucchini, roughly chopped
1 green bell pepper, cut into strips
1 carrot, sliced
2 tbsp stevia
1 tbsp parsley, chopped
2 tsp garlic, minced
6 tbsp olive oil
1 tsp mustard

In your Air Fryer, mix zucchini with bell pepper, parsnip, carrot, tomatoes, half of the oil, salt and pepper and cook at 360 degrees F for 15 minutes. In a bowl, mix the rest of the oil with salt, pepper, stevia, mustard, parsley and garlic and whisk. Pour this over veggies, toss to coat, cook for 5 minutes more at 375 degrees F, divide between plates and serve. Enjoy!

RECIPE 273: GREEN BEAN CRISPS

Serve: 4 | Total Time: 20 minutes

1 egg, beaten
1/4 cup cornmeal
1/4 cup parmesan, grated
1 tsp sea salt
1/2 tsp red pepper flakes, crushed
1 pound green beans
2 tbsp grape seed oil

In a mixing bowl, combine together the egg, cornmeal, parmesan, salt, and red pepper flakes; mix to combine well. Dip the green beans into the batter and transfer them to the cooking basket. Brush with the grape seed oil.
Cook in the preheated Air Fryer at 390 degrees F for 4 minutes. Shake the basket and cook for a further 3 minutes. Work in batches. Taste, adjust the seasonings and serve. Serve warm.

RECIPE 274: GREEN STUFFED PEPPERS

Serve: 3 | Total Time: 25 minutes

3 green bell peppers, tops, and seeds removed
1 medium-sized onion, diced
1 carrot, thinly diced
1 small cauliflower, shredded
1 tsp garlic powder
1 tsp coriander
1 tsp mixed spices
1 tsp Chinese five spice
1 tbsp olive oil
3 tbsp any soft cheese
1 zucchini, thinly diced
¼ yellow pepper, thinly diced

With the olive oil, sautè the onion in a wok over medium heat. Add the cauliflower and seasonings. Cook for 5-minutes, stir to combine. Add the vegetables (carrot, zucchini, yellow pepper) and cook for an additional 5-minutes more. Fill each of the green peppers with 1-tablespoon of soft cheese. Then stuff them with cauliflower mixture. Cap stuffed peppers with the tops and cook in Air Fryer for 15-minutes at 390°Fahrenheit.

RECIPE 275: GROUND CHICKEN MEATBALLS

Serve: 4 | Total Time: 20 minutes

1-lb. ground chicken
1/3 cup panko
1 tsp salt
2 tsp chives
1/2 tsp garlic powder
1 tsp thyme
1 egg

Toss all the meatball ingredients in a bowl and mix well. Make small meatballs out this mixture and place them in the Air Fryer basket. Press "Power Button" of Air Fry Oven and turn the dial to select the "Air Fry" mode. Press the Time button and again turn the dial to set the cooking time to 10 minutes. Now push the Temp button and rotate the dial to set the temperature at 350 degrees F. Once preheated, place the Air Fryer basket inside and close its lid. Serve warm.

RECIPE 276: GUAJILLO CHILE CHICKEN MEATBALLS

Serve: 4 | Total Time: 30 minutes

1 lb ground chicken
1 large egg
½ cup bread crumbs
1 tbsp sour cream
2 tsp brown mustard
2 tbsp grated onion
2 tbsp tomato paste
1 tsp ground cumin
1 tsp guajillo chile powder
2 tbsp olive oil

Preheat Air Fryer to 350ºF. Mix the ground chicken, egg, bread crumbs, sour cream, mustard, onion, tomato paste, cumin, and chili powder in a bowl. Form into 16 meatballs. Place the meatballs in the greased frying basket and Air Fry for 8-10 minutes, shaking once until browned and cooked through. Serve immediately.

RECIPE 277: GUILT FREE VEGETABLE FRIES

Serve: 4 | Total Time: 25 minutes

5 oz sweet potato, peeled
5 oz carrots, peeled
5 oz courgette, peeled
2 tbsp olive oil
1 tsp thyme
Pinch basil
Pinch mixed spice
Salt and ground black pepper to taste

Chop your peeled sweet potato, carrots, and courgettes into chunks of chips with different shapes. Gather them in the Air Fryer, alongside the olive oil. Allow cooking for 18 minutes at 360 F. Shake during the 5th and 12th minute to ensure even cooking. Withdraw the cooked chips from the Air Fryer and transfer them into a bowl. Add the seasoning and shake well to mix. Serve.

RECIPE 278: HALIBUT WITH COLESLAW

Serve: 4 | Total Time: 30 minutes

1 (12-oz) bag coleslaw mix
¼ cup mayonnaise
1 tsp lemon zest
1 tbsp lemon juice
1 shredded carrot
½ cup buttermilk
1 tsp grated onion
4 (6-oz) halibut fillets
Salt and pepper to taste

Combine coleslaw mix, mayonnaise, carrot, buttermilk, onion, lemon zest, lemon juice, and salt in a bowl. Let chill the coleslaw covered in the fridge until ready to use. Preheat Air Fryer at 350ºF. Sprinkle halibut with salt and pepper. Place them in the greased frying basket and Air Fry for 10 minutes until the fillets are opaque and flake easily with a fork. Serve with chilled coleslaw.

RECIPE 279: HAM AND CHEESE STUFFED CHICKEN

Serve: 4 | Total Time: 28 minutes

1 lb (454 g) chicken breasts, skinless, boneless, and cut into 4 slices
4 oz (113 g) goat cheese, crumbled
4 oz (113 g) ham, chopped
1 egg
¼ cup all-purpose flour
¼ cup grated Parmesan cheese
½ tsp onion powder
½ tsp garlic powder

Flatten the chicken breasts with a mallet. Stuff each piece of chicken with cheese and ham. Roll them up and secure with toothpicks. In a shallow bowl, mix the remaining ingredients until well combined. Dip the chicken rolls into the egg mixture. Place the stuffed chicken in the Air Fryer basket. Cook the stuffed chicken breasts at 400°F (204°C) for about 22 minutes, turning them over halfway through the cooking time. Bon appétit!

RECIPE 280: HAM AND TOMATOES OMELET

Serve: 2 | Total Time: 15 minutes

4 large eggs
1/2 cup cherry tomatoes, halved.
2 slices deli ham, chopped.
1/4 cup onions, sliced.
2-tbsp. chives, chopped.
2-tbsp. heavy cream
3-tbsp. parmesan cheese, grated.
salt and pepper, to taste

Preheat the Air Fryer to temperature of 400 degrees F. Lightly grease the Air Fryer Baking Pan with cooking spray. Salt and pepper the eggs and mix them with the heavy cream. Pour the eggs into the Air Fryer Baking Pan and add the cherry tomatoes, ham and onions. Fold in the parmesan cheese and top with the chives. Cook for 10 minutes or until desired doneness of eggs. Serve and enjoy!

RECIPE 281: HAM BREAKFAST

Serve: 6 | Total Time: 25 minutes

6 cups French bread, cubed

4 oz green chilies, chopped
10 oz ham, cubed
4 oz cheddar cheese, shredded
2 cups milk
5 eggs
1 tbsp mustard
Salt and black pepper to the taste
Cooking spray

Warmth up your Air Fryer at 350 degrees F and grease it with cooking spray. In a bowl, mix eggs with milk, cheese, mustard, salt and pepper and stir. Attach bread cubes in your Air Fryer and mix with chilies and ham. Add eggs mix, spread and cook for 15 minutes. Divide among plates and serve. Enjoy!

RECIPE 282: HAM BREAKFAST PIE

Serve: 6 | Total Time: 35 minutes

16 ounces crescent rolls dough
2 eggs, whisked
2 cups cheddar cheese, grated
1 tbsp parmesan, grated
2 cups ham, cooked and chopped
Salt and black pepper to the taste
Cooking spray

Set your Air Fryer's pan with cooking spray and press half of the crescent rolls dough on the bottom. In a bowl, mix eggs with cheddar cheese, parmesan, salt and pepper, pour well and add over dough. Scatter ham, divide the rest of the crescent rolls dough in strips, set them over ham and cook at 300 degrees F. Divide pie and serve for breakfast. Enjoy!

RECIPE 283: HAM WITH AVOCADO

Serve: 2 | Total Time: 15 minutes

1 large Hass avocado, halved and pitted
2 thin slices ham
2 large eggs
2 tbsp green onions, plus more for garnish
1/2 tsp fine sea salt
1/4 tsp ground black pepper
1/4 cup Cheddar cheese (omit for dairy-free)

Preheat the Air Fryer to 400F (205C). Place a slice of ham into the cavity of each avocado half. Crack an egg on top of the ham, then sprinkle on the green onions, salt, and pepper. Set the avocado halves in the Air Fryer cut side up and cook for 10 minutes. Top with the cheese (if using) and cook for 30 seconds more, or until the cheese is melted. Garnish with chopped green onions. Best served fresh.

RECIPE 284: HASH BROWNS

Serve: 3 | Total Time: 25 minutes

1 potato, grated
3 eggs, beaten
1 cup whole grain flour
1 tsp black pepper
1 pinch salt
1 tsp garlic powder
¼ tsp nutmeg
1 tbsp olive oil

Preheat your Airfryer to 390 degrees F. Combine the potato, eggs, flour and spices in a mixing bowl. Mix gently. (Stir by hand). Place the olive oil in a heat-safe dish. Spoon out the potato mix and flatten to form patties. Cook for 15 minutes. Serve alongside eggs for a hearty breakfast.

RECIPE 285: HAZELNUT-CRUSTED FISH

Serve: 4 | Total Time: 30 minutes

½ cup hazelnuts, ground
1 scallion, finely chopped
1 lemon, juiced and zested
½ tbsp olive oil
Salt and pepper to taste
3 skinless sea bass fillets
1 tsp Dijon mustard

Place the hazelnuts in a small bowl along with scallion, lemon zest, olive oil, salt and pepper. Mix everything until combined. Spray only the top of the fish with cooking oil, then squeeze lemon juice onto the fish. Coat the top of the fish with mustard. Spread with hazelnuts and press gently so that it stays on the fish. Preheat Air Fryer to 375°F. Air Fry the fish in the greased frying basket for 7-8 minutes or it starts browning and the fish is cooked through. Serve hot.

RECIPE 286: HEALTHY CHICKEN TENDERS

Serve: 2 | Total Time: 20 minutes

12 oz of chicken breasts
Salt and ground black pepper to taste
1 oz flour
1 egg white
1¼ oz panko bread crumbs

Before you cut the chicken breast into tenders, remove any excess fat by trimming. Use the combination of salt and pepper to season each side. Get your flour, egg, and panko breadcrumbs into different clean bowls. Then dip the chicken tenders into flour, eggs, and panko breadcrumbs respectively. Arrange the coated chicken into the basket of your Air Fryer, and spray with olive spray. Set your Air Fryer to temperature of 350 F and cook. Let the chicken cook through - for about 10 minutes.

RECIPE 287: HERBED ZUCCHINI POPPERS

Serve: 4 | Total Time: 30 minutes

1 tbsp grated Parmesan cheese
2 zucchini, sliced
1 cup breadcrumbs
2 eggs, beaten
Salt and pepper to taste
1 tsp dry tarragon
1 tsp dry dill

Preheat Air Fryer to 390°F. Place the breadcrumbs, Parmesan, tarragon, dill, salt, and pepper in a bowl and stir to combine. Dip the zucchini into the beaten eggs, then coat with Parmesan-crumb mixture. Lay the zucchini slices on the greased frying basket in an even layer. Air Fry for 14-16

minutes, shaking the basket several times during cooking. When ready, the zucchini will be crispy and golden brown. Serve hot and enjoy!

RECIPE 288: HERBY ROASTED CHERRY TOMATOES

Serve: 4 | Total Time: 20 minutes

1 tbsp dried oregano
1 tbsp dried basil
2 tsp dried marjoram
1 tsp dried thyme
1 tsp salt
2 tbsp balsamic vinegar
20 cherry tomatoes
1 tbsp olive oil

Preheat the Air Fryer to 400°F. Combine the oregano, basil, marjoram, thyme, and salt in a small bowl and mix well. Pout into a small glass jar. Poke each cherry tomato with a toothpick to prevent bursting. Put the tomatoes, balsamic vinegar and olive oil on a piece of aluminum foil and sprinkle with 1½ tsp of the herb mix; toss. Wrap the foil around the tomatoes, leaving air space in the packet, and seal loosely. Put the packet in the Air Fryer and Bake for 8-10 minutes or until the tomatoes are tender.

RECIPE 289: HOME-STYLE FISH STICKS

Serve: 4 | Total Time: 30 minutes

1 lb cod fillets, cut into sticks
1 cup flour
1 egg
¼ cup cornmeal
Salt and pepper to taste
¼ tsp smoked paprika
1 lemon

Preheat Air Fryer at 350ºF. In a bowl, add ½ cup of flour. In another medium-sized mixing bowl, beat the egg and in a third bowl, combine the remaining flour, cornmeal, salt, black pepper and paprika. Roll the sticks in the flour, shake off excess flour. Then,

dip them in the egg, shake off excess egg. Finally, dredge them in the cornmeal mixture. Place fish fingers in the greased frying basket and Air Fry for 10 minutes, flipping once. Serve with squeezed lemon.

RECIPE 290: HOMEMADE RANCH TATER TOTS

Serve: 2 | Total Time: 15 minutes

1/2 pound potatoes, peeled and shredded
1/2 tsp hot paprika
1/2 tsp dried marjoram
1 tsp Ranch seasoning mix
2 tbsp Colby cheese, finely grated about 1/3 cup
1 tsp butter, melted
Sea salt and ground black pepper, to flavor

In a mixing bowl, merge all ingredients until everything is well incorporated. Transfer your tater tots to a lightly greased Air Fryer cooking basket. Cook your tater tots in the preheated Air Fryer at 400 degrees F for 12 minutes to ensure even browning. Serve and enjoy!

RECIPE 291: HONEY DUCK BREASTS

Serve: 2 | Total Time: 32 minutes

1 duck breast, halved
1 tsp honey
1 tsp tomato paste
1 tbsp mustard
½ tsp apple vinegar

In a large bowl, mix honey with tomato paste, mustard and vinegar. Stir to combine well. Add duck breast pieces, toss to coat well. Preheat the Air Fryer to 370 F. Transfer to your Air Fryer and cook coated duck fillets for 15 minutes. Take duck breast out of the fryer, add to honey mixture, toss again, return to Air Fryer and cook at a hear of 370 degrees F for 6 minutes more. Serve and enjoy.

RECIPE 292: HONEY GLAZED SALMON

Serve: 2 | Total Time: 18 minutes

2 (6-oz.) salmon fillets
Salt, as required
2 tbsp honey

Sprinkle the salmon fillets with salt and then, coat with honey. Press "Power Button" of Air Fry Oven and turn the dial to select the "Air Fry" mode. Press the Time button and again turn the dial to set the cooking time to 8 minutes. Now push the Temp button and rotate the dial to set the temperature at 355 degrees F. Press "Start/Pause" button to start. When the unit beeps to show that it is preheated, open the lid. Arrange the salmon fillets in greased "Air Fry Basket" and insert in the oven. Serve hot.

RECIPE 293: HONEY ONIONS

Serve: 2 | Total Time: 30 minutes

2 large white onions
1 tbsp raw honey
1 tsp water
1 tbsp paprika

Peel the onions and using a knife, make cuts in the shape of a cross. Then combine the raw honey and water; stir. Add the paprika and stir the mixture until smooth. Place the onions in the Air Fryer basket and sprinkle them with the honey mixture. Cook the onions for 16 minutes at 380° F. When the onions are cooked, they should be soft. Transfer the cooked onions to serving plates and serve.

RECIPE 294: HONEY SEA BASS

Serve: 2 | Total Time: 20 minutes

2 sea bass fillets
Zest from ½ orange, grated
Juice from ½ orange
Salt and ground black pepper, to taste
2 tbsp mustard

2 tsp honey
2 tbsp olive oil
½ pound canned lentils, drained
A small bunch of dill, chopped
2 ounces watercress
A small bunch of parsley, chopped

Place fish fillets to a large bowl. Both sides should be seasoned with salt and pepper, then topped with orange zest and juice, 1 tablespoon oil, honey, and mustard. Prepare the Air Fryer to a heat of 350 degrees Fahrenheit. Place fish to the Air Fryer basket and cook for 10 minutes, turning once during cooking. Meanwhile, put lentils in a small pot, warm it up over medium heat, add the rest of the oil, watercress, dill and parsley, and stir to combine. Serve on plates, add cooked fish fillets and enjoy honey fish.

RECIPE 295: HORSERADISH SALMON

Serve: 2 | Total Time: 17 minutes

2 salmon fillets
1/4 cup breadcrumbs
2 tbsp olive oil
1 tbsp horseradish
Salt and Pepper
Fill an Air Fryer basket halfway with dehydrating trays, then place the Air Fryer basket inside an instant pot on the lowest setting. Place salmon fillets on dehydrating tray. In a small bowl, mix together breadcrumbs, oil, horseradish, pepper, and salt and spread over salmon fillets. Sealed with the Air Fryer lid, choose air fry mode and set the temperature to 400 degrees Fahrenheit and the timer for 7 minutes, and you're done! Serve and enjoy.

RECIPE 296: HOT CHICKEN WITH MUSTARD

Serve: 2 | Total Time: 17 minutes

¾ pound (340 g) chicken breasts, boneless, skinless
1 tsp minced garlic
½ cup red wine

¼ cup hot sauce
1 tbsp Dijon mustard
Sea salt and cayenne pepper, to taste

Place the chicken, garlic, red wine, hot sauce, and mustard in a ceramic bowl. Refrigerate the bowl for 3 hours to allow the chicken to marinate fully. Discard the marinade and place the chicken breasts in the Air Fryer basket. Cook the chicken breasts at 380ºF (193ºC) for 12 minutes, turning them over halfway through the cooking time. Season the chicken with the salt and cayenne pepper to taste. Bon appétit!

RECIPE 297: HOT OKRA WEDGES

Serve: 2 | Total Time: 35 minutes

1 cup okra, sliced
1 cup breadcrumbs
2 eggs, beaten
A pinch of black pepper
1 tsp crushed red peppers
2 tsp hot Tabasco sauce

Preheat Air Fryer to 350°F. Place the eggs and Tabasco sauce in a bowl and stir thoroughly; set aside. In a separate mixing bowl, combine the breadcrumbs, crushed red peppers, and pepper. Dip the okra into the beaten eggs, then coat in the crumb mixture. Lay the okra pieces on the greased frying basket. Air Fry for 14-16 minutes, shaking the basket several times during cooking. When ready, the okra will be crispy and golden brown. Serve.

RECIPE 298: INTENSE BUFFALO CHICKEN WINGS

Serve: 2 | Total Time: 40 minutes

8 chicken wings
½ cup melted butter
2 tbsp Tabasco sauce
½ tbsp lemon juice
1 tbsp Worcestershire sauce
2 tsp cayenne pepper
1 tsp garlic powder
1 tsp lemon zest

Salt and pepper to taste

Preheat Air Fryer to 350°F. Place the melted butter, Tabasco, lemon juice, Worcestershire sauce, cayenne, garlic powder, lemon zest, salt, and pepper in a bowl and stir to combine. Dip the chicken wings into the mixture, coating thoroughly. Lay the coated chicken wings on the foil-lined frying basket in an even layer. Air Fry for 16-18 minutes. Shake the basket several times during cooking until the chicken wings are crispy brown. Serve.

RECIPE 299: ITALIAN CHICKEN AND CHEESE FRITTATA

Serve: 4 | Total Time: 45 minutes

1 (1-pound) fillet chicken breast
salt and black pepper, to taste
1 tbsp olive oil
4 eggs
1/2 tsp cayenne pepper
1/2 cup Mascarpone cream
1/4 cup Asiago cheese, freshly grated
Using a meat mallet, flatten the breast. Season with salt and pepper. Preheat the olive oil in a medium frying pan. Cook for 10-12 minutes, then slice into tiny slices and reserve. Then, in a mixing bowl, thoroughly combine the eggs, and cayenne pepper; season with salt to taste. Add the cheese and stir to combine. Add the reserved chicken. And then add it to the cooking basket along with a lightly oiled pan. Cook in the preheated Air Fryer at 355 degrees F for 10 minutes, flipping over halfway through.

RECIPE 300: ITALIAN HERB STUFFED CHICKEN

Serve: 4 | Total Time: 30 minutes

2 tbsp olive oil
3 tbsp balsamic vinegar
3 garlic cloves, minced
1 tomato, diced
2 tbsp Italian seasoning
1 tbsp chopped fresh basil

1 tsp thyme, chopped
4 chicken breasts

Preheat Air Fryer to 370°F. Combine the olive oil, balsamic vinegar, garlic, thyme, tomato, half of the Italian seasoning, and basil in a medium bowl. Set aside. Cut 4-5 slits into the chicken breasts ¾ of the way through. Season with the rest of the Italian seasoning and place the chicken with the slits facing up, in the greased frying basket. Bake for 7 minutes. Spoon the bruschetta mixture into the slits of the chicken. Cook for another 3 minutes. Allow chicken to sit and cool for a few minutes. Serve and enjoy!

RECIPE 301: ITALIAN-STYLE TOMATO-PARMESAN CRISPS

Serve: 4 | Total Time: 25 minutes

4 Roma tomatoes, sliced
2 tablespoons olive oil
Sea salt and white pepper, to taste
1 teaspoon Italian seasoning mix
4 tablespoons Parmesan cheese, grated

Begin by preheating your Air Fryer, then set it to 350 degrees F. Generously grease the Air Fryer basket with nonstick cooking oil. Toss the sliced tomatoes with the remaining ingredient. Transfer them to the cooking basket without overlapping. Cook in the warmed Air Fryer for 5 minutes. Shake the cooking basket and cook an additional 5 minutes. Work in batches. Serve with Mediterranean aioli for dipping, if desired. Bon appétit!

RECIPE 302: JALAPENO POPPERS

Serve: 3 | Total Time: 50 minutes

8 oz of cream cheese
¾ cup gluten-free tortilla or bread crumbs
¼ cup fresh parsley
10 jalapeno peppers halved and deseeded

Combine the cream cheese and half of the crumbs first before adding the parsley. Fill each piece of pepper with this mixture. Press the top of each pepper into the other ¼ cup of crumbs, thus creating the top coating. Allow the peppers to cook in the Air Fryer at 370 F for 6-8 minutes. If you are using a conventional oven, just set the temperature to 375 F and the time, 20 minutes. Allow the peppers to cool before serving.

RECIPE 303: JAPANESE-INSPIRED GLAZED CHICKEN

Serve: 4 | Total Time: 25 minutes

4 chicken breasts
Chicken seasoning to taste
Salt and pepper to taste
2 tsp grated fresh ginger
2 garlic cloves, minced
¼ cup molasses
2 tbsp tamari sauce
Preheat Air Fryer to 400°F. Season the chicken breasts with seasoning. Place the chicken in the greased frying basket and Air Fry for 7 minutes, then flip the chicken. Cook for another 3 minutes. While the chicken is cooking, combine ginger, garlic, molasses, and tamari sauce in a saucepan over medium heat. Cook for 4 minutes or until the sauce thickens. Transfer all of the chicken to a serving dish. Drizzle with ginger-tamari glaze and serve.

RECIPE 304: JERK MEATBALLS

Serve: 6 | Total Time: 30 minutes

1 tsp minced habanero
1 tsp Jamaican jerk seasoning
1 sandwich bread slice, torn
2 tbsp whole milk
1 lb ground beef
1 egg
2 tbsp diced onion
1 tsp smoked paprika
1 tsp black pepper
1 tbsp chopped parsley
½ lime

Preheat Air Fryer at 350ºF. In a bowl, combine bread pieces with milk. Add in ground beef, egg, onion, smoked paprika, black pepper, habanero, and jerk seasoning, and using your hands, squeeze ingredients together until fully combined. Form mixture into meatballs. Place meatballs in the greased frying basket and Air Fry for 8 minutes, flipping once. Squeeze lime and sprinkle the parsley over.

RECIPE 305: KALE AND POTATO NUGGETS

Serve: 4 | Total Time: 35 minutes

1 tsp extra-virgin olive oil
1 clove of garlic, minced
4 cups kale, rinsed and chopped
2 cups boiled potatoes, finely chopped
1/8 cup almond milk
¼ tsp salt
1/8 tsp black pepper
cooking spray

Preheat the Air Fryer to 400F. Poke holes in the foil at the base of the Air Fryer basket to enable air to circulate. Heat the oil in a big pan and sauté the garlic for 2 minutes. Add the kale until it wilts. Transfer to a large bowl. Add the potatoes and almond milk. Season with salt and pepper to taste. Form balls and spray with cooking oil. Cook for 20 minutes or until golden brown inside the Air Fryer.

RECIPE 306: KALE CHIPS WITH WHITE HORSERADISH MAYO

Serve: 1 | Total Time: 10 minutes

2 cups loosely packed kale
1 tsp sesame oil
Sea salt and ground black pepper, to flavor
1 tsp sesame seeds, lightly toasted
1 ounce mayonnaise
1 tsp prepared white horseradish

Toss the kale pieces with sesame oil, salt and black pepper. Cook the kale pieces at 370 degrees F for 2

minutes; shake the basket and continue to cook for 2 minutes more. Meanwhile, make the horseradish mayo by whisking the mayonnaise and prepared horseradish. Let cool slightly, kale chips will crisp up as it cools. Sprinkle toasted sesame seeds over the kale chips. Serve the kale chips with the horseradish mayo. Enjoy!

RECIPE 307: KENTUCKY-STYLE PORK TENDERLOIN

Serve: 2 | Total Time: 30 minutes

1 lb pork tenderloin, halved crosswise
1 tbsp smoked paprika
2 tsp ground cumin
1 tsp garlic powder
1 tsp shallot powder
¼ tsp chili pepper
Salt and pepper to taste
1 tsp Italian seasoning
2 tbsp butter, melted
1 tsp Worcestershire sauce
Preheat Air Fryer to 350ºF. In a shallow bowl, combine all spices. Set aside. In another bowl, whisk butter and Worcestershire sauce and brush over pork tenderloin. Sprinkle with the seasoning mix. Place pork in the lightly greased frying basket and Air Fry for 16 minutes, flipping once. Let sit onto a cutting board for 5 minutes before slicing. Serve immediately.

RECIPE 308: KIDNEY BEANS IN AIR FRYER

Serve: 4 | Total Time: 55 minutes

2 cups kidney beans, pre-soaked
2 large red onion, chopped
Oil spray, for greasing the pan
2 garlic cloves, minced or paste
1 inch or tsp ginger, paste
Salt, to taste
1/3 tsp turmeric
1 tsp Red chili powder, to taste
4 cups water

Soak the beans for one hour before starting the cooking. Add oil in an Air Fryer pan along with red onions, ginger, garlic, turmeric,

chili, and salt. Cook for 6 minutes. Then open the Air Fryer and add the pre-soaked beans along with four cups of water. Cook for 18 minutes. The beans will become soft and tender. Serve with whole wheat bread or rice.

RECIPE 309: LAMB RACK WITH LEMON CRUST

Serve: 5 | Total Time: 35 minutes

1.7 lbs. frenched rack of lamb
Salt and black pepper, to taste
0.13-lb. dry breadcrumbs
1 tsp grated garlic
1/2 tsp salt
1 tsp cumin seeds
1 tsp ground cumin
1 tsp oil
1/2 tsp Grated lemon rind
1 egg, beaten

Place the lamb rack in a baking tray and pour the whisked egg on top. Whisk rest of the crusting ingredients in a bowl and spread over the lamb. Choose "Power Button" of Air Fry Oven and turn the dial to select the "Air Fry" mode. Choose the Time button and again turn the dial to set the cooking time to 25 minutes. Now press the Temp button and rotate the dial to set the temperature at 350 degrees F. Once preheated, set the lamb baking tray in the oven and close its lid. Slice and serve warm.

RECIPE 310: LAYERED CHEESE AND HAM CASSEROLE

Serve: 4 | Total Time: 25 minutes

¼ cup minced peeled sweet onion
1/3 cup shredded cheddar
5 eggs
Salt and pepper to taste
1 tsp Dijon mustard
1 tsp ground coriander
1 mashed clove of garlic
¼ cup diced cooked ham
2 bread slices, diced

Preheat Air Fryer at 325ºF. Combine the eggs, salt, black

pepper, coriander, garlic, mustard, onion, ham, cheddar cheese, and bread in a bowl. Pour it into a greased cake pan. Place cake pan in the frying basket and Air Fry for 14 minutes. Let cool onto a cooling rack for 5 minutes before slicing. Serve immediately.

RECIPE 311: LEMON DRUMSTICKS

Serve: 2 | Total Time: 38 minutes

½ cup hot sauce
2 tbsp butter
½ cup water
1/3 cup lemon juice
1 pound of drumstick

Add all the ingredients into the cook and crisp basket and place the basket inside the Air Fryer. Attaching the pressure cooker cover to the pot and turning the pressure valve to the seal position are the next steps. Set the pressure cooker function to high heat and set the timer for 5 minutes. Immediately after the cooking is done, release the pressure quickly by carefully opening the steamer valve. Serve it while hot.

RECIPE 312: LEMON GARLIC CHICKEN BREAST

Serve: 2 | Total Time: 30 minutes

1 pound chicken breasts, boneless and skinless
4 cloves of garlic, minced
1-2-inch ginger, minced
2 lemons
2 tbsp olive oil
Salt, to taste
Black pepper, to taste
¼ tsp turmeric

Combine garlic, ginger, lemons, olive oil, salt, pepper and turmeric in a bowl. Dump the chicken pieces in it and rub the chicken with the spices for perfect coating. Leave the chicken for 2 hours to marinate. Heat the Air Fryer for 5 minutes, and then place the chicken into the Air Fryer. Cook for 20 minutes at 375 degrees F.

Once the chicken turns golden, serve.

RECIPE 313: LEMON GARLIC PRAWNS WRAPPED IN BACON

Serve: 2 | Total Time: 31 minutes

6 large tiger prawns, peeled and deveined. but leave on the tails
6 rashers bacon
1 tbsp. ghee, melted.
1 tbsp. flat-leaf parsley leaves, chopped.
¼ tsp. lemon juice
1 tsp. garlic, minced

Preheat the Air Fryer to temperature of 350 degrees F. Mix together the melted ghee, minced garlic, lemon juice and chopped parsley. Brush the ghee mixture on the prawns and season with some pepper. Wrap the prawns with the slices of bacon and chill for 15 minutes. Arrange the prawns in the Air Fryer Basket and use the Air Fryer Double Layer Rack if needed. Cook for 6 minutes or until the prawns are cooked through. Serve and enjoy!

RECIPE 314: LEMON GARLIC SCALLOPS

Serve: 4 | Total Time: 18 minutes

1 lb sea scallops, pat dry with paper towels
1 tsp fresh thyme
1 garlic clove, minced
2 tbsp fresh lemon juice
1/4 cup olive oil
Pepper
Salt
Season scallops with pepper and salt. Using cooking spray, coat the Air Fryer basket. Add scallops into the Air Fryer basket and cook at 400°F for 5–8 minutes or until the internal temperature of scallops reaches 120°F. Transfer scallops to the serving bowl. Heat olive oil in a pan on medium heat. Add garlic and sauté until garlic softens. Add lemon juice and whisk until sauce is heated through. Pour olive oil

mixture overcooked scallops. Garnish with thyme and serve.

RECIPE 315: LEMON PEPPER TILAPIA FILLETS

Serve: 4 | Total Time: 20 minutes

4 tilapia fillets
1 tsp garlic powder
1 tsp paprika
1 tsp dried basil
Lemon-pepper seasoning, to taste

Heat the Air Fryer to 400F (205C). Add the olive oil, garlic powder, paprika, basil, lemon-pepper seasoning, fillets to a large bowl, and toss well to coat the fillets thoroughly. Transfer the coated fillets to the Air Fryer basket. Cook in the warmed Air Fryer for 8 minutes. Flip the fillets and cook for 7 minutes more until the fish flakes easily with a fork. Divide the fillets among four serving plates and serve hot.

RECIPE 316: LEMON PEPPER TURKEY

Serve: 6 | Total Time: 55 minutes

3 lbs. turkey breast
2 tbsp oil
1 tbsp Worcestershire sauce
1 tsp lemon pepper
1/2 tsp salt

Whisk everything in a bowl and coat the turkey liberally. Place the turkey in the Air Fryer basket. Press "Power Button" of Air Fry Oven and turn the dial to select the "Air Fry" mode. Press the Time button and again turn the dial to set the Cooking Time to 45 minutes. Now push the Temp button and rotate the dial to set the temperature at 375 degrees F. Once preheated, place the Air Fryer basket inside and close its lid. Serve warm.

RECIPE 317: LEMON TURKEY WINGS

Serve: 5 | Total Time: 45 minutes

2 pounds (907 g) turkey wings
2 tbsp olive oil
½ tsp garlic powder
½ tsp onion powder
1 tsp poultry seasoning mix
2 tbsp roughly chopped fresh parsley
1 lemon, cut into slices

Toss the turkey wings with the olive oil, garlic powder, onion powder, and poultry seasoning mix. Cook the turkey wings at 400°F (204°C) for 40 minutes, turning them over halfway through the cooking time. Reserving 10 minutes before slicing and serving Garnish the turkey wings with the parsley and lemon slices. Bon appétit!

RECIPE 318: LEMONY CHICKEN WITH BARBECUE SAUCE

Serve: 6 | Total Time: 22 minutes

6 boneless, skinless chicken thighs
2 tablespoons lemon juice
¼ cup barbecue sauce, gluten-free
2 cloves garlic, minced

In a medium bowl, mix the chicken, cloves, barbecue sauce, and lemon juice. Set aside for 10 minutes to marinate. Transfer the marinated chicken thighs into the Air Fryer basket, shaking off excess sauce. You may need to work in batches to avoid overcrowding. Put the Air Fryer lid on and grill in the preheated instant pot at 375°F for 12 minutes. Flip the chicken thighs when it shows 'TURN FOOD' on the lid screen halfway through cooking time or until the chicken registers at least 165°F using a meat thermometer inserted into the center of the chicken. Repeat this with remaining chicken thighs. Serve warm.

RECIPE 319: LEMONY LAMB CHOPS

Serve: 2 | Total Time: 35 minutes

2 medium lamb chops
1/4 cup lemon juice

Liberally rub the lamb chops with lemon juice. Place the lemony chops in the Air Fryer basket. Choose "Power Button" of Air Fry Oven and turn the dial to select the "Air Fry" mode. Choose the Time button and again turn the dial to set the cooking time to 25 minutes. Now press the Temp button and rotate the dial to set the temperature at 350 degrees F. Close the oven door after preheating the Air Fryer basket. Flip the chops when cooked halfway through then resume cooking. Serve warm.

RECIPE 320: LIME CHICKEN

Serve: 4 | Total Time: 25 minutes

2 pounds chicken breasts, boneless and skinless
2 cloves of garlic, minced
1-inch ginger, minced
4 limes, zest, and juice
4 tbsp vegetable oil
Salt, to taste
Black pepper, to taste
1/3 tsp red chilies
1 cup yogurt
1/3 tsp cumin
½ tsp white pepper

Combine garlic cloves, ginger, lime zest, lime juice, vegetable oil, salt, black pepper, red chills, yogurt, cumin and white pepper in a bowl. Marinade the chicken for 1 hour. Now preheat the Air Fryer to 375 degrees F. Place the chicken in the Air Fryer basket and cook it for 25 minutes. Once brown, serve and enjoy.

RECIPE 321: LOBSTER TAILS WITH GREEN OLIVES

Serve: 5 | Total Time: 17 minutes

2 pounds (907 g) fresh lobster tails, cleaned and halved, in shells
1 tsp onion powder
1 tsp cayenne pepper
2 garlic cloves, minced

1 cup of green olives

Warm the Air Fryer to 390°F (199°C) and spray the basket with cooking spray. Put all the ingredients except for the green olives in a sealable plastic bag. Seal the bag and shake until the lobster tails are coated completely. Arrange the coated lobster tails in the greased basket. Cook in batches in the preheated Air Fryer for 6 to 7 minutes, shaking the basket halfway through. Remove from the basket and serve with green olives.

RECIPE 322: MARINATED SCALLOPS WITH BUTTER AND BEER

Serve: 4 | Total Time: 67 minutes

2 pounds sea scallops
1/2 cup beer
4 tablespoons butter
2 sprigs rosemary, only leaves
salt and cracked black pepper, to taste
In a ceramic dish, mix the sea scallops with beer; let it marinate for 1 hour. Meanwhile, preheat your Air Fryer to temperature of 400 degrees f. Melt the butter and add the rosemary leaves. Stir for a few minutes. Discard the marinade and transfer the sea scallops to the Air Fryer basket. Season with salt and black pepper. Cook the scallops in the preheated Air Fryer for 7 minutes, shaking the basket halfway through the cooking time. Work in batches.

RECIPE 323: MASHED SWEET POTATO TOTS

Serve: 6 | Total Time: 12 minutes

1 cup cooked mashed sweet potatoes
1 egg white, beaten
⅛ tsp ground cinnamon
1 dash nutmeg
2 tbsp chopped pecans
1½ tsp honey
salt
½ cup panko breadcrumbs

oil for misting or cooking spray

Preheat Air Fryer to 390°F. Mix the potatoes, egg white, cinnamon, nutmeg, nuts, honey, and salt to taste. Put panko crumbs on wax paper. For each tot, use about 2 teaspoons of sweet potato mixture. To shape, drop the measure of potato mixture onto panko crumbs and push crumbs up and around potatoes to coat edges. Then turn tot over to coat other side with crumbs. Mist tots with oil or cooking spray and place in Air Fryer basket in single layer. Cook at 390°F for 12 minutes, until browned and crispy. Repeat steps 5 and 6 to cook remaining tots.

RECIPE 324: MEATBALLS IN TOMATO SAUCE

Serve: 2 | Total Time: 20 minutes

2 green onions, minced
2 tsp garlic cloves, minced
1 egg, cooked
½ cup saltine cracker crumbs
Pinch salt, to taste
1 tsp freshly ground black pepper
1 pound beef, ground
Olive oil for misting
2 cups pasta sauce
1 tsp mustard paste
2 green chilies

Combine green onions, cooked egg, garlic, cracker crumbs, green chilies, salt, and pepper in a bowl and mix well. Mix in the ground beef. Form the 3-inch meatballs of the prepared mixture. Now mist the meatballs with olive oil. Cook for 15 minutes in an Air Fryer basket. Meanwhile, combine pasta sauce with mustard paste. Open the Air Fryer after 15 minutes and add in the pasta sauce. Cook for 4 more minutes. Then serve it over cooked rice.

RECIPE 325: MEDITERRANEAN AIR FRIED VEGGIES

Serve: 4 | Total Time: 16 minutes

1 large zucchini, sliced

1 cup cherry tomatoes, halved
1 parsnip, sliced
1 green pepper, sliced
1 carrot, sliced
1 tsp mixed herbs
1 tsp mustard
1 tsp garlic purée
6 tbsp olive oil
Salt and ground black pepper, to taste

Preheat the Air Fryer oven to 400°F (204ºC). Combine all the ingredients in a bowl, making sure to coat the vegetables well. Press "Power Button" turn the dial to select "air fry". Push "Temp" to set the temperature at 400°F. Press "Timer" to set the cooking time to 6 minutes and air fry, ensuring the vegetables are tender and browned. Serve immediately.

RECIPE 326: MEXICAN CHEESY ZUCCHINI BITES

Serve: 4 | Total Time: 25 minutes

1 large-sized zucchini, thinly sliced
1/2 cup flour
1/4 cup yellow cornmeal
1 egg, whisked
1/2 cup tortilla chips, crushed
1/2 cup Queso Añejo, grated
Salt and cracked pepper, to taste

Pat dry the zucchini slices with a kitchen towel. Mix the remaining ingredients in a shallow bowl; mix until everything is well combined. Dip each zucchini slice in the prepared batter. Cook in the preheated Air Fryer at 400 degrees F for 12 minutes, shaking the basket halfway through the cooking time. Work in batches until the zucchini slices are crispy and golden brown. Enjoy!

RECIPE 327: MEXICAN CHICKEN ROLL-UPS

Serve: 4 | Total Time: 35 minutes

½ red bell pepper, cut into strips
½ green bell pepper, cut into strips
2 chicken breasts

½ lime, juiced
2 tbsp taco seasoning
1 spring onion, thinly sliced

Preheat Air Fryer to 400°F. Cut the chicken into cutlets by slicing the chicken breast in half horizontally in order to have 4 thin cutlets. Drizzle with lime juice and season with taco seasoning. Divide the red pepper, green pepper, and spring onion equally between the 4 cutlets. Roll up the cutlets. Secure with toothpicks. Place the chicken roll-ups in the Air Fryer and lightly spray with cooking oil. Bake for 12 minutes, turning once. Serve warm.

RECIPE 328: MEXICAN CRUNCHY CHEESE STRAWS

Serve: 3 | Total Time: 15 minutes

1/2 cup almond flour
1/4 tsp xanthan gum
1/4 tsp shallot powder
1/4 tsp garlic powder
1/4 tsp ground cumin
1 egg yolk, whisked
1 ounce Manchego cheese, grated
2 ounces Cotija cheese, grated

Merge all ingredients until everything is well incorporated. Twist the batter into straw strips and place them on a baking mat inside your Air Fryer. Cook the cheese straws in your Air Fryer at 360 degrees F for 5 minutes; turn them over and cook an additional 5 minutes. Let the cheese straws cool before serving. Enjoy!

RECIPE 329: MEXICAN TACO CHICKEN FINGERS

Serve: 4 | Total Time: 20 minutes

1 egg, whisked
1/2 cup parmesan cheese, preferably freshly grated
1/2 cup tortilla chips, crushed
1/2 tsp onion powder
1/2 tsp garlic powder
1 tsp red chili powder
1 1/2 pounds chicken breasts, boneless skinless cut into strips

Whisk the egg in a shallow bowl. In a separate bowl, whisk the parmesan cheese, tortilla chips, onion powder, garlic powder, and red chili powder. Dip the chicken pieces into the egg mixture. Then, roll the chicken pieces over the breadcrumb mixture. Cook the chicken at 380 degrees F for 12 minutes, turning them over halfway through the cooking time. Bon appétit!

RECIPE 330: MIGHTY MEATBALLS

Serve: 8 | Total Time: 70 minutes

1 cup of onion minced
1 lb. Ground-based beef
3 egg yolks
Mozzarella 1 cup, shredded
1 tbsp. Extra Virgin Olive Oil

Pre-heat the fryer at 375 degrees F. Grease yourself with olive oil. In a bowl, put the onion and ground beef and season as desired. Combine your hands with the egg yolks. Take a handful of beef and with your palm, press it flat out. Place a small amount of cheese on the meat to form a ball and wrap the meat around it. Make the majority of the cheese and beef. In the fryer, place all the meatballs and cook for ten minutes. Serve it wet.

RECIPE 331: MINI SWEET PEPPER POPPERS

Serve: 4 | Total Time: 23 minutes

8 mini sweet peppers
4 ounces full-fat cream cheese, softened
4 slices sugar-free bacon, cooked and crumbled
¼ cup shredded pepper jack cheese

Remove the tops from the peppers and portion each one in half lengthways. Practice a small knife to eliminate seeds and membranes. In a small bowl, blend cream cheese, bacon, and pepper jack. Place three teaspoons of the mix into each sweet pepper and press

down smooth. Put it into the fryer basket. Regulate the temperature to 400°F and set the timer for 8 minutes. Serve warm.

RECIPE 332: MINCED BEEF KETO BREAKFAST SANDWICH

Serve: 2 | Total Time: 16 minutes

6-ounces minced beef
4 lettuce leaves
1 tsp flax seeds
1 tsp olive oil
½ tsp ground black pepper
½ tsp chili flakes
½ tomato, sliced
½ avocado, pitted, sliced

Combine the chili flakes with the minced beef and salt. Add the flax seeds and stir the meat mixture using a fork. Preheat your Air Fryer to 370°Fahrenheit. Pour the olive oil into the Air Fryer basket tray. Make 2 burgers from the beef mixture and place them in the Air Fryer basket. Cook the burgers for 8-minutes on each side. Meanwhile, slice the avocado and tomato. Place the avocado and tomato onto 2 lettuce leaves. Add the cooked minced beef burgers and serve them hot!

RECIPE 333: MINI PEPPERS WITH GOAT CHEESE

Serve: 8 | Total Time: 20 minutes

8 mini or snack peppers
1 tsp freshly ground black pepper
½ tbsp olive oil
4 oz soft goat cheese, in eight pieces

Ensure that your Air Fryer is preheated to 390 F. Get rid of the membrane, seeds, and the caps of the mini peppers. In a deep mixing dish, combine the Italian herbs, the olive oil, and the pepper. Place the pieces of goat cheese in the mixture one after the other. Withdraw and transfer each piece into each of the mini pepper. Arrange the goat cheese-filled mini peppers in the basket, placing them next to

each other. Return the basket into the Air Fryer. Allow baking for 8 minutes, or until you have the cheese all melted. Serve the mini peppers by placing them in small dishes. They are best eaten as snacks or appetizers.

RECIPE 334: MINI SHRIMP FRITTATA

Serve: 4 | Total Time: 35 minutes

1 tsp olive oil, plus for spraying
½ small red bell pepper, finely diced
1 tsp minced garlic
1 (4-ounce) can of tiny shrimp, Dry out
Salt
Freshly ground black pepper
4 eggs, beaten
4 tsp ricotta cheese

Spray four ramekins with olive oil. 1 teaspoon olive oil, heated in a medium-sized pan over medium-low heat. Add the bell pepper and garlic and sauté until the pepper is soft, about 5 minutes. Add the shrimp, season with salt and pepper, and cook until warm, 1 to 2 minutes Remove from the heat. Add the eggs and stir to combine. Pour one quarter of the mixture into each ramekin. Place 2 ramekins in the fryer basket and cook for 6 minutes. Remove the fryer basket from the Air Fryer and stir the mixture in each ramekin. Top each frittata with 1 teaspoon of ricotta cheese. Return the fryer basket to the Air Fryer and cook until eggs are set and the top is lightly browned, 4 to 5 minutes. Repeat with the remaining two ramekins.

RECIPE 335: MOJITO FISH TACOS

Serve: 4 | Total Time: 30 minutes

1 ½ cups chopped red cabbage
1 lb cod fillets
2 tsp olive oil
3 tbsp lemon juice
1 large carrot, grated
1 tbsp white rum

½ cup salsa
1/3 cup Greek yogurt
4 soft tortillas

Preheat Air Fryer to 390°F. Rub the fish with olive oil, then a splash with a tablespoon of lemon juice. Place in the fryer and Air Fry for 9-12 minutes. The fish should flake when done. Mix the remaining lemon juice, red cabbage, carrots, salsa, rum, and yogurt in a bowl. Take the fish out of the fryer and tear into large pieces. Serve with tortillas and cabbage mixture. Enjoy!

RECIPE 336: MOLTEN SWEET POTATO HASH

Serve: 2 | Total Time: 20 minutes

1 cup mozzarella cheese, grated.
1/2 cup cheddar cheese, grated.
2 eggs
2 cups sweet potatoes, grated.
2 tbsp. spring onions, chopped.
1 tsp. garlic salt
pepper, to taste

Preheat the Air Fryer to temperature of 350 degrees F. Whisk the eggs with the garlic salt and pour into the Air Fryer Baking Pan. Add the grated sweet potatoes and spring onions and mix well to combine. Top with the grated cheddar cheese and season with the pepper. Press the mixture lightly to the Air Fryer Baking Pan to remove any air bubbles. Place the Air Fryer Baking Pan in the Air Fryer Basket and cook for 13 minutes. Top with the grated mozzarella and cook for 2 more minutes. Serve and enjoy!

RECIPE 337: MOLTEN SWEET PURPLE POTATOES

Serve: 2 | Total Time: 23 minutes

2 cups baby potatoes, halved.
1/4 cup feta cheese, crumbled.
1/2 cup parmesan, shavings.
1 cup purple yam, cubed.
1/2 cup mozzarella cheese, grated.
1 tbsp. chives, chopped.
1 tbsp. of olive oil

1 tsp. onion powder
1 tsp. paprika
1 tsp. garlic powder
salt and pepper, to taste

Preheat the Air Fryer to 350 degrees F. Season the potatoes and purple yam with the olive oil, paprika, garlic powder, onion powder, salt and pepper and place in the Air Fryer Basket. Cook for 15 minutes and give the vegetables a shake halfway through the cooking time. Top with the mozzarella cheese and feta cheese and return to the Air Fryer for 2 more minutes or until the cheese has melted. Top with the parmesan cheese and chives. Serve and enjoy!

RECIPE 338: MOUTHWATERING TUNA MELTS

Serve: 8 | Total Time: 35 minutes

1/8 tsp. salt
1/3 cup, onion, chopped
16 1/3 oz. Biscuits, refrigerated, flaky layer
10 oz. tuna, water packed, drained
1/3 cup mayonnaise.
1/8 tsp. pepper
4 oz. cheddar cheese, shredded
Tomato, chopped
Sour cream
Lettuce, shredded

Preheat the Air Fryer at 325 degrees Fahrenheit. Mist cooking spray onto a cookie sheet. Mix tuna with mayonnaise, pepper, salt, and onion. Separate dough so you have 8 biscuits; press each into 5-inch rounds. Arrange 4 biscuit rounds on the sheet. Fill at the center with tuna mixture before topping with cheese. Cover with the remaining biscuit rounds and press to seal. Air-fry for fifteen to twenty minutes. Slice each sandwich into halves. Serve each piece topped with lettuce, tomato, and sour cream.

RECIPE 339: MUSHROOM LEEK FRITTATA

Serve: 4 | Total Time: 42 minutes

6 eggs
6 oz mushrooms, sliced
1 cup leeks, sliced
Salt

Preheat the Air Fryer to 325 F. Grease the Air Fryer baking dish with cooking spray and set aside. Heat another pan over medium heat. Spray pan with cooking spray. Cook for 6 minutes after adding the mushrooms, leeks, and salt to a pan. Break the eggs into a bowl and whisk vigorously. Place the sautéed mushroom and leek mixture into the baking dish that has been prepared. Pour egg over mushroom mixture. Put the dish in the Air Fryer and cook for 32 minutes. Serve and enjoy.

RECIPE 340: MUSHROOM TURKEY PATTIES

Serve: 6 | Total Time: 20 minutes

6 medium mushrooms
1 tbsp Maggi seasoning sauce
1 tsp garlic powder
1 tsp onion powder
1/2 tsp salt substitute
1/2 tsp ground black pepper
1 lb ground turkey

Puree washed mushrooms in a food processor until smooth. Add seasoning sauce, pepper, salt, and onion powder. Mix well, then add this mushroom mixture to the turkey ground. Combine the mixture well then make five patties out of it. Place these patties in the Air Fryer's Basket and spray them with cooking oil. Return the basket to its fryer and cook them for 10 minutes at 320 F. Serve warm.

RECIPE 341: MUSTARD AIR CHICKEN

Serve: 6 | Total Time: 70 minutes

4 garlic cloves
8 chicken slices
1 tbsp. thyme leaves
½ cup, dry wine vinegar

Salt as needed
½ cup Dijon mustard
2 cups almond meal
2 tbsp. melted butter
1 tbsp. lemon zest
2 tbsp. olive oil

Preheat your Air Fryer to 350 temperature of degrees F. Take a bowl and add garlic, salt, cloves, almond meal, pepper, olive oil, melted butter, and lemon zest. Take another bowl and mix mustard and wine. Place chicken slices in the wine mixture and then in the crumb mixture. Transfer prepared chicken to your Air Fryer cooking basket and cook for 40 minutes. Serve and enjoy!

RECIPE 342: MUSTARD MARINA TED BEEF

Serve: 6 | Total Time: 55 minutes

3 lb. beef roast
6 bacon strips
1-3/4 beef stock
2 tbsp. butter
3/4 cup red wine
1 tbsp. horseradish
3 cloves garlic (minced)
1 tbsp. mustard
Salt and pepper, to taste

Preheat the Air Fryer to 400F. In a bowl, add the butter, horseradish, mustard, garlic, salt, garlic, and mix. Rub the beef with the mixture. Arrange the bacon on a cutting board, add the meat on top and wrap the beef with the bacon strips. Put it into the Air Fryer then cook for 15 minutes. Remove the beef roast and transfer to a pan. Immediately add the stock and wine to the pan and reduce the heat to 300F, where it will simmer for 30 minutes. Carve the beef and serve.

RECIPE 343: MUTTON CHOPS

Serve: 4 | Total Time: 20 minutes

3 tbsp of oil
1 tsp of garam masala
½ tsp of salt

½ tsp of pepper
1 tbsp of ginger
1 tbsp of garlic
3 tablespoon of red chili pepper
2 eggs
2 cups of bread crumbs
2 lbs of mutton chops

Preheat the Air Fryer for 320F and sprinkle the frying basket with oil. In a large mixing bowl combine red chili pepper, garlic, ginger, pepper, salt and garam masala. Stir to combine. After that rub meat with the mixture. In a shallow bowl beat eggs. In another shallow bowl place bread crumbs. Take meat, place it in egg and after that in the cup of bread crumbs. Transfer coated meat to the Air Fryer basket and cook for 5-6 minutes. Then put meat on the other side. Cook for 5 minutes more. Serve warm with salad or vegetables. Enjoy with this snack.

RECIPE 344: NUTMEG PORK CUTLETS

Serve: 2 | Total Time: 15 minutes

6 oz of tinned salmon
1 large egg
3 tbsp olive oil
5 tbsp wheat germ
½ tsp garlic powder
1 tsp dill, fresh, chopped
4 tbsp spring onion, diced
4 tbsp celery, diced

Preheat your Air Fryer to 370°Fahrenheit.
Combine the salmon, egg, celery, onion, dill, and garlic in a large mixing bowl.
Shape the mixture into golf ball size balls and roll them in the wheat germ.
In a small pan, warm olive oil over medium-low heat.
Add the salmon balls and slowly flatten them.
Transfer them to your Air Fryer and cook for 10-minutes.

RECIPE 345: NUTTY ASPARAGUS

Serve: 4 | Total Time: 16 minutes

1 ½ lb Asparagus, ends trimmed
Salt and Pepper, to taste
1 cup Water
1 tbsp butter
½ cup chopped Pine Nuts

Open the cooker, pour the water in, and fit the reversible rack at the bottom. Place the asparagus on the rack, close the crisping lid, select Air Fry mode, and set the time to 8 minutes on 380 F. Press Start. At the 4-minute mark, carefully turn the asparagus over. When ready, remove to a plate, sprinkle with salt and pepper, and set aside. Select Sear/Sauté on your cooker, set to Medium and melt the butter. Put the pine nuts and cook for 2-3 minutes until golden. Scatter over the asparagus the pine nuts, and drizzle olive oil.

RECIPE 346: OLD BAY COD FISH

Serve: 2 | Total Time: 30 minutes

1 lb cod, cut into 4 strips
Salt, to taste
Freshly ground black pepper, to taste
½ cup all-purpose flour
1 large egg, beaten
2 cups panko bread crumbs
1 tsp Old Bay seasoning
Lemon wedges, for serving
Tartar sauce, for serving

Rub the fish with salt and black pepper. Add flour in one shallow bowl, beat eggs in another bowl and mix panko with Old Bay in a shallow bowl. First coat the fish with flour, then dip it in the eggs and finally coat with the panko mixture. Place the seasoned cod fish in the Air Fryer basket and cook for 12 minutes at 400 F. Flip the fish once cooked halfway then resume cooking. Serve warm and fresh with tartar sauce and lemon wedges.

RECIPE 347: OLD BAY CRISPY CHICKEN WINGS

Serve: 4 | Total Time: 40 minutes

3 lbs. bone-in chicken wings
¾ cup almond flour
1 tbsp Old Bay seasoning
2 fresh lemons, juiced
4 tbsp butter

In a bowl, mix the Old Bay seasoning and flour. Add chicken wings and toss well to combine. Preheat your Air Fryer to 375°Fahrenheit. Take off excess flour and transfer the chicken wings into Air Fryer. Work in batches does not overcrowd. Cook for 40-minutes and often shake while cooking. Melt butter in a sauté pan over low heat. Squeeze the lemon juice from the two lemons into melted butter and to blend. Serve hot wings and pour the lemon butter over them. Serve hot!

RECIPE 348: OMELET WITH ONION AND CHEESE

Serve: 1 | Total Time: 25 minutes

2 eggs
Ground black pepper to taste
Soy sauce to taste
Cooking spray
1 medium onion, sliced
Cheddar cheese, grated

Get a clean bowl and crack open the eggs in it. Add the pepper and soy sauce (as seasoning). Spritz some cooking spray lightly into the pan. Transfer the sliced onions in the oiled pan at air fry for 8-10 minutes at 360 F. Withdraw when the onion is softened. Transfer the egg mixture into the pan, and add bits of Cheddar Cheese. Air fry until the eggs are fully cooked - about 3 to 5 minutes. Serve.

RECIPE 349: ONION LAMB KEBABS

Serve: 4 | Total Time: 30 minutes

18 oz. lamb kebab
1 tsp chili powder
1 tsp cumin powder
1 egg
2 oz. onion, chopped
2 tsp sesame oil

Whisk onion with egg, chili powder, oil, cumin powder, and salt in a bowl. Add lamb to coat well then thread it on the skewers. Place these lamb skewers in the Air Fryer basket. Choose "Power Button" of Air Fry Oven and turn the dial to select the "Air Fry" mode. Choose the Time button and again turn the dial to set the cooking time to 20 minutes. Now press the Temp button and rotate the dial to set the temperature at 395 degrees F. Close the oven door after preheating the Air Fryer basket. Slice and serve warm.

RECIPE 350: ONION GREEN BEANS

Serve: 2 | Total Time: 22 minutes

11 oz green beans
1 tbsp onion powder
1 tbsp olive oil
½ tsp salt
¼ tsp chili flakes

Wash the green beans carefully and place them in the bowl. Sprinkle the green beans with the onion powder, salt, chili flakes, and olive oil. Shake the green beans carefully. Preheat the Air Fryer to 400 F. Put the green beans in the Air Fryer and cook for 8 minutes. After this, shake the green beans and cook them for 4 minutes more at 400 F. When the time is over – shake the green beans. Serve the side dish and enjoy!

RECIPE 351: OREGANO CHICKEN BREAST

Serve: 6 | Total Time: 35 minutes

2 lbs. chicken breasts, minced
1 tbsp avocado oil
1 tsp smoked paprika
1 tsp garlic powder
1 tsp oregano
1/2 tsp salt
Black pepper, to taste

Toss all the meatball ingredients in a bowl and mix well. Make small meatballs out this mixture and place them in the Air Fryer basket.

Press "Power Button" of Air Fry Oven and turn the dial to select the "Air Fry" mode. Press the Time button and again turn the dial to set the cooking time to 25 minutes. Now push the Temp button and rotate the dial to set the temperature at 375 degrees F. Once preheated, place the Air Fryer basket inside and close its lid. Serve warm.

RECIPE 352: PANKO CHICKEN TENDERS

Serve: 4 | Total Time: 15 minutes

1 ½ pounds (680 g) chicken tenders
1 tbsp olive oil
1 egg, whisked
1 tsp minced fresh parsley
1 tsp minced garlic
Sea salt and black pepper, to taste
1 cup bread crumbs

Pat the chicken dry with kitchen towels. In a bowl, thoroughly combine the oil, egg, parsley, garlic, salt, and black pepper. Dip the chicken tenders into the egg mixture. Then, roll the chicken over the bread crumbs. Cook the chicken tenders at 360°F (182°C) for 10 minutes, shaking the basket halfway through the cooking time. Bon appétit!

RECIPE 353: PARMESAN HADDOCK FILLETS

Serve: 2 | Total Time: 18 minutes

1/2 cup Parmesan cheese, freshly grated
1 tsp dried parsley flake
1 egg
1/4 tsp cayenne pepper
2 haddock fillets patted dry

Warm the Air Fryer to 360F (182C). Stir together the Parmesan cheese and parsley flakes in a shallow dish. Beat the egg with the cayenne pepper, sea salt, and pepper in a bowl. Dunk the haddock fillets into the egg, and then roll over the Parmesan mixture until fully coated on both sides. Handover the fillets to the Air Fryer basket and drizzle with the olive oil. Cook in the preheated Air Fryer for 11 to 13 minutes, or until the flesh is opaque. Remove from the basket to a plate and serve.

RECIPE 354: PARMESAN STICKS

Serve: 3 | Total Time: 25 minutes

1/4 tsp black pepper
4 tbsp almond flour
1 egg
1/2 cup heavy cream
8 ounces parmesan cheese

Crack your egg into a bowl, beating it. Add in your almond flour and cream, mixing well. Sprinkle your cream mixture with black pepper, whisking well. Cut your cheese into short, thick sticks, and then dip it in the cream mixture. Place these sticks in a plastic bag and place them in the freezer. Let them freeze. Turn your Air Fryer to 400, and then place your frozen sticks on the Air Fryer rack, and then cook for eight minutes.

RECIPE 355: PARTY BUFFALO CHICKEN DRUMETTES

Serve: 6 | Total Time: 30 minutes

16 chicken drumettes
1 tsp garlic powder
1 tbsp chicken seasoning
Black pepper to taste
¼ cup Buffalo wings sauce
2 spring onions, sliced

Preheat Air Fryer to 400°F. Sprinkle garlic, chicken seasoning, and black pepper on the drumettes. Place them in the fryer and spray with cooking oil. Air Fry for 10 minutes, shaking the basket once. Transfer the drumettes to a large bowl. Drizzle with Buffalo wing sauce and toss to coat. Place in the fryer and Fry for 7-8 minutes, until crispy. Allow to cool slightly. Top

with spring onions and serve warm.

RECIPE 356: PASTRAMI ONION WRAPS

Serve: 2 | Total Time: 15 minutes

8 slices pastrami
4 wraps (or soft tortillas)
1 onion, sliced into rings
1 cup cream cheese
1 cup cheddar cheese
1 tbsp garlic powder
1 tomato, sliced

Preheat your Air Fryer to 390 degrees F. Mix the cream cheese, cheddar cheese and garlic powder. Spread onto each wrap. Place two slices of pastrami onto each wrap. Add the tomato and onion. Roll up. Fry for 15 minutes.

RECIPE 357: PECAN-CRUSTED CATFISH FILLETS

Serve: 4 | Total Time: 17 minutes

1/2 cup pecan meal
4 (4-ounce / 113-g) catfish fillets, rinsed and patted dry
Fresh oregano, for garnish (optional)
Pecan halves, for garnish (optional)

Warm the Air Fryer to 375F (190C). Grease the Air Fryer basket with half of the avocado oil and set aside. Stir together the pecan meal, salt, and pepper in a large bowl. Roll the fillets with the mixture, pressing, so the fish is well coated. Brush the fillets with the remaining avocado oil and transfer to the Air Fryer basket. Cook in the preheated Air Fryer for 12 minutes, flipping the fillets halfway through, or until the fish flakes easily with a fork. Remove from the basket to a large plate. Sprinkle the oregano and pecan halves on top for garnish, if desired.

RECIPE 358: PEPPERED GARLIC MUSHROOM CAPS

Serve: 2 | Total Time: 20 minutes

4 large shiitake mushrooms, stems removed.
1 cup breadcrumbs
1 tbsp. fresh parsley, finely chopped.
1 tbsp. garlic, minced.
1 tsp. garlic powder
1 tsp. paprika
salt and pepper, to taste

Preheat the Air Fryer to temperature of 400 degrees F. Season the mushrooms with salt and pepper and spray with a little cooking spray. Mix together the breadcrumbs, garlic, garlic powder, paprika and parsley. Fill the mushrooms with the breadcrumbs mixture. Arrange the mushrooms in the Air Fryer Basket and cook for 10 minutes. Serve and enjoy!

RECIPE 359: PERFECT ASPARAGUS

Serve: 3 | Total Time: 10 minutes

1 pound Very thin asparagus spears
2 tbsp olive oil
1 tsp sea salt
¾ tsp Finely grated lemon zest

Preheat the Air Fryer to 400°F. Trim the asparagus spears just enough to fit in the basket. Put the spears on a large plate and drizzle them with some of the olive oil. Turn them over and drizzle more olive oil, working to get all the spears coated. When the machine is at temperature, place the spears in one direction in the basket. They may be touching. Air-fry for 10 minutes, tossing and rearranging the spears twice, until tender. Dump the contents of the basket on a serving platter. Spread out the spears. Sprinkle them with the salt and lemon zest while still warm. Serve at once.

RECIPE 360: PHILADELPHIA HERBY CHICKEN BREASTS

Serve: 2 | Total Time: 30 minutes

2 chicken breasts
Mixed herbs chicken seasoning
Salt and ground black pepper to taste
2 tbsp soft cheese

Ensure that your Air Fryer is preheated to 355 F. Slice midway into the breasts to create ample space to accommodate the seasoning. Add salt and pepper into the spaces created. Cover the entire chicken with soft cheese; use your hands to ensure a nice creamy layer. Have the seasoned chicken breasts rolled in the mixed herbs. Place them on a reusable baking mat and transfer into the Air Fryer. Cook until the chicken breasts are cooked in the middle (for about 15 minutes). Serve.

RECIPE 361: PICKLE FRIES

Serve: 12 | Total Time: 25 minutes

1 1/2 (16 oz.) jars spicy dill pickle spears
1 cup all-purpose flour
1/2 tsp paprika
1/4 cup milk
1 egg, whisked
1 cup bread crumbs
cooking spray

After draining the pickles, pat them dry completely. Thoroughly mix flour with paprika in one bowl and beat egg with milk in another. Spread the breadcrumbs in another shallow bowl. Preheat your Air Fryer machine on Air fry mode at 400 F in 3 minutes. Dip the pickle sticks first in the flour mixture then in egg and finally in the panko crumbs. Arrange them on the crisper plate of the fryer basket and insert it back. Select Air fry mode for 14 minutes at 400 F. Press Start/Pause button after 7 minutes and flip the pickles in the basket. Resume cooking for another 7 minutes. Serve warm.

RECIPE 362: PIGS IN A BLANKET

Serve: 8 | Total Time: 45 minutes

1 can (8 oz) of crescent rolls
1 pack (12 oz) of cocktail franks or mini smoked sausages

Withdraw and drain the cocktail franks from the package. To get rid of any remaining moisture, dry with a paper towel. Remove the crescent rolls dough from the can, and form eight triangles from it. Make two thin triangles from each of the eight triangles. In the end, you will have 16 triangles. Place one frank on the triangle (on the widest part) and roll up. Do the same for the other franks and triangles. Transfer about 8 "Pigs in a Blanket" into the Air Fryer basket, and air fry for 8 minutes at 330 F. Do the same for the other 8. Serve the fried Pigs in a Blanket alongside hot ketchup, gesso dip, salsa, or mustard.

RECIPE 363: PIZZA DOGS

Serve: 2 | Total Time: 17 minutes

2 hot dogs
4 slices pepperoni, halved
½ cup pizza sauce
2 hot dog buns
¼ cup shredded mozzarella cheese
2 tsp sliced olives

Ensure that your Air Fryer is preheated to 390 F. Cut four slits into each hot dog, and place them into the basket of the Air Fryer. Allow cooking for 3 minutes before withdrawing onto a cutting board using tongs. Put a pepperoni half in each of the slits in the hot dogs. Divide the pizza sauce between the buns, and fill with the olives, hot dogs, and mozzarella cheese. Place the hot dogs in the basket of the Air Fryer and allow to cook, again. Remove when cheese has melted and buns are crisp.

RECIPE 364: PIZZA PEPPERS

Serve: 2 | Total Time: 18 minutes

4 medium bell peppers
8 slices deli ham
1 cup cheddar cheese
1 cup pineapple chunks
1/4 cup onions, finely chopped.
1 cup tomato sauce
1/2 cup feta cheese, crumbled.
1 cup mozzarella cheese, grated.
2-tbsp. fresh basil, finely chopped

Preheat the Air Fryer to temperature of 400 degrees F. Slice off the tops of the bell peppers and remove the seeds. Place two slices of deli ham inside each bell pepper. Divide the cheddar cheese, pineapple chunks and onions between the bell peppers. Divide the tomato sauce between the bell peppers and top with the feta cheese and mozzarella cheese. Top with the fresh basil and arrange the peppers inside the Air Fryer Basket. Cook for 8 minutes. Serve and enjoy!

RECIPE 365: PIZZA TOAST

Serve: 4 | Total Time: 10 minutes

6 Slices Chicken Breast
2-3 Eggs
1/3 Red Bell Pepper, Sliced
1/3 Avocado, Sliced
1 Cup of Grated Mozzarella Cheese
2 tbsp Salsa
Salt & Pepper, to taste
4 Tortillas wrap

Salt and pepper eggs in a basin. Pour the egg mixture into a shallow tin and place into the Air Fryer basket. Cook the eggs in the Air Fryer at 400 degrees F for 4 minutes. Then remove the tin from the Air Fryer and remove the eggs from the tin. Fill the tortilla with egg mixture, chicken slices, pepper, avocado, and cheese. Apply salsa, to taste. Wrap it up. Line the Air Fryer with aluminum foil and place wraps on top. Cook for 4 minutes at 350 degrees. Once tortillas become toasted, serve while hot.

RECIPE 366: PORK BACON BITES

Serve: 6 | Total Time: 35 minutes

1 tsp olive oil
1 tbsp apple cider vinegar
1/2 tsp red pepper
1 tsp turmeric
1 tsp sea salt, fine
1 lb. pork brisket
6 ounces bacon, sliced

Start by cutting your pork into bite size pieces, and then place your pork bites into a mixing bowl. Sprinkle with red pepper, apple cider vinegar, turmeric and salt and mix well. Allow this to marinate for ten minutes, and then wrap each one in a slice of bacon. Secure them with toothpicks, and then heat your Air Fryer to 370. Cook for eight minutes, and then flip them over. Cook for another six minutes. Allow them to cool down before serving.

RECIPE 367: PORK BELLY WITH PEANUTS

Serve: 6 | Total Time: 35 minutes

5 oz. of peanut
1 lb. of pork belly
1 cup of chicken stock
1 tbsp. of salt
1 tsp. of ground black pepper
1 garlic cloves
1 tsp. of onion powder
1 tsp. of paprika
1 tbsp. of cilantro
3 tbsp. of fresh rosemary

Rub the pork belly with salt, ground black pepper, onion powder, paprika, and cilantro. Set pressure cooker to Pressure mode. Put the pork belly into the cooker followed by rosemary and chicken stock. Close pressure cooker lid and cook for about 25 minutes. Crush the peanuts. When the cooking time ends, open pressure cooker lid and remove the pork belly. Towel dry the pork belly. After that, slice it and sprinkle crushed peanuts before serving.

RECIPE 368: PORK CHOPS

Serve: 2 | Total Time: 30 minutes

2 pork chops
½ tsp minced garlic
¼ tsp ground black pepper
1/3 tsp salt
¼ tsp ground paprika

Beat the pork chops gently. After this, combine the ground black pepper, salt, and ground paprika in the bowl. Shake it to make it homogeneous. Then rub the pork chops with the minced garlic from both sides. Then sprinkle the pork chops with the spices. Preheat the Air Fryer to 360 F. Cook the pork chops for 20 minutes. When the time is over – remove the pork chops from the Air Fryer and serve them. Enjoy!

RECIPE 369: PORK CHOPS WITH STIR-FRIED JALAPENO PEPPERS

Serve: 4 | Total Time: 22 minutes

1 lb. pork chops, chopped
¾ cup cornstarch
½ tsp sea salt
¼ tsp black pepper
1 egg white
2 tbsp olive oil
½ tsp sea salt
¼ tsp black pepper
2 scallions, sliced

Coat the frying basket of your Air Fryer with cooking spray. In a mixing bowl, beat egg white with pepper and salt until foamy. Add pork chop to egg mixture and set aside for 20-minutes. Coat marinated pork chops with cornstarch and place in Air Fryer basket. Cook the pork chops at 360°Fahrenheit for 12-minutes. Shake the basket halfway through. Flip pork chops over and cook at 400°Fahrenheit for an additional 6-minutes. Heat the olive oil in a pan over medium heat. Add jalapeno, scallions, pepper, and salt into pan and cook for about 1-minute. Add air fried pork chop pieces into pan and toss to coat.

RECIPE 370: PORK CHUNKS WITH SWEET AND SOUR SAUCE

Serve: 2 | Total Time: 15 minutes

1 cup cornstarch
½ tsp spice mix
¼ cup sweet and sour sauce
2 lbs. pork, chunked
3 tbsp olive oil
2 large eggs, beaten
½ tsp sea salt
¼ tsp black pepper

In a bowl, combine spice mix, cornstarch, pepper, and salt. In another bowl add beaten eggs. Coat pork chunks with cornstarch mixture then dip in eggs and again into cornstarch. Grease Air Fryer basket with olive oil and preheat to 340°Fahrenheit. Place the coated pork chunks into Air Fryer basket and cook for 10-minutes. Shake the basket half way through. Place the air fried pork chunks on serving dish and drizzle with sweet and sour sauce.

RECIPE 371: PORK CORDON BLEU

Serve: 2 | Total Time: 22 minutes

2 pork steaks; pounded
2 slices deli ham
2 slices cheese
1 egg; beaten
3-tbsp. breadcrumbs
1-tsp. paprika
1-tsp. garlic powder
salt and pepper, to taste

Preheat the Air Fryer to temperature of 350 degrees F. Mix together the breadcrumbs, paprika, and garlic powder. Salt and pepper the eggs. Place a slice of ham and a slice of cheese onto a slice of pork and fold them in half. Dip into the egg mixture and then coat evenly in breadcrumbs. Shake off the excess breadcrumbs and arrange in the Air Fryer Basket. Cook for 12 minutes. Serve and enjoy!

RECIPE 372: PORK KABOBS WITH PINEAPPLE

Serve: 4 | Total Time: 30 minutes

2 (8-oz) cans juice-packed pineapple chunks, juice reserved
1 green bell pepper, cut into ½-inch chunks
1 red bell pepper, cut into ½-inch chunks
1 lb pork tenderloin, cubed
Salt and pepper to taste
1 tbsp honey
½ tsp ground ginger
½ tsp ground coriander
1 red chili, minced

Preheat the Air Fryer to 375°F. Mix the coriander, chili, salt, and pepper in a bowl. Add the pork and toss to coat. Then, thread the pork pieces, pineapple chunks, and bell peppers onto skewers. Combine the pineapple juice, honey, and ginger and mix well. Use all the mixture as you brush it on the kebabs. Put the kebabs in the greased frying basket and Air Fry for 10-14 minutes or until cooked through. Serve and enjoy!

RECIPE 373: PORK KATSU

Serve: 1 | Total Time: 8 minutes

1 -2 cups soy sauce
½ cup miso
2-3 pork cutlets
1-2 cups flour
2-3 eggs, beaten
1-2 cups panko breadcrumbs

Mix the soy sauce and the miso together to desired consistency. Add more soy sauce or miso as needed. Marinate the pork cutlets into the soy sauce-miso mix for 30 minutes. Once done, dip the cutlets first into the flour, then into the egg, then into the panko. Then, place the cutlets in one layer into the Air Fryer and cook for 13 minutes at 400°F, checking for doneness. Rest for a few minutes before serving.

RECIPE 374: PORK SATAY WITH PEANUT SAUCE

Serve: 4 | Total Time: 21 minutes

1 tsp ground ginger
2 tsp hot pepper sauce
2 cloves garlic, crushed
3 tbsp sweet soy sauce
3 ½ ounces unsalted peanuts, ground
¾ cup coconut milk
1 tsp ground coriander
2 tbsp vegetable oil
14-ounces lean pork chops, in cubes of 1-inch

In a large mixing bowl, combine hot sauce, ginger, half garlic, oil and soy sauce. Place the meat into the mixture and leave for 15-minutes to marinate. Place the meat into wire basket of your Air Fryer. Cook at 390°Fahrenheit for 12-minutes. Turn over halfway through cook time. For the peanut sauce, place the oil into a skillet and heat it up. After adding the garlic and coriander, cook for 5 minutes, stirring often. Add the coconut milk, peanuts, hot pepper sauce and soy sauce to the pan and bring to boil. Stir often. Remove the pork from Air Fryer and pour sauce over it and serve warm.

RECIPE 375: POTATO FRITTERS

Serve: 8 | Total Time: 30 minutes

1 cup diced yellow potatoes
2 cups cauliflower, chopped
1 ¼ cups chickpea flour
¾ cup of water
½ red onion, chopped
1 tbsp salt
1 garlic clove, minced
1 tsp curry powder
1 tsp coriander
½ tsp ground cayenne pepper
½ tsp cumin
Cooking spray

Prepare the cauliflower, potatoes and chickpea flour with water, salt, garlic and curry powder. Rest for 10 minutes. Preheat your Air Fryer machine to 350 F. Spray the basket of the Air Fryer with cooking spray. Add 2 tbsp of cauliflower mixture to a tray, lined with parchment paper, and flatten it. Continue doing so to get as many fritters as you can. Place the

fritters in the Air Fryer basket in batches and cook each batch for 8 minutes at 350 F. Flip the fritters and continue cooking for another 8 minutes. Serve warm.

RECIPE 376: POTATO GRATIN

Serve: 3 | Total Time: 35 minutes

1 pound potato, pilled
4 tbsp milk
4 tbsp cream
A Pinch of freshly ground pepper
Nutmeg to taste
2 oz cheese, grated
Salt to taste

Slice potatoes. Milk and cream are whisked together in a large mixing basin. Season to taste with salt, ground pepper, and nutmeg. Add in potato slices and stir to combine well. Preheat the Air Fryer to 370°F. Transfer covered potato slices to the quiche pan. Pour the remaining milk mixture over the potatoes. Evenly cover the potatoes with grated cheese. Place the quiche pan into the Air Fryer and cook for 15-20 minutes until nicely golden.

RECIPE 377: POTATO WITH CRISPY SKIN

Serve: 5 | Total Time: 60 minutes

6 potatoes (medium size)
2 tbsp. canola oil
1 ½ tsp paprika
Salt and pepper to taste

Clean potato under the cold and running water. Put it in salted water. Boil potatoes for 40 minutes and when you sure that they are tender, cool in a refrigerator for 30 minutes. Mix paprika and canola oil. Add salt and pepper to taste. Paprika is the spice which will make your potato red and crispy. Potatoes cut into quarters or medium cubes and mix with the oil and spices. Put into the fryer, be careful to not overcrowd. Fryer can't work if it's too loaded, and it can be dangerous. Cook the potatoes for 14-16 minutes on the

390°F. You'll recognize when it's finished, potatoes should be golden brown with crispy skin.

RECIPE 378: PRAWN PASTE CHICKEN WINGS

Serve: 2 | Total Time: 16 minutes

1 tbsp prawn/shrimp paste
2 tbsp olive oil
1 tsp liquid Stevia
1 tsp sesame oil
½ tsp dried ginger
2/3 lb. chicken wings

Except the chicken wings, put all ingredients in a big bowl. Stir well, then place the chicken on top. Leave for at least an hour. Preheat your Air Fryer to 350°Fahrenheit. Remove the wings from the marinade, lightly brush them with oil and place into your Air Fryer. Cook wings for 8-minutes at 350°Fahrenheit. Pull out the tray and using a pair of tongs flip over the wings and place tray back into Air Fryer for another 8-minutes. Serve the cooked chicken wings on paper towels.

RECIPE 379: QUICK BACON HASH

Serve: 4 | Total Time: 20 minutes

2 large sweet potato, small cubes
2 slices bacon, small pieces
2 tbsp olive oil
1 tbsp smoked paprika
1 tsp sea salt
1 tsp ground black pepper
1 tsp dried dill weed

At 400 F, preheat your Air Fryer. Add sweet potato, dill weed, black pepper, salt, olive oil, smoked paprika, and bacon to a large bowl. Toss them well to coat and spread the potato cubes in the Air Fryer Basket. Return the fryer basket to the Air Fryer and cook for 16 minutes. Shake the potatoes after every 5 minutes and resume cooking. Serve.

RECIPE 380: RANCH CHIPS

Serve: 2 | Total Time: 30 minutes

1 tsp dry ranch seasoning
Salt and pepper to taste
2 cups sliced potatoes
2 tsp olive oil
¼ cup white wine vinegar

Preheat Air Fryer at 400°F. In a bowl, combine ranch mix, salt, and pepper. Reserve ½ tsp for garnish. In another bowl, mix sliced fingerling potatoes with the vinegar and stir around. Let soak in the vinegar water for at least thirty minutes then drain the potatoes and pat them dry. Place potato chips and spread with olive oil until coated. Sprinkle with the ranch mixture and toss to coat. Place potato chips in the frying basket and Air Fry for 16 minutes, shaking 4 times. Transfer it into a bowl. Sprinkle with the reserved mixture and let sit for 15 minutes. Serve immediately.

RECIPE 381: RASPBERRY CRUMBLE

Serve: 3 | Total Time: 40 minutes

1 (6 oz) tub fresh raspberries
1 tsp cornstarch
1 tbsp white granulated sugar
4 tbsp (1/2 stick) of cold butter, chopped into small cubes
¼ cup light brown sugar
1/3 cup old fashioned oats
¼ cup all-purpose flour
Whipped cream or ice cream to serve

Pat dry the washed raspberries, before moving them into the bowl containing the cornstarch and white sugar. Leave for about 10 minutes for the mixture to macerate. Meanwhile, place the cubes of cold butter, brown sugar, oats and the all-purpose flour in the food processor and pulse until the mixture appears like crumbs. Make two mini pie pans out of the macerating raspberries and the juices released (4-inches each). Top each pie with the oat-butter crumble and transfer them into the Air Fryer basket. Allow air frying at 350 F for 15 minutes. Serve while warm,

alongside ice cream or whipped cream and some more berries.

RECIPE 382: RED WINE TURKEY WINGS

Serve: 5 | Total Time: 45 minutes

2 pounds (907 g) turkey wings, bone-in
2 garlic cloves, minced
1 small onion, chopped
1 tablespoon Dijon mustard
½ cup red wine
salt and black pepper, to taste
1 teaspoon poultry seasoning

Place the turkey wings, garlic, onion, mustard, and wine in a ceramic bowl. Cover the bowl and let the turkey marinate in your refrigerator overnight. Discard the marinade and toss the turkey wings with the salt, black pepper, and poultry seasoning. Cook the turkey wings at 400°F (204°C) for 40 minutes, turning them over halfway through the cooking time. Bon appétit!

RECIPE 383: RESTAURANT-STYLE CHICKEN THIGHS

Serve: 4 | Total Time: 30 minutes

1 lb boneless, skinless chicken thighs
¼ cup barbecue sauce
2 cloves garlic, minced
1 tsp lemon zest
2 tbsp parsley, chopped
2 tbsp lemon juice

Coat the chicken with barbecue sauce, garlic, and lemon juice in a medium bowl. leave to marinate for 10 minutes. Preheat Air Fryer to 380°F. When ready to cook, remove the chicken from the bowl and shake off any drips. Arrange the chicken in the Air Fryer and Bake for 16-18 minutes, until golden and cooked through. Serve topped with lemon zest and parsley. Enjoy!

RECIPE 384: RIB EYE BITES WITH MUSHROOMS

Serve: 4 | Total Time: 30 minutes

1 ¼ lb boneless rib-eye or sirloin steak, cubed
8 oz button mushrooms, halved
4 tbsp rapeseed oil
1 onion, chopped
2 garlic cloves, minced
Salt and pepper to taste
2 tsp lime juice
1 tsp dried marjoram
2 tbsp chopped parsley

Preheat the Air Fryer to 400°F. Combine the rapeseed oil, onion, mushrooms, garlic, steak cubes, salt, pepper, lime juice, marjoram, and parsley in a baking pan. Put it in the frying basket and Bake for 12-15 minutes, stirring once or twice to ensure an even cooking, and until golden brown. The veggies should be tender. Serve hot.

RECIPE 385: RICE WINE CHICKEN BREASTS

Serve: 4 | Total Time: 20 minutes

1 pound (454 g) chicken breasts, boneless, skinless
½ cup rice wine
1 tbsp stone-ground mustard
1 tsp minced garlic
1 tsp whole black peppercorns
1 tsp chili powder
¼ tsp sea salt, or more to taste

Place the chicken, wine, mustard, garlic, and whole peppercorns in a ceramic bowl. Refrigerate the chicken for 3 hours. Then put the chicken breasts in. Cook the chicken breasts at 380°F (193°C) for 12 minutes, turning them over halfway through the cooking time. Season the chicken with the chili powder and salt. Serve immediately and enjoy!

RECIPE 386: RISOTTO WITH ZUCCHINI AND RED CAPSICUM

Serve: 4 | Total Time: 55 minutes

1 ½ tsp vegetable spice
2 cups water
1 tin tomato purée 13 oz
3 medium red capsicum
1 large zucchini
1/2 cup of rice
1 large onion
4 garlic cloves

Wash all vegetables. Cut zucchini in cubes, capsicum in 1-inch squares, dice onion, chop garlic. Preheat Air Fryer to 330°F and heat 1 tablespoon of oil in 2 minutes. Put diced onion and cook for 5 minutes until golden, then put chopped garlic and cook another 3-5 minutes. Combine vegetable spice with water, tomato puree and rice. Cook in Air Fryer for 10 minutes. Add zucchini and capsicum and some water, cook for 20-25 minutes. You can add extra water depending on the consistency you like.

RECIPE 387: ROAST LAMB SHOULDER

Serve: 2 | Total Time: 15 minutes

1 lb. boneless lamb shoulder roast
4 cloves garlic, minced
1 tbsp rosemary, chopped
2 tsp thyme leaves
3 tbsp olive oil, divided
Salt
Black pepper
2 lb. baby potatoes halved

Toss potatoes with all the herbs, seasonings, and oil in a baking tray. Choose "Power Button" of Air Fry Oven and turn the dial to select the "Air Roast" mode. Choose the Time button and again turn the dial to set the cooking time to 60 minutes. Now rest the Temp button and rotate the dial to set the temperature at 370 degrees F. Once preheated, set the lamb baking tray in the oven and close its lid. Slice and serve warm.

RECIPE 388: ROASTED BUTTERNUT PUMPKIN WITH NUTS AND BALSAMIC VINAIGRETTE

Serve: 4 | Total Time: 20 minutes

1 butternut pumpkin, cut into 1-inch slices
Sprigs of thyme for garnishing
2 ½ tbsp toasted pine nuts
Sea salt and pepper to taste
1 ½ tbsp olive oil

Vinaigrette:
6 tbsp olive oil
1 tbsp Dijon mustard
Sea salt and black pepper to taste
2 tbsp balsamic vinegar

Preheat Air Fryer to 390°Fahrenheit for 5-minutes. Cover the slices of pumpkin with olive oil and season with thyme, salt, and pepper. Set the Air Fryer to cook for 20-minutes, and place seasoned pumpkin slices into Air Fryer. Prepare the vinaigrette by combining all the vinaigrette ingredients in a bowl. Serve pumpkin covered with vinaigrette, sprinkle top with toasted pine nuts and sprigs of thyme.

RECIPE 389: ROASTED CITRUS TURKEY DRUMSTICKS

Serve: 3 | Total Time: 85 minutes

3 medium turkey drumsticks, bone-in skin-on
1/2 butter stick, melted
salt and black pepper, to taste
1 tsp cayenne pepper
1 tsp fresh garlic, minced
1 tsp dried parsley flakes
1 tsp onion powder
Zest of one orange
1/4 cup orange juice

Rub all ingredients onto the turkey drumsticks. Preheat your Air Fryer to temperature of 400 degrees F. Cook the turkey drumsticks for 16 minutes in the preheated Air Fryer. Loosely cover with foil and cook for an additional 24 minutes. Once cooked, let it rest for 10 minutes before slicing and serving. Bon appétit!

RECIPE 390: ROASTED RACK OF LAMB WITH MACADAMIA CRUST

Serve: 4 | Total Time: 35 minutes

1 garlic clove, minced
1 1/3 lbs. rack of lamb
1 tbsp olive oil
Salt and pepper to taste

Macadamia Crust:
3-ounces macadamia nuts, raw and unsalted
1 egg, beaten
1 tbsp fresh rosemary, chopped
1 tbsp breadcrumbs

In a small mixing bowl, mix garlic and olive oil. Brush all over lamb and season with salt and pepper. In your food processor, chop macadamia nuts and mix with breadcrumbs and rosemary. Be careful not to make the nuts into a paste. Stir in egg. Coat lamb with nut mixture. Preheat your Air Fryer to 220°Fahrenheit. Place the lamb in Air Fryer and cook for 30-minutes. Raise the temperature to 390°Fahrenheit and cook for an additional 5-minutes. Remove the meat, cover it loosely with foil for 10-minutes. Serve warm.

RECIPE 391: ROSEMARY CITRUS CHICKEN

Serve: 2 | Total Time: 15 minutes

1 lb. chicken thighs
1/2 tsp rosemary, fresh, chopped
1/8 tsp thyme, dried
½ cup tangerine juice
2 tbsp white wine
1 tsp garlic, minced
Salt and pepper to taste
2 tbsp lemon juice

Place the chicken thighs in a mixing bowl. In another bowl, mix tangerine juice, garlic, white wine, lemon juice, rosemary, pepper, salt, and thyme. Pour the mixture over chicken thighs and place in the fridge for 20-minutes. Preheat your Air Fryer to 350°Fahrenheit and place your marinated chicken in Air Fryer basket and cook for 15-minutes. Serve hot and enjoy!

RECIPE 392: ROSEMARY LEMON CHICKEN

Serve: 2 | Total Time: 19 minutes

¾ lb. chicken
½ fresh lemon, cut into wedges
1 tbsp oyster sauce
1 tsp liquid stevia
1 tbsp rosemary, fresh, chopped
1 tbsp soy sauce
½ tbsp olive oil
1 tsp fresh ginger, minced

In a bowl, mix chicken, soy sauce, oil, and ginger. Put the marinated chicken inside of fridge for 30-minutes. Preheat your Air Fryer to 390°Fahrenheit for 3 minutes. Add marinated chicken into baking pan and set inside Air Fryer and cook for 6-minutes. In a small bowl, mix stevia, rosemary and oyster sauce. Pour the rosemary mixture over the chicken, then place lemon wedges over chicken. Continue to cook for an additional 13-minutes and flip the chicken over halfway through the cook time.

RECIPE 393: SAGE PORK WITH POTATOES

Serve: 4 | Total Time: 30 minutes

2 cups potatoes
2 tsp olive oil
1 lb pork tenderloin, cubed
1 onion, chopped
1 red bell pepper, chopped
2 garlic cloves, minced
½ tsp dried sage
½ tsp fennel seeds, crushed
2 tbsp chicken broth

Preheat Air Fryer to 370°F. Add the potatoes and olive oil to a bowl and toss to coat. Transfer them to the frying basket and Air Fry for 15 minutes. Remove the bowl. Add the pork, onion, red bell pepper, garlic, sage, and fennel seeds, to the potatoes, add chicken broth and stir gently. Return the bowl to the frying basket and cook for 10 minutes. Be sure to shake the basket at least once. The pork should be cooked through and the potatoes soft and crispy. Serve immediately.

RECIPE 394: SALMON CROQUETTES

Serve: 4 | Total Time: 10 minutes

14 oz tin of red salmon, drained
2 free-range eggs
5 tbsp olive oil
½ cup breadcrumbs
2 tbsp spring onions, chopped
Salt and pepper to taste
Pinch of herbs

Add drained salmon into a bowl and mash well. Break in the egg, add herbs, spring onions, salt, pepper, and mix well. In another bowl, combine breadcrumbs and oil and mix well. Take a spoon of the salmon mixture and shape it into a croquette shape in your hand. Place it in the Air Fryer after rolling it in breadcrumbs. Set your Air Fryer to 390°Fahrenhiet for 10-minutes.

RECIPE 395: SALMON IN PAPILLOTE WITH ORANGE

Serve: 4 | Total Time: 50 minutes

600g salmon fillet
4 oranges
2 cloves of garlic
Chives to taste
1 lemon

Pour the freshly squeezed orange juice, the lemon juice, the zest of the two oranges into a bowl. Add two tablespoons of oil, salt, and garlic. Dip the previously washed salmon fillet and leave it in the marinade for one hour, preferably in the refrigerator. Place the steak and part of your marinade on a sheet of foil. Salt and sprinkle with chives and a few slices of orange. Set to 160C. Simmer for 30 minutes. Open the sheet let it evaporate, and serve with a nice garnish of fresh orange.

RECIPE 396: SALMON PATTIES

Serve: 4 | Total Time: 15 minutes

1 tsp chili powder

2 tbsp full-fat mayonnaise
¼ cup ground pork rinds
2 x 5-oz pouches of cooked pink salmon
1 egg

Stir everything together to prepare the patty mixture. If the mixture is dry or falling apart, add in more pork rinds as necessary. Take equal-sized amounts of the mixture to form four patties, before placing the patties in the basket of your Air Fryer. Cook at 400°F for eight minutes. Halfway through cooking, flip the patties over. Once they are crispy, serve with the toppings of your choice and enjoy.

RECIPE 397: SALMON WITH CREAMY ZUCCHINI

Serve: 4 | Total Time: 25 minutes

2 5-6 oz salmon fillets, skin on
1 tsp olive oil
salt and pepper to taste
2 large zucchini, trimmed and spiralizer
1 avocado, peeled and roughly chopped
½ garlic clove, minced
small handful parsley, roughly chopped
small handful cherry tomatoes, halved
small handful black olives, chopped
2 tbsp pine nuts, toasted

Briefly preheat your Air Fryer to 350F. After coating the salmon with olive oil, season it with salt and pepper. Place the salmon in the Fryer and cook until the skin is crisp, about 10 minutes. While the salmon cooks, prepare the vegetables: blend the avocado, garlic, and parsley in a food processor until smooth. Toss in a large bowl with the zucchini, tomatoes, and olives. Divide the vegetables between two plates, top each portion with a salmon fillet, sprinkle with pine nuts, and serve.

RECIPE 398: SALT AND VINEGAR CHICKPEAS

Serve: 2 | Total Time: 55 minutes

1 (15 oz) can chickpeas, drained and rinsed
1 cup white vinegar
½ tsp sea salt
1 tbsp olive oil

Get a clean small saucepan, and in it, combine chickpeas and vinegar. Bring to a simmer over high heat. Once simmering, withdraw and allow to stand for 30 minutes. Drain the chickpeas and get rid of all loose skins. Ensure that your Air Fryer is preheated to 390 F. With the chickpeas spread evenly in the Air Fryer basket, allow cooking for about 4 minutes or until the chickpeas dry out. Move the dried chickpeas into a heat-proof bowl. Drizzle with sea salt and oil and stir to coat evenly. Place the coated chickpeas into the Air Fryer again and allow cooking for about 8 minutes. Endeavor to shake the basket at 2 or 3 minutes intervals. Withdraw once you have lightly browned chickpeas. Serve instantly.

RECIPE 399: SALTED LEMON ARTICHOKES

Serve: 2 | Total Time: 60 minutes

1 lemon
2 artichokes
1 tsp kosher salt
1 garlic head
2 tsp olive oil

Cut off the edges of the artichokes. Cut the lemon into the halves. Peel the garlic head and chop the garlic cloves roughly. Then place the chopped garlic in the artichokes. Sprinkle the artichokes with the olive oil and kosher salt. Then squeeze the lemon juice into the artichokes. Wrap the artichokes in the foil. Preheat the Air Fryer to 330 F. Place the wrapped artichokes in the Air Fryer and cook for 45 minutes. When the artichokes are cooked – discard the foil and serve. Enjoy!

RECIPE 400: SAUCE CHICKEN THIGHS

Serve: 4 | Total Time: 35 minutes

8 boneless, skinless chicken thighs
1 tbsp Italian seasoning
Salt and pepper to taste
2 garlic cloves, minced
½ tsp apple cider vinegar
½ cup honey
¼ cup Dijon mustard

Preheat Air Fryer to 400°F. Season the chicken with Italian seasoning, salt, and black pepper. Place in the greased frying basket and Bake for 15 minutes, flipping once halfway through cooking. While the chicken is cooking, add garlic, honey, vinegar, and Dijon mustard in a saucepan and stir-fry over medium heat for 4 minutes or until the sauce has thickened and warmed through. Transfer the thighs to a serving dish and drizzle with honey-mustard sauce. Serve and enjoy!

RECIPE 401: SAUSAGE BALLS

Serve: 5 | Total Time: 8 minutes

8-ounces ground chicken
1 egg white
1 tsp paprika
1 tbsp olive oil
2 tbsp almond flour
½ tsp ground black pepper
½ tsp salt
1 tbsp parsley, dried

Whisk the egg white and combine it with the ground chicken in a mixing bowl. Add parsley and salt to the mixture. Add paprika and ground black pepper to mixture and stir. With wet hands make small sausage balls from the ground chicken mixture. Sprinkle each sausage ball with almond flour. Preheat your Air Fryer to 380°Fahrenheit. Olive oil the interior of the Air Fryer basket tray. Place the sausage balls into the basket and cook for 8-minutes. Turn the balls to brown all sides during the cooking process.

Transfer the cooked sausage balls into serving plates. Serve warm.

RECIPE 402: SAUSAGE CHEESE BURRITOS

Serve: 6 | Total Time: 20 minutes

6 medium flour tortillas
6 scrambled eggs
½ lb ground sausage – browned
½ bell pepper – minced
1/3 cup bacon bits
½ cup shredded cheese
Cooking spray

In a mixing bowl, add scrambled eggs, bell pepper, cooked sausage, cheese, and bacon bits. Mix well to combined. Place a tortilla on the working surface and add about ½ cup of the eggs filling at the center of the tortilla. First, fold the sides of the tortilla and then roll it to make a burrito. Use the remaining filling and tortillas to make more burritos. Place half of the burritos in the Air Fryer Basket, spray them with cooking oil and cook them for 5 minutes at 330 F in the Air Fryer. Repeat the same steps to cook the remaining burritos. Serve warm.

RECIPE 403: SAUSAGE EGG CUP

Serve: 6 | Total Time: 25 minutes

12 ounces (340 g) ground pork breakfast sausage
6 large eggs
1/2 tsp salt
1/4 tsp ground black pepper
1/2 tsp crushed red pepper flakes

Place sausage in six 4-inch ramekins (about 2 ounces (57 g) per ramekin) greased with cooking oil. Press sausage down to cover bottom and about 1/2-inch up the sides of ramekins. Beat one egg into each ramekin and sprinkle evenly with salt, black pepper, and red pepper flakes. Place ramekins into Air Fryer basket. Adjust the temperature to 350F (180C) and set the timer for 15 minutes. Egg cups will be done when sausage is fully

cooked to at least 145F (63C) and the egg is firm. Serve warm.

RECIPE 404: SCOTCH EGGS

Serve: 6 | Total Time: 30 minutes

6 hard-boiled eggs
600 g minced chicken or turkey
3 raw eggs
300 g dried breadcrumbs
100 g flour
Some oil

Peel the hard-boiled eggs and set aside. In a large bowl, mix well the minced chicken, 1 raw egg and 100 g breadcrumbs. Divide the ingredients into six equal portions and roll each into a tiny oval ball. In a shallow bowl, whisk the remaining 2 raw eggs. Then roll the hard-boiled eggs in flour and coat with the minced chicken mixture. Sprinkle the coated egg with flour, dip in the beaten eggs and finally roll in the breadcrumbs. Brush the container of the Air Fryer with oil and place the breaded eggs in the container. Fry at 185 degrees for about 6-7 minutes, then turn and fry for another 6-7 minutes.

RECIPE 405: SCRAMBLED PANCAKE HASH

Serve: 7 | Total Time: 10 minutes

1 egg
¼ cup heavy cream
5 tbsp butter
1 cup coconut flour
1 tsp ground ginger
1 tsp salt
1 tsp apple cider vinegar
1 tsp baking soda

Combine the salt, baking soda, ground ginger and flour in a mixing bowl. In a separate bowl crack, the egg into it. Add butter and heavy cream. Mix well using a hand mixer. Combine the liquid and dry mixtures and stir until smooth. Preheat your Air Fryer to 400°Fahrenheit. Pour the pancake mixture into the Air Fryer basket

tray. Cook the pancake hash for 4-minutes. After this, scramble the pancake hash well and continue to cook for another 5-minutes more. When dish is cooked, transfer it to serving plates, and serve hot!

RECIPE 406: SEA SALTED CARAMEL COOKIE CUPS

Serve: 6 | Total Time: 12 minutes

⅓ cup butter
¼ cup brown sugar
1 tsp vanilla extract
1 large egg
1 cup all-purpose flour
½ cup old-fashioned oats
½ tsp baking soda
¼ tsp salt
⅓ cup sea-salted caramel chips

Preheat the Air Fryer to 300°F. Cream the butter, brown sugar, and vanilla. Whisk in the egg and set aside. Dissolve the baking soda and salt in the flour. Then gently mix the dry ingredients into the wet. Fold in the caramel chips. Divide the batter into 12 silicon muffin liners. Place the cookie cups into the Air Fryer basket and cook for 12 minutes or until a toothpick inserted in the center comes out clean. Remove and cool before serving.

RECIPE 407: SEAFOOD TOSTADAS

Serve: 4 | Total Time: 20 minutes

18 shrimps, peeled and deveined.
1/4 cup sour cream
1/4 cup cheese sauce
1/2 cup tomatoes, diced.
12 ounces nacho chips
2 tbsp. olives, sliced.
1 tsp. garlic powder
1 tsp. paprika
salt and pepper, to taste

Preheat the Air Fryer to temperature of 350 degrees F. Season the shrimps with the garlic powder, paprika, salt and pepper. Place the prepared and seasoned shrimps in the Air Fryer Basket and cook for 3 to 5 minutes or until the shrimps are cooked through. Remove the cooked shrimps from the Air Fryer and set aside. Place the nachos into the Air Fryer Basket and cook for 3 to 5 minutes or until they are well toasted. Remove the chips from the Air Fryer and arrange them on a serving plate. Top the nachos with the shrimps, tomatoes and olives. Dollop with the sour cream and cheese sauce. Serve and enjoy!

RECIPE 408: SEED PORRIDGE

Serve: 3 | Total Time: 12 minutes

1 tbsp butter
¼ tsp nutmeg
1/3 cup heavy cream
1 egg
¼ tsp salt
3 tbsp sesame seeds
3 tbsp chia seeds

Place the butter in your Air Fryer basket tray. Add the chia seeds, sesame seeds, heavy cream, nutmeg, and salt. Stir gently. Beat the egg in a cup and whisk it with a fork. Add the whisked egg to Air Fryer basket tray. Stir the mixture with a wooden spatula. Preheat your Air Fryer to 375°Fahrenheit. Place the Air Fryer basket tray into Air Fryer and cook the porridge for 12-minutes. During cooking, stir it 3 times. Remove the porridge from Air Fryer basket tray immediately and serve hot!

RECIPE 409: SEEDY RIB EYE STEAK BITES

Serve: 4 | Total Time: 20 minutes

1 lb rib eye steak, cubed
2 garlic cloves, minced
2 tbsp olive oil
1 tbsp thyme, chopped
1 tsp ground fennel seeds
Salt and pepper to taste
1 onion, thinly sliced

Preheat Air Fryer to 380°F. Place the steak, garlic, olive oil, thyme, fennel seeds, salt, pepper, and onion in a bowl. Mix until all of the beef and onion are well coated. Put the seasoned steak mixture into the frying basket. Roast for 10 minutes, stirring once. Let sit for 5 minutes. Serve.

RECIPE 410: SEMOLINA VEGGIE CUTLETS

Serve: 2 | Total Time: 23 minutes

1 cup semolina
Olive oil for frying
Salt and pepper to taste
1 ½ cups of your favorite veggies
5 cups milk

Stir and warm the milk in a saucepan over medium heat. Add vegetables when it becomes hot and cook until they are softened for about 3-minutes. Season with salt and pepper. Add the semolina to milk mixture and cook for another 10-minutes. Remove from heat and spread thin across a piece of parchment on a baking sheet, and chill for 4 hours in the fridge. Take out the baking sheet from the fridge, cut semolina mixture into cutlets. Preheat your Air Fryer to 350°Fahrenheit. Brush the cutlets with oil and bake for 10-minutes in your Air Fryer and serve with hot sauce!

RECIPE 411: SESAME-CRUSTED TUNA STEAK

Serve: 2 | Total Time: 13 minutes

2 (6-ounce) tuna steaks
1 tbsp coconut oil, melted
1/2 tsp garlic powder
2 tsp white sesame seeds
2 tsp black sesame seeds

Brush each tuna steak with coconut oil and sprinkle with garlic powder. In a large bowl, mix sesame seeds and then press each tuna steak into them, covering the steak as completely as possible. Place tuna steaks into the Air Fryer basket. Adjust the temperature to 400F and set the timer for 8 minutes. Flip the steaks halfway through the cooking time. Steaks will be well-done at 145F internal temperature. Serve warm.

RECIPE 412: SESAME FLAVORED CHICKEN BREAST

Serve: 5 | Total Time: 20 minutes

2 tbsp sesame seeds
4 tbsp sesame oil
2 tbsp coconut sugar
2 tbsp soy sauce
Salt, to taste
2 tbsp lemon juice
1 tbsp ginger garlic paste
2 pounds chicken breast, pieces

Combine sesame seeds, sesame oil, coconut sugar, soy sauce, lemon juice, salt, and ginger garlic paste in a large bowl. Pour in the chicken breasts. Transfer the pieces to a zip lock plastic bag and freeze in the refrigerator for 2 hours. Preheat the Air Fryer at 392 degrees F for 2 minutes. Place marinated chicken pieces into the Air Fryer basket. Let them cook for 18-25 minutes. Once golden brown, serve and enjoy.

RECIPE 413: SHREDDED CHICKEN

Serve: 2 | Total Time: 20 minutes

1 tsp honey
1 tsp mustard
1 tsp garlic puree
2 large chicken breasts
Salt and ground black pepper to taste

Combine the whole marinade ingredients into the baking pan of the Air Fryer and stir very well. Immerse the chicken breasts into the marinade, while seasoning the top of the chicken breasts with pepper and salt. Allow the seasoned chicken to cook for 15 minutes in the Air Fryer, at 360 F. After the first five minutes of cooking, slice the chicken breasts into thirds and pour some marinade into the openings. This is to ensure that the breasts cook fast and are well-flavored. Transfer the well-cooked chicken into a chopping board and leave for about two minutes. Chop the cooked chicken into small pieces using a knife and fork. Serve.

RECIPE 414: SHRIMPS FRIED WITH CELERY

Serve: 2 | Total Time: 20 minutes

4 stalks celery
1 small carrot
10-12 fresh shrimps
3 clove garlic, finely chopped
1 tbsp olive oil
1 tbsp oyster sauce
1 tbsp soy sauce
1 tsp sugar
1 tsp cornstarch
3/4 to 1 cup water

Preheat the Air Fryer to 350 F. Put chopped garlic, sliced celery and sliced carrot diagonally into the Air Fryer, pour with oil and cook for 7 minutes. Mix oyster sauce, soy sauce, sugar, cornstarch and water in a bowl. Add this mixture into the Air Fryer and cook for another 1-2 minutes. Add shrimps and cook for another 5 minutes.

RECIPE 415: SIMPLY FRIED CHICKEN THIGHS

Serve: 4 | Total Time: 30 minutes

1 tsp kosher salt
½ cup all purpose flour
1 egg beaten
4 small chicken thighs
1½ tbsp Old Bay cajun seasoning

Ensure that your Air Fryer is preheated to 390 F. Combine the salt, flour, and the Old Bay, and mix the mixture. Submerge the chicken in the flour mixture, and into the egg, before taking it back into the flour mixture again. Remove all excess flour by shaking them off. Transfer the four chicken thighs into the cooking compartment of your Air Fryer - preferably at the bottom. Allow to cook for 25 minutes in this position, or until the chicken reaches the temperature of 180 F.

Once either of this happens, it means the chicken is ready. Remove and serve.

RECIPE 416: SKIRT STEAK WITH HORSERADISH CREAM

Serve: 2 | Total Time: 20 minutes

1 cup heavy cream
3 tbsp horseradish sauce
1 lemon, zested
1 (12-oz) skirt steak, halved
2 tbsp olive oil
Salt and pepper to taste

Mix together the heavy cream, horseradish sauce, and lemon zest in a small bowl. Let chill in the fridge. Preheat Air Fryer to 400ºF. Brush steak halves with olive oil and sprinkle with salt and pepper. Place steaks in the frying basket and Air Fry for 10 minutes or until you reach your desired doneness, flipping once. Let sit onto a cutting board for 5 minutes. Thinly slice against the grain and divide between 2 plates. Drizzle with the horseradish sauce over. Serve and enjoy!

RECIPE 417: SMOKED PAPRIKA SWEET POTATO FRIES

Serve: 4 | Total Time: 35 minutes

2 sweet potatoes, peeled
1 ½ tbsp cornstarch
1 tbsp canola oil
1 tbsp olive oil
1 tsp smoked paprika
1 tsp garlic powder
Salt and pepper to taste
1 cup cocktail sauce

Cut the potatoes lengthwise to form French fries. Put in a resealable plastic bag and add cornstarch. Seal and shake to coat the fries. Combine the canola oil, olive oil, paprika, garlic powder, salt, and pepper fries in a large bowl. Add the sweet potato fries and mix to combine. Preheat Air Fryer to 380ºF. Place fries in the greased basket and fry for 20-25 minutes, shaking the basket once

until crisp. Drizzle with Cocktail sauce to serve.

RECIPE 418: SMOKY ROASTED VEGGIE CHIPS

Serve: 4 | Total Time: 40 minutes

2 tbsp butter
2 tsp smoked paprika
1 tsp dried dill
Salt and pepper to taste
2 carrots, cut into rounds
1 parsnip, cut into rounds
1 tbsp chopped fresh dill

Preheat the Air Fryer to 375ºF. Combine the butter, paprika, dried dill, salt, and pepper in a small pan, over low heat until the butter melts. Put the carrots and parsnip in the frying basket, top with the butter mix, and toss. Air Fry for 20-25 minutes or until the veggies are tender and golden around the edges. Toss with fresh dill and serve.

RECIPE 419: SPAGHETTI SQUASH FRITTERS

Serve: 4 | Total Time: 23 minutes

2 cups cooked spaghetti squash
2 tbsp unsalted butter, softened
1 large egg
1/4 cup finely ground almond flour
2 stalks green onion, sliced
1/2 tsp garlic powder
1 tsp dried parsley

Detach excess moisture from the squash using a cheesecloth or kitchen towel. Mix all ingredients in a large bowl. Form into four patties. Divide a piece of parchment to fit your Air Fryer basket. Place each patty on the parchment and place into the Air Fryer basket. Adjust the temperature to 400F and set the timer for 8 minutes. Turn over the patties halfway through the cooking time. Serve warm.

RECIPE 420: SPICED CHICKEN BREASTS

Serve: 4 | Total Time: 20 minutes

½ tsp dried oregano
½ tsp granulated garlic
½ tsp granulated onion
½ tsp chili powder
¼ tsp sweet paprika
Salt and pepper to taste
1 lb chicken breasts, sliced
2 tbsp yellow mustard

Preheat Air Fryer to 375°F. Mix together oregano, salt, garlic, onion, chili powder, paprika, and black pepper in a small bowl. Coat the chicken with mustard in a bowl. Sprinkle the seasoning mix over the chicken. Place the chicken in the greased frying basket and Air Fry for 7-8, flipping once until cooked through. Serve immediately.

RECIPE 421: SPICED CHICKEN WINGS IN AIR FRYER

Serve: 4 | Total Time: 45 minutes

1 kg chicken wings
Salt
Ground pepper
Extra virgin olive oil
Spices, I put roasted chicken or roast chicken spices.

We clean the wings and chop, throw the tip and place in a bowl the other two parts of the wings that have more meat. We season and add some extra virgin olive oil threads. Sprinkle with spices, we can put whatever we want, put spices for roast chicken that they sell as is in supermarkets, in regular spice cans. We flirt well and leave for 30 minutes to rest in the refrigerator. We put the wings in the basket of the Air Fryer and select 180 degrees, about 30 minutes. From 20 minutes, we are checking if we have to remove them before. From time to time, we shake the basket so that the wings move and are made all over their faces. Serve

RECIPE 422: SPICED MEXICAN STIR-FRIED CHICKEN

Serve: 4 | Total Time: 30 minutes

1 lb chicken breasts, cubed
2 green onions, chopped
1 red bell pepper, chopped
1 jalapeño pepper, minced
2 tsp olive oil
2/3 cup canned black beans
½ cup salsa
2 tsp Mexican chili powder

Preheat Air Fryer to 400°F. Combine the chicken, green onions, bell pepper, jalapeño, and olive oil in a bowl. Transfer to a bowl to the frying basket and Air Fry for 10 minutes, stirring once during cooking. When done, stir in the black beans, salsa, and chili powder. Air Fry for 7-10 minutes or until cooked through. Serve.

RECIPE 423: SPICY CAJUN BABY CORNS

Serve: 2 | Total Time: 25 minutes

9 ounces baby corns; boiled
1 cup all-purpose flour
1/4 cup water
1 tsp. Cajun seasoning
2 tsp. ginger, minced.
1 tsp. olive oil
1/8 tsp. baking soda
chili flakes, to taste.
salt and pepper, to taste
Preheat the Air Fryer to temperature of 350 degrees F. Mix together the flour, baking soda and water to make a thin batter. Mix in the minced ginger, Cajun seasoning, chili flakes and olive oil. Coat the baby corns with the batter and arrange them in Air Fryer Basket. Cook for 10 minutes. Allow the baby corns to cool in the Air Fryer. Season with salt and pepper to taste. Serve and enjoy!

RECIPE 424: SPICY CHEESE LINGS

Serve: 3 | Total Time: 25 minutes

1 cup flour + extra for kneading
4 tbsp. grated cheese + extra for rolling
½ tsp. baking powder
3 tsp. butter

¼ tsp. chili powder
A pinch of salt

Take a bowl and, mix cheese, flour, baking powder, chili powder, butter and salt. Add some water and mix well to get a dough. Remove the dough on a flat floured surface. Using a rolling pin, roll the dough out into a thin sheet. Cut the dough into lings' shape. Add the cheese lings to the basket and cook for 6 minutes at 350 degrees F, flipping once halfway through.

RECIPE 425: SPICY FRIED CHICKEN

Serve: 4 | Total Time: 35 minutes

500g chicken breast
125ml whole milk
40g whey protein powder
45g grated parmesan
¼ tsp salt
½ tsp paprika
1 tsp ground cayenne pepper
2 eggs
2 tbsp olive oil

Preheat your Air Fryer to 240 degrees Celsius and line the Air Fryer tray or baking pan with foil. Place the chicken breast and whole milk in a large bowl. Cover and marinate in the fridge overnight. Toss the protein powder, parmesan, salt, cayenne pepper, and paprika in a shallow bowl. Whisk the egg in a separate bowl. After dipping the chicken in the egg, coat it with the protein powder mixture. Place the chicken breast on the prepared sheet tray and, once they are all dipped, drizzle with the olive oil. Bake in the Air Fryer for 15 minutes or until the tenders are golden brown. Serve.

RECIPE 426: SPICY SRIRACHA CAULIFLOWER

Serve: 4 | Total Time: 35 minutes

1 cauliflower head, cut into florets
¾ cup onion white, sliced
5 garlic cloves, finely sliced
1 ½ tbsp tamari

1 tbsp rice vinegar
½ tsp coconut sugar
1 tbsp sriracha
2 scallions, for garnish

Add cauliflower to the Air Fryer's Basket. Return the fryer basket to the Air Fryer and cook on air fry mode for 10 minutes at 350 F. Toss the cauliflower then add the onion. Cook again for 10 minutes on air fry mode. Add garlic and then cook for 5 minutes in the fryer. Whisk tamari, sugar, salt, pepper, sriracha, and rice vinegar in a small bowl. Pour this mixture over the cauliflower and cook on air fry mode for 5 minutes. Garnish with scallions. Enjoy.

RECIPE 427: SPICY SWEET POTATO WEDGES

Serve: 2 | Total Time: 30 minutes

2 large sweet potatoes, peeled
1 tsp chilli powder
1 tsp cumin
1 tsp mustard powder
1 tbsp mexican seasoning
Salt and ground black pepper to taste
1 tbsp olive oil

Chop the peeled sweet potatoes into the shape of wedges. Ensure that your Air Fryer is preheated to 360 F for 5 minutes. Get a clean mixing bowl and in it, combine your seasonings and mix thoroughly. Toss in the potato wedges until they are evenly coated. Transfer the coated wedges into the Air Fryer, add some olive oil and allow cooking for 20 minutes. Shake the basket at 5 minutes' intervals until the cooking is complete. Serve the cooked sweet potatoes alongside a thousand island dip and sprinkles of a little extra chili powder.

RECIPE 428: SPINACH AND TOMATO EGG

Serve: 4 | Total Time: 25 minutes

2 cups 100% liquid egg whites

3 tbsp salted butter, melted
1/4 tsp salt
1/4 tsp onion powder
1/2 medium Roma tomato, cored and diced
1/2 cup chopped fresh spinach leaves

In a large bowl, merge egg whites with butter, salt, and onion powder. Stir in tomato and spinach, and then pour evenly into four 4-inch ramekins greased with cooking spray. Place ramekins into Air Fryer basket. Adjust the temperature to 300F (150C) and set the timer for 15 minutes. Eggs will be fully cooked and firm in the center when done. Serve warm.

RECIPE 429: SPINACH PIE

Serve: 4 | Total Time: 25 minutes

7 oz flour
2 tbsp butter
7 oz spinach
1 tbsp olive oil
2 eggs
2 tbsp milk
3 oz cottage cheese
Salt and black pepper to the taste
1 yellow onion, chopped

In your food processor, mix flour with butter, 1 egg, milk, salt and pepper, blend well, transfer to a bowl, knead, cover and leave for 10 minutes. Over medium high heat, heat the oil in a skillet, then add the onion and spinach, mix, and cook for 2 minutes. Add salt, pepper, the remaining egg and cottage cheese, stir well and take off heat. Divide dough in 4 pieces, roll each piece, place on the bottom of a ramekin, add spinach filling over dough, place ramekins in your Air Fryer's basket and cook at 360 degrees F for 15 minutes. Serve warm, enjoy!

RECIPE 430: SQUASH WITH CUMIN AND CHILI

Serve: 2 | Total Time: 25 minutes

2 butternut squash

4 tbsp cumin seeds
1 tsp chili flakes
2 tbsp olive oil
2 cups plain Greek yogurt
½ cup pine nuts

Wash and slice the squash and remove the seeds. Cut into small chunks. Place the squash into a bowl. Sprinkle cumin seed, chili flakes, olive oil, and nuts. Heat an Air Fryer to 350 degrees F. Place squash pieces in the basket and cook for 20 minutes. Remember to turn the squash, two or three times during the cooking process. Serve the cooked squash with a dollop of yogurt. Enjoy.

RECIPE 431: STEAK AND CABBAGE

Serve: 4 | Total Time: 25 minutes

2 pounds sirloin steak, sliced
4 tbsp cornstarch
4 tbsp peanut oil
3 cups cabbage
1 bell pepper
2 onions, chopped
4 cloves garlic, sliced
½ cup soy sauce

Preheat the Air Fryer to temperature of 400 degrees F. Coat the steak with cornstarch and set aside. In a mixing bowl, add oil and cabbage. Place cabbage in the Air Fryer basket and cook for 5 minutes. Afterward, add the steak, pepper, garlic, and onions. Cook for 15 minutes. After 15 minutes, add the soy sauce and let it cook for 5 more minutes. Serve.

RECIPE 432: STEAMED SALMON WITH DILL SAUCE

Serve: 2 | Total Time: 15 minutes

Sea salt about 2 pinches
2 tsp olive oil
2 tbsp dill, chopped
½ cup plain Greek yogurt
½ cup light sour cream
12-ounce salmon fillet

First, set your Air Fryer to 300°Fahrenheit. Add one cup of water to the bottom of air fryer. Cut the salmon into pieces and sprinkle one tablespoon of olive oil in the bowl and mix with a pinch of salt. Add the pieces of salmon to the Air Fryer and cook for 12 minutes. Combine the chopped dill, salt, yogurt, sour cream in a bowl. Save a teaspoon of chopped dill to garnish the top of the salmon.

RECIPE 433: STUFFED CUTTLEFISH

Serve: 4 | Total Time: 50 minutes

8 small cuttlefish
50 g of breadcrumbs
Garlic to taste
Parsley to taste
1 egg
Clean the cuttlefish, cut, and separate the tentacles. In a blender, pour the breadcrumbs, the parsley (without the branches), the egg, the salt, a drizzle of olive oil, and the sepia tentacles. Blend until you get a dense mixture. Fill the sepia with the mixture obtained. Place the cuttlefish in the bowl. Set the Air Fryer to 150C and cook for 20 minutes. At the end of cooking, add a drizzle of olive oil and serve.

RECIPE 434: STUFFED PEPPERS WITH CHEESE AND BACON

Serve: 2 | Total Time: 18 minutes

1/4 cup bacon, chopped.
2 large bell peppers
1/2 cup mozzarella cheese, grated.
1/2 cup tomatoes, diced.
2 cloves garlic, minced.
1-tsp. paprika
Salt and pepper, to taste

Preheat the Air Fryer to temperature 350 degrees F. Cut the tops off the bell peppers. Remove the seeds and the rest of the insides of the bell peppers, so they are completely hollow. Mix together the bacon, mozzarella cheese, garlic, tomatoes, paprika,

salt and pepper in a medium size bowl. Fill both bell peppers with the bowl mixture. Place all of the prepared the bell peppers in the Air Fryer Basket and cook for 8 minutes. Serve and enjoy!

RECIPE 435: SUPER SIMPLE FISHERMAN'S FISHCAKES

Serve: 4 | Total Time: 60 minutes

3 cups white fish boned and cooked
1 cup mashed potatoes
1 tsp parsley
1 tsp sage
Salt and ground black pepper
3 tbsp butter
3 tbsp milk
3 tsp flour
Mix the fish, potatoes, and spices in a large mixing dish. Mix very well and add the butter and milk. Mix again until you have a uniform mixture. You may need to add more milk to ensure a nice consistency. Add a little flour to the mixture and make patty cakes from it. Transfer the cakes into the fridge and leave for three hours. This solidifies the cakes. Cook the cakes in the Air Fryer for 15 minutes at 390 F. 6. Serve.

RECIPE 436: SWEET AND SOUR SESAME TOFU
Serve: 2 | Total Time: 55 minutes

2 tsp apple cider vinegar
1 tbsp coconut sugar
1 tbsp soy sauce
3 tsp lime juice
1 tsp ground ginger
1 tsp garlic powder
½ block firm tofu
1 tsp corn starch
2 green onions, chopped

In a mixing bowl, mix together the first six ingredients. Mix until well combined. Marinate the tofu in the sauce for at least 30 minutes. Strain the marinated tofu and save the sauce. Place the tofu in a preheated Air Fryer and cook at 400F for 20 minutes or until crisp. Meanwhile, pour the remaining

sauce in a saucepan and add cornstarch. Turn on the flame and allow to thicken under medium low heat. Toss the air fried tofu in the thickened sauce and add green onions and sesame seeds. Serve with rice.

RECIPE 437: SWEET CREAM CHEESE WONTONS

Serve: 8 | Total Time: 25 minutes

1 egg mixed with a bit of water
Wonton wrappers
½ C. powdered erythritol
8 ounces softened cream cheese
Olive oil

Preparing the Ingredients. Mix sweetener and cream cheese together. Lay out 4 wontons at a time and cover with a dish towel to prevent drying out. Place ½ of a teaspoon of cream cheese mixture into each wrapper. Dip finger into egg/water mixture and fold diagonally to form a triangle. Seal edges well. Repeat with remaining ingredients. Air Frying. Place filled wontons into the Instant Vortex Air Fryer oven and cook 5 minutes at 400 degrees, shaking halfway through cooking.

RECIPE 438: SWEET MUSTARD COCONUT SHRIMP

Serve: 2 | Total Time: 20 minutes

½ cup breadcrumbs
Salt and black pepper to taste
½ cup shredded coconut, unsweetened
½ tsp cayenne pepper
8-ounces coconut milk
8 large shrimps
1 tablespoon sugar-free syrup
¼ tsp hot sauce
½ cup orange jam, sugar-free
1 tsp mustard

Preheat your Air Fryer to 350°Fahrenheit. Place breadcrumbs, coconut, salt, pepper, and cayenne pepper in a bowl and mix. Dip the shrimp in coconut milk first, then in breadcrumb mixture. Line baking sheet and arrange shrimp on it. Place in Air Fryer and cook for 20-minutes. Whisk the orange jam, mustard, syrup, and hot sauce. Add the shrimp to a serving platter and drizzle with sauce and serve.

RECIPE 439: SWEET POTATO AND TUNA CHIPS

Serve: 2 | Total Time: 85 minutes

4 large sweet potatoes; peeled and sliced
1 cup canned tuna; in water
1/4 cup celery, chopped.
1/4 cup onions, chopped.
2-tbsp. yogurt
1/4-tsp. cayenne pepper
salt and pepper, to taste.
pepper, to taste

Preheat the Air Fryer to temperature of 350 degrees F. Soak the sweet potatoes in water for 30 minutes. Drain and pat dry. Season the sweet potatoes with salt and pepper and spray with some cooking spray. Place the sweet potatoes in the Air Fryer Basket and cook for 30 minutes or until the sweet potatoes are fried and crispy. Mix together the tuna, yogurt, cayenne powder, onions and celery and season with pepper. Serve the tuna with the sweet potato chips. Enjoy!

RECIPE 440: SWEET POTATO CHIPS

Serve: 2 | Total Time: 25 minutes

1 medium sweet potato, peeled and sliced crossways into 1/8-inch slices
1 tsp avocado oil
½ tsp Creole seasoning, or to taste

Ensure that your Air Fryer is preheated to 400 F. Get a large bowl, and place the sweet potato slices in it, add the avocado oil and stir well to ensure that each piece is well coated. Pour the creole seasoning and stir to make it mix with the potato. Transfer the coated slices into a thin layer on the Air Fryer basket's base. Allow

cooking for 7 minutes, after which you turn and shake the fries to ensure even cooking. Resume cooking until the fries are crisp according to your taste - this may take 6 minutes or more. Place the cooked potato slices on a rack and allow to cool. Serve.

RECIPE 441: SWEET POTATO CRISPS

Serve: 6 | Total Time: 35 minutes

2 medium sized sweet potatoes, sliced
¼ cup of olive oil
1 tsp of ground cinnamon
Black pepper and salt to taste

Slice the sweet potatoes. Soak the sweet potato slices in a bowl filled with cold water for 30 minutes approximately. Drain and pat dry all the potato slices. Toss the sweet potato slices with black pepper, olive oil, and salt, and cinnamon. Grease the air fry basket. Add sweet potatoes slices to the Air Fryer basket and cook them in batches at 390F for 22 minutes approximately, toss the chips after every 5 minutes. Serve warm.

RECIPE 442: SWEET POTATO FRIES

Serve: 5 | Total Time: 25 minutes

3 Large Sweet Potatoes, Peeled
1 Tbsp Olive Oil
A Pinch Tsp Sea Salt

Turn on your Air Fryer to 390. Start by cutting your sweet potatoes in quarters, cutting them lengthwise to make fries. Combine the uncooked fries with a tbsp of sea salt and olive oil. Make sure all of your fries are coated well. Place your sweet potato pieces in your basket, cooking for 12 minutes. Cook for two to three minutes more if you want it to be crispier. Add more salt to taste, and serve when cooled.

RECIPE 443: SWEET POTATO HASH BROWNS

Serve: 4 | Total Time: 30 minutes

4 sweet potatoes
2 minced garlic cloves
1 tsp cinnamon
1 tsp paprika
2 tsp olive oil
Salt and black pepper, to taste

Peel and grate all the sweet potatoes with the help of a cheese grater. Add sweet potato shreds to a bowl filled with cold water and leave it soaked for 25 minutes. Drain the water and place the sweet potato shreds in a plate lined with a paper towel. Transfer the shreds to a dry bowl and add olive oil, paprika, garlic, and black pepper. Mix well then spread the potato mixture in the Air Fryer Basket. Return the fryer basket to the Air Fry and cook for 10 minutes at 400 F. Shake the potatoes in the basket and toss in onions and pepper. Return the fryer basket again to the Fryer and continue cooking for another 10 minutes on the same temperature. Once done, serve warm.

RECIPE 444: SWEET POTATO TOTS

Serve: 24 | Total Time: 10 minutes

2 sweet potatoes, peeled
1/2 tsp Cajun seasoning
Salt

In a large pot, add water to bring to a boil. Add sweet potatoes to the pot and boil for 15 minutes. Drain well. Grated boil sweet potatoes into a large bowl using a grated. Add Cajun seasoning and salt in grated sweet potatoes and mix until well combined. Spray Air Fryer basket with cooking spray. Make a tiny tot of sweet potato mixture and place it in an Air Fryer basket. Cook at 400 F for 8 minutes. Turn tots to another side and cook for 8 minutes more. Serve and enjoy.

RECIPE 445: SWEETS AND TREATS

Serve: 8 | Total Time: 30 minutes

2 free-range eggs
1 1/2 cups milk
1/4 cup butter
1 1/2 tsp vanilla extract
1 cup shredded coconut
1/2 cup Monk Fruit sweetener
1/2 cup coconut flour

Heat the Air Fryer to 350F and oil a 6 inches pie plate with any oil of your choice. Set aside. Attach all the ingredients to a large bowl. Mix properly to combine. Pour the mixture into the pie plate and place in your Air Fryer. Let it cook properly for 10-12 minutes. Serve and enjoy!

RECIPE 446: TACO DOGS

Serve: 2 | Total Time: 17 minutes

2 jumbo hot dogs
1 tsp taco seasoning mix
2 hot dog buns
1/3 cup guacamole
4 tbsp salsa
6 pickled jalapeno slices

Ensure that your Air Fryer is preheated at 390 F for at least four minutes. Make five slits into each hot dog, and rub ½ teaspoon taco seasoning over each hot dog. Allow all the hot dogs to cook in the Air Fryer for 5 minutes before transferring them to the bus. This time around, cook until the buns are toasted and hot dogs crisp. This takes about 4 minutes or more. Top the hot dogs with guacamole, salsa, and jalapenos - all in equal amounts.

RECIPE 447: TANDOORI CHICKEN WITH MINT YOGURT

Serve: 4 | Total Time: 20 minutes

2-ounces of chicken breast
2 tbsp tandoori paste, divided
4 tbsp + ¾ cup
Greek yogurt, divided
3 sprigs of mint, minced
Salt and pepper to taste
1 tbsp olive oil

2 cups cooked basmati rice
Mint leaves for garnishing
Combine 1 tablespoon of tandoori paste and 2 tablespoons of yogurt in a bowl. Coat the chicken breast with mixture. Marinate for 2-hours in the fridge. Preheat your Air Fryer to 360°Fahrenheit for 5-minutes. Set Air Fryer timer to 15-minutes and place the chicken inside. Prepare the mint yogurt sauce by mixing the minced mint with 2 tablespoons of yogurt. Season with salt and pepper and stir well. Prepare tandoori sauce: heat the olive oil in a pan over medium heat and sauté 1 tablespoon tandoori paste for 3-minutes. Add remaining ¾ cup of yogurt and sauté for another 2-minutes. Slice the chicken breast and serve with basmati rice. Cover meat with tandoori sauce and mint yogurt sauce on top. Garnish with mint leaves.

RECIPE 448: TANGY COD FILLETS

Serve: 2 | Total Time: 35 minutes

½ tbsp sesame oil
1/2 heaping tsp dried parsley flakes
1/3 tsp fresh lemon zest, finely grated
medium-sized cod fillets
1 tsp sea salt flakes
A pinch of salt and pepper
1/3 tsp ground black pepper, or more to savor
1/2 tbsp fresh lemon juice

Set the Air Fryer to cook at 375 degrees f. Season each cod fillet with sea salt flakes, black pepper, and dried parsley flakes. Now, drizzle them with sesame oil. Place the seasoned cod fillets in a single layer at the bottom of the cooking basket; air-fry for approximately 10 minutes. While the fillets are cooking, prepare the sauce by mixing the other ingredients. Serve cod fillets on four individual plates garnished with the creamy citrus sauce.

RECIPE 449: TASTY BREAKFAST CUPS

Serve: 2 | Total Time: 14 minutes

1/2 cup spring onions, sliced.
2 slices bread
6 rashers bacon
4 eggs
3 tbsp. low-fat mayonnaise, optional.
2 tbsp. tomatoes, diced.
salt and pepper, to taste

Preheat the Air Fryer to temperature of 350 degrees F. Lightly spray 4 muffin cups with cooking spray. Cut 4 bread circles to fit the base of the muffin cups. Bacon should be used to line the sides of the muffin cups. Fill the cups with tomatoes and spring onions. Add a dollop of mayonnaise in each cup, if desired. Salt and pepper each egg cup. Place the muffin cups in the Air Fryer Basket and cook for 4 minutes, or until the bacon is crisp and the eggs are of your desired doneness. Serve and enjoy!

RECIPE 450: TASTY BRUSSELS SPROUTS WITH GUANCIALE

Serve: 4 | Total Time: 50 minutes

3 guanciale slices, halved
1 lb Brussels sprouts, halved
2 tbsp olive oil
¼ tsp salt
¼ tsp dried thyme

Preheat Air Fryer to 350°F. Air Fry Lay the guanciale in the Air Fryer, until crispy, 10 minutes. Remove and drain on a paper towel. Give the guanciale a rough chop and Set aside. Coat Brussels sprouts with olive oil in a large bowl. Add salt and thyme, then toss. Place the sprouts in the frying basket. Air Fry for about 12-15 minutes, shake the basket once until the sprouts are golden and tender. Top with guanciale and serve.

RECIPE 451: TASTY CHEESY OMELET

Serve: 2 | Total Time: 25 minutes

1 large onion, chopped
2 tbsp cheddar cheese, grated
3 eggs
½ tsp soy sauce
Salt to taste
Pepper powder to taste
Cooking spray

Combine the eggs, salt, pepper, and soy sauce in a mixing bowl. Spray a small pan, which fits inside the Air Fryer with cooking spray. Place the pan inside the Air Fryer and add the onions, spreading them out evenly. Air fry at 355F for 6-7 minutes or until onions are translucent. Pour the beaten egg mixture all over the onions. Sprinkle cheese all over it. Air fry for another 5-6 minutes. Place the chicken on toasted multigrain bread after removing it from the Air Fryer.

RECIPE 452: TASTY COD PATTIES

Serve: 3 | Total Time: 90 minutes

4 cod fillets
1 raw egg, lightly beaten.
2 tbsp. chives, chopped.
2 tbsp. fresh parsley, chopped.
1 tbsp. lemon juice
2 tbsp. olive oil
1 tsp. red pepper flakes
1 tsp. lemon zest
1 tsp. tabasco
salt and pepper, to taste

Preheat the Air Fryer to temperature 300 degrees F. Season the cod fillets with salt and pepper and place in the Air Fryer Basket. Cook for 5 minutes. Remove the fillets from the Air Fryer and mash them with a fork. Mix in the pepper flakes, lemon zest, lemon juice, parsley, chives, salt and pepper. Add the tabasco, egg and olive oil. Patties for an hour or overnight. Preheat the Air Fryer to temperature of 300 degrees F. Put patties in the Air Fryer and spray with some cooking spray. Cook for 15 minutes. Serve and enjoy!

RECIPE 453: TASTY ROASTED KIDNEY BEANS AND PEPPERS

Serve: 4 | Total Time: 20 minutes

2 (15-oz) cans kidney beans
1 green bell pepper, diced
1 shallot, diced
3 garlic cloves, minced
1 tbsp olive oil
Salt and pepper to taste
1 rosemary sprig
1 bay leaf

Preheat Air Fryer to 360°F. Combine the beans, bell pepper, shallot, garlic, olive oil, salt, and pepper in a bowl. Pour the bean mixture into a greased casserole dish, put the rosemary and bay leaf on top, and then place the casserole dish into the Air Fryer. Roast for 15 minutes. Remove the rosemary and bay leaves, then stir. Serve.

RECIPE 454: TAWA VEGGIES

Serve: 4 | Total Time: 25 minutes

¼ cup okra
2 tsp garam masala
1 tsp red chili powder
1 tsp amchur powder
¼ cup taro root
¼ cup potato
¼ cup eggplant
Salt to taste
Olive oil for brushing

Cut potato and taro root into fries and soak in salt water for 10 minutes. Cut okra and eggplant into four pieces. Rinse potatoes and taro root and pat dry. Add the spices to potatoes, taro roots, okra, and eggplant. Brush pan with oil and preheat to 390°Fahrenheit and cook for 10-minutes. Lower the heat to 355°Fahrenheit and cook for an additional 15-minutes.

RECIPE 455: TENDER COCONUT SHRIMPS

Serve: 4 | Total Time: 25 minutes

2 pounds (12-15) raw shrimps

1 cup egg whites
1 cup dried coconut, unsweetened
1 cup breadcrumbs
1 cup all-purpose flour
½ tsp salt

Prepare shrimps and set aside. In the large mixing bowl combine breadcrumbs and coconut. Season with salt lightly. In another bowl place flour and in the third bowl place egg whites. Meanwhile, preheat the Air Fryer to 340F. Dip each shrimp into the flour, then into egg whites and then into breadcrumbs mixture. Transfer shrimps to a fryer and cook for about 8-10 minutes, shaking occasionally. Serve with dipping sauce you prefer.

RECIPE 456: TENDER STEAK WITH SALSA VERDE

Serve: 4 | Total Time: 20 minutes

1 (2-lb) flank steak, halved
1 ½ cups salsa verde
½ tsp black pepper

Toss steak and 1 cup of salsa verde in a bowl and refrigerate covered for 2 hours. Preheat Air Fryer to 400°F. Add steaks to the lightly greased frying basket and Air Fry for 10-12 minutes or until you reach your desired doneness, flipping once. Let sit onto a cutting board for 5 minutes. Thinly slice against the grain and divide between 4 plates. Spoon over the remaining salsa verde and serve sprinkled with black pepper to serve.

RECIPE 457: TERIYAKI BEEF STRIPS

Serve: 2 | Total Time: 33 minutes

3/4-lb. beef loin, cut into strips.
1/2 cup teriyaki sauce
2 cups bean sprouts
2 tbsp. spring onions, chopped.
2 tbsp. garlic, minced.
2 tbsp. olive oil
1 tsp. sesame seeds
salt and pepper, to taste

Preheat the Air Fryer to temperature of 350 degrees F. Season the beef strips with salt and pepper. Marinate the beef strips with the teriyaki sauce, olive oil, garlic and sesame seeds for 10 minutes. Place the beef and marinade in the Air Fryer Baking Pan and place the Air Fryer Baking Pan in the Air Fryer Basket. Cook for 15 minutes. Add the bean sprouts to the Air Fryer Baking Pan and cook for 3 more minutes. Top with the spring onions. Serve and enjoy!

RECIPE 458: TERIYAKI GLAZED STEAK

Serve: 2 | Total Time: 20 minutes

1.5 pounds Halibut Steak
1/2 cup Soy Sauce
1 cup Japanese cooking wine
¼ cup Brown Sugar
1 tbsp Lime Juice
1/3 cup Orange Juice
1/3 tsp Ginger, ground
½ tsp garlic
2 cups boiled rice
Combine all the Teriyaki glaze ingredients in a bowl. Mix to make a sauce. Add the halibut steak to the sauce and place it in the refrigerator for 2 hours. Now, preheat the Air Fryer at 392 degrees F for 5 minutes. Place the steak in the Air Fryer and cook for 16 minutes. Serve over white rice. Enjoy.

RECIPE 459: THYME SIRLOIN FINGER STRIPS

Serve: 2 | Total Time: 25 minutes

½ lb top sirloin strips
1 cup breadcrumbs
½ tsp garlic powder
½ tsp steak seasoning
2 eggs, beaten
Salt and pepper to taste
½ tbsp dried thyme

Preheat Air Fryer to 350°F. Put the breadcrumbs, garlic powder, steak seasoning, thyme, salt, and pepper in a bowl and stir to combine. Add

in the sirloin steak strips and toss to coat all sides. Dip into the beaten eggs, then dip again into the dry ingredients. Lay the coated steak pieces on the greased frying basket in an even layer. Air Fry for 16-18 minutes, turning once. Serve and enjoy!

RECIPE 460: THYME STEAK FINGER STRIPS

Serve: 2 | Total Time: 25 minutes

½ lb top sirloin strips
1 cup breadcrumbs
½ tsp garlic powder
½ tsp steak seasoning
2 eggs, beaten
Salt and pepper to taste
½ tbsp dried thyme

Preheat Air Fryer to 350°F. Put the breadcrumbs, garlic powder, steak seasoning, thyme, salt, and pepper in a bowl and stir to combine. Add in the sirloin steak strips and toss to coat all sides. Dip into the beaten eggs, then dip again into the dry ingredients. Lay the coated steak pieces on the greased frying basket in an even layer. Air Fry for 16-18 minutes, turning once. Serve and enjoy!

RECIPE 461: THYME SWEET POTATO WEDGES

Serve: 4 | Total Time: 30 minutes

2 peeled sweet potatoes, cubed
¼ cup grated Parmesan
1 tbsp olive oil
Salt and pepper to taste
½ tsp dried thyme
½ tsp ground cumin

Preheat Air Fryer to 330°F. Add sweet potato cubes to the frying basket, then drizzle with oil. Toss to gently coat. Season with salt, pepper, thyme, and cumin. Roast the potatoes for about 10 minutes. Shake the basket and continue roasting for another 10 minutes. Shake the basket again, this time adding Parmesan cheese. Shake and return to the Air Fryer. Roast

until the potatoes are tender, 4-6 minutes. Serve and enjoy!

RECIPE 462: THYME TURKEY BREAST

Serve: 4 | Total Time: 50 minutes

2 lb. turkey breast
Salt, to taste
Black pepper, to taste
4 tbsp butter, melted
3 cloves garlic, minced
1 tsp thyme, chopped
1 tsp rosemary, chopped

Mix butter with salt, black pepper, garlic, thyme, and rosemary in a bowl. Rub this seasoning over the turkey breast liberally and place in the Air Fryer basket. Turn the fryer dial to select the "Air Fry" mode. Hit the Time button and again use the dial to set the cooking time to 40 minutes. To adjust the temperature to 375 degrees F, press the Temp button and move the dial. Once preheated, place the Air Fryer basket inside the oven. Slice and serve fresh.

RECIPE 463: TRUFFLE VEGETABLE CROQUETTES

Serve: 4 | Total Time: 40 minutes

2 cooked potatoes, mashed
1 cooked carrot, mashed
1 tbsp onion, minced
2 eggs, beaten
2 tbsp melted butter
1 tbsp truffle oil
½ tbsp flour
Salt and pepper to taste

Preheat Air Fryer to 350°F. Sift the flour, salt, and pepper in a bowl and stir to combine. Add the potatoes, carrot, onion, butter, and truffle oil to a separate bowl and mix well. Shape the potato mixture into small bite-sized patties. Dip the potato patties into the beaten eggs, coating thoroughly, then roll in the flour mixture to cover all sides. Arrange the croquettes in the greased frying basket and Air Fry for 14-16 minutes. Halfway through cooking, shake the basket. The croquettes should be crispy and golden. Serve hot and enjoy!

RECIPE 464: TUNA VEGGIE STIR-FRY

Serve: 4 | Total Time: 27 minutes

1 tbsp olive oil
1 red bell pepper, chopped
1 cup green beans, divide into 2-inch pieces
1 onion, sliced
2 cloves garlic, sliced
2 tbsp low-sodium soy sauce
1 tbsp honey
1/2 pound fresh tuna, cubed

In a 6-inch metal bowl, combine the olive oil, pepper, green beans, onion, and garlic. Cook in the Air Fryer for 4 to 6 minutes, stirring once, until crisp and tender. Add soy sauce, honey, and tuna, and stir. Cook for another 3 to 6 minutes, stirring once, until the tuna is cooked as desired. Tuna can be served rare or medium-rare, or you can cook it until well done.

RECIPE 465: TURKEY AND AVOCADO BURRITO

Serve: 2 | Total Time: 10 minutes

4 free-range eggs
8-slices turkey breast, cooked
4 tbsp salsa
¼ cup mozzarella cheese, grated
½ cup avocado, sliced
½ red bell pepper, sliced
2 x tortillas
Salt and pepper to taste

Whisk the eggs, then add some salt and pepper. Spray the inside of your Air Fryer tray with cooking spray and pour in the egg mixture. Cook for 5-minutes at 390° Fahrenheit. Scrape into a clean bowl. Divide the eggs between the two tortillas, followed by the turkey, avocado, pepper, cheese, and salsa. Roll up carefully. Spray inside of the Air Fryer again and place the burritos inside of it.

Cook at 350°Fahrenheit for 5-minutes. Serve warm.

RECIPE 466: TURKEY AND CHEESE CALZONE

Serve: 4 | Total Time: 10 minutes

1 free-range egg, beaten
¼ cup mozzarella cheese, grated
1 cup cheddar cheese, grated
1-ounce bacon, diced, cooked
Cooked turkey, shredded
4 tbsp tomato sauce
Salt and pepper to taste
1 tsp thyme
1 tsp basil
1 tsp oregano
1 package frozen pizza dough

Roll the pizza dough out into small circles, the same size as a small pizza. Add thyme, oregano, basil into a bowl with tomato sauce and mix well. Pour a small amount of sauce onto your pizza bases and spread across the surface. Add the turkey, bacon, and cheese. Brush the edge of dough with beaten egg, then fold over and pinch to seal. Brush the outside with more egg. Place into Air Fryer and cook at 350°Fahrenehit for 10-minutes. Serve warm.

RECIPE 467: TURKEY AND CHICKEN MEATBALLS

Serve: 2 | Total Time: 85 minutes

5 ounces ground chicken
1/2 cup breadcrumbs
1/4 cup feta cheese, crumbled.
5 ounces ground turkey
1 tbsp. fresh basil, finely chopped.
1 tsp. onion powder
1 tsp. paprika
salt and pepper, to taste

Combine the ground turkey and ground chicken with the breadcrumbs. Add the feta cheese, fresh basil, paprika and onion powder. Season with salt and pepper. Knead well and form the meatballs with wet palms. Chill for 1 hour. Preheat the Air Fryer to 450 degrees F. Cook for 10

minutes in the Air Fryer Basket. Serve and enjoy!

RECIPE 468: TURKEY AND MUSHROOM SANDWICHES

Serve: 1 | Total Time: 15 minutes

1/3 cup shredded leftover turkey
1/3 cup sliced mushrooms
1 hamburger bun
2 tomato slices
1 tbsp. butter, divided
½ tsp. red pepper flakes
¼ tsp. salt
¼ tsp. black pepper

Half of the butter should be melted before adding the mushrooms. Cook for 4 minutes. Cut the bun in half and spread the remaining butter on the outside of the bun. Place the turkey on one half of the bun. Arrange mushroom slices on top of the turkey. Place the tomato slices over the mushrooms. Red pepper flakes, salt the other bun half. Cook it for about at least 5 minutes at 350 degrees F.

RECIPE 469: TURKEY BACON WITH SCRAMBLED EGGS

Serve: 4 | Total Time: 45 minutes

1/2-pound turkey bacon
4 eggs
1/3 cup milk
2 tbsp yogurt
1/2 tsp sea salt
1 bell pepper, finely chopped
2 green onions, finely chopped
1/2 cup Colby cheese, shredded

Place the turkey bacon in the cooking basket. Cook at 360 degrees F for 9 to 11 minutes. Work in batches. Reserve the fried bacon. In a mixing bowl, thoroughly whisk the eggs with milk and yogurt. Add salt, bell pepper, and green onions. Brush the sides and bottom of the baking pan with the reserved 1 teaspoon of bacon grease. Place the egg mixture in the pan. Cook at 355 degrees F for about 5 minutes. Top with shredded Colby cheese and cook for 5 to 6 minutes more. Serve the scrambled eggs with the reserved bacon and enjoy!

RECIPE 470: TURKEY BREAST WITH MAPLE MUSTARD GLAZE

Serve: 6 | Total Time: 49 minutes

5 lbs. turkey breast
1 tbsp unsalted butter
2 tbsp Dijon mustard
¼ cup sugar-free maple syrup
½ tsp black pepper
1 tsp sea salt
½ tsp paprika
1 tsp dried thyme
1 tbsp olive oil
½ tsp sage

Preheat your Air Fryer to 350° Fahrenheit. Prepare the turkey breast by brushing it with olive oil. Combine salt, pepper, paprika, sage, thyme in a bowl. Cover the turkey breast with this mixture. Place the turkey breast inside Air Fryer and cook for 25-minutes. Turn and cook for another 12-minutes. Turn once more and cook for an additional 12-minutes. Use a small saucepan to mix mustard, melted butter, and maple syrup, stir well. When turkey breast is done cooking, cover with sauce. Then air-fry for another 5-minutes. Take the turkey out of Air Fryer and set aside for at least 5-minutes, covering with aluminum foil. Slice turkey and serve.

RECIPE 471: TURKEY BURRITO

Serve: 2 | Total Time: 40 minutes

4 slices turkey breast already cooked
1/2 red bell pepper, sliced
2 eggs
1 small avocado, peeled, pitted and sliced
2 tbsp salsa
Salt and black pepper
1/8 cup mozzarella cheese, grated
Tortillas for serving

In a bowl, merge eggs with salt and pepper to the taste, set them in a pan and set it in the Air Fryer's basket. Cook at 400 degrees F, take pan out of the device and transfer eggs to a plate. Set tortillas on a working surface, divide eggs on them, also divide turkey meat, bell pepper, cheese, salsa and avocado. Roll your burritos and Set them in your device after you've lined it with some tin foil. Set up the burritos at 300 degrees F, divide them on plates and serve. Enjoy!

RECIPE 472: TURKEY CORDON BLEU

Serve: 2 | Total Time: 25 minutes

4 slices of turkey breast
2 slices of ham
1 cup Gruyere or another type of aged cheese
2 eggs, beaten
2 cups breadcrumbs

Preheat your Airfryer to 390 degrees F. Top one of the turkey slices with ham and half of the cheese. Place another slice of turkey on top. Repeat the procedure with the other two turkey slices and the rest of the cheese and ham. Tip one stack first into the egg mixture, and then into the breadcrumbs. Coat well. Repeat. Place in a heat safe dish and cook for 25 minutes.

RECIPE 473: TURKEY CURRY SAMOSAS

Serve: 2 | Total Time: 10 minutes

2 oz shredded turkey wing meat
1 tsp coriander
1 tsp turmeric
1 tsp garam masala
Salt and ground black pepper to taste
Coconut milk
1 small egg beaten
2 pastry sheets

Get a clean mixing bowl and combine the turkey and all the seasonings. Mix well. To get a soft and creamy mixture that would not dry out, put a little coconut milk to the mixture. Transfer the contents onto your pastry sheets. Fold the sheet over to appear like samosa in shape. Beat your eggs into a bowl, and brush the folded sheets until they have a golden glow. Set your Air Fryer to 320 F and allow to cook for 3 minutes. Serve.

RECIPE 474: TURKEY HUMMUS WRAPS

Serve: 2 | Total Time: 7 minutes

4 large whole wheat wraps
½ cup hummus
16 thin slices deli turkey
8 slices provolone cheese
1 cup fresh baby spinach (or more to taste)

To assemble, place 2 tablespoons of hummus on each wrap and spread to within about a half inch from edges. Top with 4 slices of turkey and 2 slices of provolone. Finish with ¼ cup of baby spinach —or pile on as much as you like. Roll up each wrap. You don't need to fold or seal the ends. Place 2 wraps in Air Fryer basket, seam side down. Cook at 360°F for 4 minutes to warm filling and melt cheese. If you like, you can continue cooking for 3 more minutes, until the wrap is slightly crispy. Repeat step 4 to cook remaining wraps.

RECIPE 475: TURKEY PATTIES

Serve: 6 | Total Time: 18 minutes

1 pound ground turkey
½ pound fresh mushrooms
2 garlic cloves, minced
1 small onion, chopped
Salt and black pepper to taste
Cooking spray

First, you need to prepare mushrooms. Rinse them well, place into food processor and make a puree. Season with salt and pepper, add minced garlic and chopped onion and pulse for 30 seconds more. On a large dish, combine the ground turkey and mushroom combination. Combine well with spoon or hands. Divide the mixture to six equal pieces and shape patties. Prepare the Air Fryer to a temperature of 340 degrees Fahrenheit and add the patties to the frying basket. Cook for 10 minutes until patties become tender. Serve hot with mashed potatoes or steamed rice.

RECIPE 476: TURKEY SAUSAGE PATTIES

Serve: 2 | Total Time: 6 minutes

1 tsp olive oil
1 small onion, diced
1 large garlic clove, chopped
Salt and pepper to taste
1 tbsp vinegar
1 tbsp chives, chopped
¾ tsp paprika
Pinch of nutmeg
1 lb. lean ground turkey
1 tsp fennel seeds

Preheat your Air Fryer to 375° Fahrenheit. Add half of the oil along with onion and garlic to Air Fryer. Air fry for 1-minute then add fennel seeds then transfer to plate. In a mixing bowl, mix paprika, ground turkey, nutmeg, chives, vinegar, salt pepper, and onion. Mix well and form patties. Add the remaining oil to your Air Fryer and air fry patties for 3-minutes. Serve on buns.

RECIPE 477: TUSCAN STUFFED CHICKEN

Serve: 4 | Total Time: 30 minutes

1/3 cup ricotta cheese
1 cup Tuscan kale, chopped
4 chicken breasts
1 tbsp chicken seasoning
Salt and pepper to taste
1 tsp paprika

Preheat Air Fryer to 370°F. Soften the ricotta cheese in a microwave-safe bowl for 15 seconds. Combine in a bowl along with Tuscan kale. Set aside. Cut 4-5 slits in the top of each chicken breast about ¾ of

the way down. Season with chicken seasoning, salt, and pepper. Place the chicken with the slits facing up in the greased frying basket. Lightly spray the chicken with oil. Bake for 6-8 minutes. Slide-out and stuff the cream cheese mixture into the chicken slits. Sprinkle ½ tsp of paprika and cook for another 3 minutes. Serve and enjoy!

RECIPE 478: TWISTED DEVILED EGGS

Serve: 6 | Total Time: 20 minutes

2 tbsp. crumbled feta cheese
3 tbsp. mayonnaise
6 large eggs
1 tsp. Dijon mustard
1 tsp. white wine vinegar
1/4 tsp. turmeric powder
1 tbsp smoked paprika
1 red chili, minced
1 tbsp. chopped parsley

Place the eggs in boiling salted water in a pot over medium heat and boil them for 10 minutes. Transfer to an ice water bath. Let cool for 5 minutes, peel, and slice in half. Remove the yolks to a bowl and put the whites on a plate. Fork-mashed yolks with mustard, mayonnaise, vinegar, feta, turmeric, and chili. Fill an egg white piping bag with the mixture. Garnish with parsley and paprika.

RECIPE 479: VEGAN CROUTONS

Serve: 2 | Total Time: 15 minutes

2 heaping cups of cubed baguette (or your preferred bread), cut in 1 inch pieces
2 tsp extra virgin olive oil
2 tsp lemon juice
½ tsp dried basil
½ tsp granulated garlic
½ tsp dried oregano
Salt and ground black pepper to taste

Get a clean large mixing bowl, and in it, add the cubed baguette, drizzles of extra virgin olive oil,

and lemon juice across the bread. Then sprinkle the dried basil, garlic granules, dried oregano, salt, and pepper. With your hands, coat the cubed bread evenly by tossing it into the spices mixture. For easy coating, ensure that the spices are on the bread instead of being stuck on the sides of the bowl. Transfer the bread into the Air Fryer, and allow cooking for 5 minutes at 400 F. Shake the basket once or twice within this cooking time. Serve as toppings for your favorite salad.

RECIPE 480: VEGAN FRENCH TOAST

Serve: 4 | Total Time: 15 minutes

1 ripe banana, mashed
¼ cup protein powder
½ cup milk
2 tbsp ground flaxseed
4 bread slices
2 tbsp agave syrup

Preheat Air Fryer to 370°F. Combine the banana, protein powder, milk, and flaxseed in a shallow bowl and mix well Dip bread slices into the mixture. Place the slices on a lightly greased pan in a single layer and pour any of the remaining mixture evenly over the bread. Air Fry for 10 minutes, or until golden brown and crispy, flipping once. Serve warm topped with agave syrup.

RECIPE 481: VEGAN STUFFED BELL PEPPERS

Serve: 6 | Total Time: 50 minutes

2 tsp dried mixed herbs
2 cloves garlic, minced
1 carrot, diced
1 small onion, diced
½ cup peas
1 potato, diced
1 vegan bread roll, diced
6 green bell peppers
1/3 cup shredded vegan cheese

In a clean bowl, combine the mixed herbs, garlic, carrot, onion, peas, potato, and bread. After dicing the tops of the green bell pepper, toss them into the bowl. Mix thoroughly. Ensure that your Air Fryer is preheated to 350 F. Stuff the peppers equally with the filling. Transfer the stuffed peppers into the Air Fryer basket. Allow cooking until tender and hot throughout - this takes about 20 minutes. Stir in the shredded vegan cheese and cook until melted - this takes an additional 5 minutes.

RECIPE 482: VEGETABLE EGG CUPS

Serve: 4 | Total Time: 30 minutes

4 eggs
1 tbsp cilantro, chopped
4 tbsp half and half
1 cup cheddar cheese, shredded
1 cup vegetables, diced
Pepper
Salt

Sprinkle four ramekins with cooking spray and set aside. In a mixing bowl, whisk eggs with cilantro, half and half, vegetables, 1/2 cup cheese, pepper, and salt. Pour egg mixture into the four ramekins. Place ramekins in Air Fryer basket and cook at 300 F for 12 minutes. Top with remaining 1/2 cup cheese and cook for 2 minutes more at 400 F. Serve and enjoy.

RECIPE 483: VEGETABLE EGG PANCAKE

Serve: 2 | Total Time: 15 minutes

1 cup almond flour
½ cup milk
1 tbsp parmesan cheese, grated
3 eggs
1 potato, grated
1 beet, peeled and grated
1 carrot, grated
1 zucchini, grated
1 tbsp olive oil
¼ tsp nutmeg
1 tsp onion powder
1 tsp garlic powder
½ tsp black pepper

Preheat your Air Fryer to 390° Fahrenheit. Mix the zucchini, potato, beet, carrot, eggs, milk, almond flour and parmesan in bowl. Place olive oil into oven-safe dish. Form patties with vegetable mix and flatten to form patties. Place patties into oven-safe dish and cook in Air Fryer for 15-minutes. Serve with sliced tomatoes, sour cream, and toast.

RECIPE 484: VEGETABLE EGG SOUFFLE

Serve: 4 | Total Time: 30 minutes

4 large eggs
1 tsp onion powder
1 tsp garlic powder
1 tsp red pepper, crushed
1/2 cup broccoli florets, chopped
1/2 cup mushrooms, chopped

Sprinkle four ramekins with cooking spray and set aside. In a bowl, whisk eggs with onion powder, garlic powder, and red pepper. Add mushrooms and broccoli and stir well. Pour egg mixture into the prepared ramekins and place ramekins into the Air Fryer basket. Cook at 350 F for 15 minutes Make sure soufflé is cooked if soufflé is not cooked then cook for 5 minutes more. Serve and enjoy.

RECIPE 485: VEGETABLE QUICHE

Serve: 6 | Total Time: 35 minutes

8 eggs
1 cup of coconut milk
1 cup tomatoes, chopped
1 cup zucchini, chopped
1 tbsp butter
1 onion, chopped
1 cup Parmesan cheese, grated
1/2 tsp pepper
1 tsp salt

Preheat the Air Fryer to 370 F. Thaw butter in a pan then add onion and sauté until onion lightly brown. Add tomatoes and zucchini to the pan and sauté for 4-5 minutes. Transfer cooked vegetables into the Air Fryer baking dish. Beat eggs with cheese, milk, pepper, and salt in a bowl. Pour egg mixture over vegetables in a baking dish. Put it in the Air Fryer then cook for 24 minutes or until eggs are set. Slice and serve.

RECIPE 486: VEGETABLE ROLLS FOR LUNCH

Serve: 5 | Total Time: 15 minutes

1 cup mushrooms, sliced
1 /3 cup grated carrots, grated
1/4 cup zucchini, chopped
1 cup red bell pepper, chopped
2 green onions, chopped
4 tbsp soy sauce
10 egg roll wrappers
1 tbsp cornstarch
2 eggs, beaten

Combine all the vegetables in a medium-sized bowl and drizzle soy sauce. Stir to combine well. Place the wrap on a flat working space and top each roll with 2 tbsp mixture. In a medium bowl, combine the cornstarch and egg. Mix well. Roll up the wrapper by brushing the egg mixture on edges of the wrappers. Then seal the wrappers. Cook for 10 minutes in the Air Fryer until slightly browned. Serve and enjoy.

RECIPE 487: VEGETABLE SKEWERS

Serve: 6 | Total Time: 27 minutes

8 wooden skewers
2 zucchinis, cut into 1-inch slices
2 yellow squash, cut into 1-inch slices
½ pound whole fresh mushrooms
1 red onion, cut into chunks
12 cherry tomatoes
1 fresh pineapple, cut into chunks
1 red bell pepper, cut into chunks
⅓ cup olive oil
1 ½ tsp dried basil
¾ tsp dried oregano
½ tsp salt
⅛ tsp ground black pepper

Toss all the veggies with spices and herbs in a large suitable bowl. Alternately thread the veggies on the skewers and place half of them in the Air Fryer basket. Air fry them for 7 minutes per side at 350 F. Cook the remaining skewers in the same way and serve warm.

RECIPE 488: VEGETARIAN HASH BROWNS

Serve: 8 | Total Time: 19 minutes

4 large potatoes, peeled, shredded
1 tsp onion powder
1 tsp garlic powder
2 tsp chili flakes
Salt and pepper to taste
2 tbsp corn flour
2 tsp olive oil
Cooking spray as needed

Drain and re-soak potatoes in cold water. Add a teaspoon of olive oil into skillet and cook potatoes over medium heat for 4-minutes. Place potatoes on plate to cool once they are cooked. In a large mixing bowl, add flour, potatoes, salt, pepper and other seasonings and combine well. Place bowl in fridge for 20-minutes. Preheat your Air Fryer to 350°Fahrenheit. Remove hash browns from fridge and cut into size pieces you desire. Spray the wire basket of your Air Fryer with some oil, add the hash browns and fry them for 15-minutes. Halfway through flip them to help cook them all over. Serve hot!

RECIPE 489: VEGGIE BALLS

Serve: 4 | Total Time: 25 minutes

2 heads cauliflower; cut into florets
1 cup cornstarch
1/4 cup onions, minced.
1 tbsp. garlic, minced.
1 tsp. paprika
1 tsp. onion powder
1 tsp. garlic powder
salt and pepper, to taste

Pulse the cauliflower florets in a food processor until they resemble a grain-like texture. Mix the ground cauliflower, onions, garlic, garlic powder, onion powder, paprika, salt and pepper. Cover with a plastic wrap and chill overnight. Preheat the Air Fryer to temperature of 400 degrees F. Season the cornstarch with salt and pepper. Form balls from the mixture and dust them with the cornstarch. Arrange the balls in the Air Fryer and cook for 15 minutes. Serve and enjoy!

RECIPE 490: VEGGIE BURRITO WITH TOFU

Serve: 8 | Total Time: 25 minutes

16 ounces tofu, crumbled
1 green bell pepper, chopped
¼ cup scallions, chopped
15 oz canned black beans, drained
1 cup vegan salsa
½ cup water
¼ tsp cumin, ground
½ tsp turmeric powder
½ tsp smoked paprika
A pinch of salt and black pepper
¼ tsp chili powder
3 cups spinach leaves, torn
8 vegan tortillas for serving

In your Air Fryer, mix tofu with bell pepper, scallions, black beans, salsa, water, cumin, turmeric, paprika, salt, pepper and chili powder, stir, cover and cook at 370 degrees F for 20 minutes. Add spinach, toss well, divide this on your vegan tortillas, roll, wrap them and serve for breakfast. Enjoy!

RECIPE 491: VEGGIE CASSEROLE WITH CASHEW

Serve: 4 | Total Time: 26 minutes

2 tsp onion powder
¾ cup cashews, soaked for 30 minutes
¼ cup nutritional yeast
1 tsp garlic powder
½ tsp sage, dried
Salt and black pepper to the taste
1 yellow onion, chopped
2 tbsp parsley, chopped

3 garlic cloves, minced
1 tbsp olive oil
4 red potatoes, cubed
½ tsp red pepper flakes

In your blender, mix cashews with onion powder, garlic powder, nutritional yeast, sage, salt and pepper and pulse really well. Add oil to your Air Fryer's pan and preheat the machine to 370 degrees F. Arrange potatoes, pepper flakes, garlic, onion, salt, pepper and parsley in the pan. Add cashews sauce, toss, cover and cook for 16 minutes. Divide between plates and serve for breakfast. Enjoy!

RECIPE 492: VERY BERRY BREAKFAST PUFFS

Serve: 3 | Total Time: 20 minutes

3 pastry dough sheets
2 cups cream cheese
2 tbsp. mashed strawberries
1 tbsp. honey
2 tbsp. mashed raspberries
1/4-tsp. vanilla extract

Preheat your Air Fryer to temperature of 375 degrees F. Divide the cream cheese between the dough sheets and spread it evenly. In a small bowl, combine the berries, honey and vanilla. Divide the mixture between the pastry sheets. Pinch the ends of the sheets, to form puff. Place the puffs on a lined baking dish. Place the dish in the Air Fryer and cook for 15 minutes.

RECIPE 493: ZESTY RANCH FISH FILLETS

Serve: 4 | Total Time: 17 minutes

3/4 cup of bread crumbs or panko
130g packet of dry ranch-style dressing mix
2 1/2 tbsp. of vegetable oil
2 eggs beaten
4 tilapia salmon or other fish fillets
Lemon wedges to garnish

Preheat your Air-fryer at 180 °C. Merge the panko/breadcrumbs and the ranch dressing mix together. Attach in the oil and keep stirring until the mixture becomes loose and crumbly. After that, soak the fish fillets into the egg, letting the excess drip off, dip the fish fillets into the crumb mixture, making sure they are coated evenly and thoroughly. Now place fish fillets into your Air-fryer carefully and cook for 12 to 13 minutes, depending on the thickness of the fillets. Remove and serve immediately. Press the lemon wedges over the fish if desired.

RECIPE 494: ZUCCHINI AND BELL PEPPER STIR-FRY

Serve: 4 | Total Time: 25 minutes

1 zucchini, cut into rounds
1 red bell pepper, sliced
3 garlic cloves, sliced
2 tbsp olive oil
1/3 cup vegetable broth
1 tbsp lemon juice
2 tsp cornstarch
1 tsp dried basil
Salt and pepper to taste

Preheat the Air Fryer to 400°F. Combine the veggies, garlic, and olive oil in a bowl. Put the bowl in the frying basket and Air Fry the zucchini mixture for 5 minutes, stirring once; drain. While the veggies are cooking, whisk the broth, lemon juice, cornstarch, basil, salt, and pepper in a bowl. Pour the broth into the bowl along with the veggies and stir. Air Fry for 5-9 more minutes until the veggies are tender and the sauce is thick. Serve and enjoy!

RECIPE 495: ZUCCHINI, CARROTS AND YELLOW SQUASH

Serve: 4 | Total Time: 35 minutes

½ lb carrots, diced
1 lime, cut into wedges
½ tsp ground white pepper
1 lb. zucchini, trim stem and root ends, cut into ¾ inch semicircles

1 lb. yellow squash, with roots and stems, trimmed
6 tsp olive oil, divided
1 tsp sea salt
1 tbsp tarragon leaves, chopped

In a bowl add carrots and cover with 2 teaspoons of oil and stir. Put the carrots in fryer basket and set to 400°Fahrenheit and cook for 5-minutes. Place the zucchini and yellow squash into a bowl. Cover with the remaining 4 teaspoons of olive oil. Season with pepper and salt. When Air Fryer timer goes off, stir in zucchini and yellow squash with carrots. Cook for 30-minutes. Stir from time to time. Garnish with lime wedges and tarragon leaves.

RECIPE 496: ZUCCHINI CHIPS

Serve: 2 | Total Time: 20 minutes

1 cup panko bread crumbs
¾ cup grated Parmesan cheese
1 medium zucchini, thinly sliced
1 large egg, beaten
Cooking spray

Preheat an Air Fryer to 350 F before you begin preparing the zucchini. Mix panko breadcrumbs with Parmesan cheese on a plate. Dip a zucchini slice into the whisked egg and then coat it with panko mixture. Place the coated zucchini slices on a wire rack and spray them with cooking oil. Add zucchini slices to an Air Fryer's basket in a single, in batches, and cook for about 10 minutes. Flip them with tongs. Cook for another 2 minutes. Repeat the same cooking steps with remaining zucchini slices. Serve warm.

RECIPE 497: ZUCCHINI CORN FRITTERS

Serve: 4 | Total Time: 15 minutes

2 medium zucchinis, grated
1 cup corn kernel
1 medium potato cooked
2 tbsp chickpea flour
2 garlic finely minced

2 tsp olive oil
Salt and black pepper

For Serving:
Yogurt tahini sauce

In a colander, combine shredded zucchini and salt for 15 minutes. Seize their water. Squeeze out their excess water. Mash the cooked potato in a large-sized bowl with a fork. Add zucchini, corn, garlic, chickpea flour, salt, and black pepper to the bowl. Mix these fritters ingredients together and make 2 tbsp-sized balls out of this mixture and flatten them lightly. Place the fritters in the Air Fryer's basket in a single layer and spray them with cooking. Air fry them for 8 minutes, then flip and continue cooking for 4 minutes. Cook all the fritters in batches and serve warm.

RECIPE 498: ZUCCHINI CUBES

Serve: 2 | Total Time: 15 minutes

1 zucchini
½ tsp ground black pepper
1 tsp oregano
2 tbsp chicken stock
½ tsp coconut oil

Chop the zucchini into cubes. Combine the ground black pepper, and oregano; stir the mixture. Sprinkle the zucchini cubes with the spice mixture and stir well. After this, sprinkle the vegetables with the chicken stock. Place the coconut oil in the Air Fryer basket and preheat it to 360° F for 20 seconds. Then add the zucchini cubes and cook the vegetables for 8 minutes at 390° F, stirring halfway through. Transfer to serving plates and enjoy!

RECIPE 499: ZUCCHINI CURLY FRIES

Serve: 2 | Total Time: 25 minutes

1 zucchini
1 egg, whisked
1 cup panko bread crumbs

1 tsp Italian seasoning
½ cup Parmesan cheese, grated
nonstick cooking spray
Prepare an Air Fryer with a heat of 400 F. Cut zucchini into spirals using a spiralizer fitted with the large blade. Place egg in a shallow dish. Mix bread crumbs, with Italian seasoning and Parmesan cheese, in a large Ziplock plastic bag. Coat 1/2 of the spiralized zucchini in the whisked egg and then transfer them to the breadcrumbs bag to coat. Spray the Air Fryer's basket with cooking spray. Spread the breaded zucchini fries in the prepared basket in a single layer. Spray the fries with cooking spray. Cook for about 10 minutes until crispy, flip them when cooked halfway through. Prepare and cook the remaining fries in a similar way. Serve warm.

RECIPE 500: ZUCCHINI FRIES AND ROASTED GARLIC AIOLI

Serve: 4 | Total Time: 12 minutes

Roasted Garlic Aioli:
½ cup mayonnaise
Sea salt and pepper to taste
1 tsp roasted garlic, pureed
2 tbsp olive oil
½ lemon, juiced

Zucchini Fries:
Sea salt and pepper to taste
½ cup almond flour
2 eggs, beaten
1 cup breadcrumbs
1 large zucchini, cut into ½-inch sticks
1 tbsp olive oil
Cooking spray

Take three bowls and line them up on the counter. In the first, combine flour, salt, and pepper. Place eggs in the second bowl. Place breadcrumbs combined with salt and pepper in the third bowl. Take zucchini sticks and dip first into flour, then in the eggs, and then into crumbs. Preheat your Air Fryer to 400°Fahrenheit.

RECIPE 501: ZUCCHINI HASH

Serve: 2 | Total Time: 20 minutes

1 large zucchini, grated.
1 tbsp. spring onions, chopped.
1/4 cup cheddar cheese, grated.
½ tsp. garlic salt
1 egg
pepper, to taste
Preheat the Air Fryer to temperature of 350 degrees F. Whisk the egg with the garlic salt and pour into the Air Fryer Baking Pan. Add the grated zucchinis and spring onions to the Air Fryer Baking Pan and press lightly to the Air Fryer Baking Pan to release any air bubbles. Season with pepper and grated cheese on top. Place the Air Fryer Baking Pan in the Air Fryer Basket and cook for 15 minutes. Serve and enjoy!

CHAPTER 2: 250 RECIPES FOR GRILL

RECIPE 502: AIR FRIED TURKEY BREAST WITH BASIL

Serve: 4 | Total Time: 50 minutes

2 pounds turkey breasts, bone-in skin-on
2 tbsp. olive oil
Coarse sea salt and ground black pepper, to taste
1 tsp. fresh basil leaves, chopped
2 tbsp. lemon zest, grated

Preheat the PowerXL Air Fryer Grill by selecting air fry mode. Adjust the temperature to 330°F, set Time to 5 minutes. Rub olive on all sides of the turkey breast. Sprinkle with salt, pepper, lemon zest, and basil. Arrange on the PowerXL grill Pizza rack. Transfer to the PowerXL Air Fryer Grill. Air fry for 30 minutes. Flip and air fry for another 28 minutes. Enjoy!

RECIPE 503: AIR FRIED WHOLE CHICKEN

Serve: 10 | Total Time: 35 minutes

1 Whole chicken
1 tbsp. oil
1 tsp. garlic powder
1 tsp. onion powder
1 tsp. paprika
1 tsp. Italian seasoning
Salt or pepper to taste
1-1/2 cup chicken broth

Truss and Wash up chicken. Preheat the PowerXL Air Fryer Grill by selecting Air fry/grill mode. Adjust the temperature to 390°F, set Time to 5 minutes. Mix the season and rub the chicken with half of it. Place the chicken in the baking tray, add the broth. Transfer to the PowerXL Air Fryer Grill. Air fry for 25 minutes. Flip the chicken and rub with the remaining seasoning. Air fry for another 10 minutes. Enjoy.

RECIPE 504: AIR FRYER BABY BACK RIBS

Serve: 4 | Total Time: 30 minutes

1rack baby back ribs
1 tbsp garlic powder
1 tsp freshly ground black pepper
2 tbsp salt
1 cup barbecue sauce (any type)

Dry the ribs with a paper towel. Season the ribs with garlic powder, pepper, and salt. Place the seasoned ribs into the Air Fryer. Set the temperature of your Pro Breeze AF to 400°F. Set the timer and grill for 10 minutes. Using tongs, flip the ribs. Reset the timer and grill for another 10 minutes. Once the ribs are cooked, use a pastry brush to brush on the barbecue sauce, then set the timer and grill for a final 3 to 5 minutes.

RECIPE 505: AIR FRYER GRILLED CHICKEN BREASTS

Serve: 4 | Total Time: 19 minutes

1/2 tsp. garlic powder
salt and black pepper to taste
1 tsp. dried parsley
2 tbsp. olive oil, divided
3 boneless, skinless chicken breasts

Combine the garlic powder, salt, pepper, and parsley in a small bowl. 1 tbsp olive oil and half of the spice combination on each chicken breast. Place the chicken breast in the Air Fryer basket. Set the temperature of your Cuisinart AF to 370°F. Set the Timer and grill for 7 minutes. Using tongs, flip the chicken and brush the remaining olive oil and spices onto the chicken. Reset the Timer and grill for 7 minutes more. Check that the chicken has reached an internal temperature of 165°F. Add Cooking Time if needed. Serve the cooked chicken in a serving dish.

RECIPE 506: AIR-GRILLED HONEY-GLAZED SALMON

Serve: 2 | Total Time: 70 minutes

2 pcs Salmon Fillets
6 tbsp Honey
6 tsp Soy Sauce
3 tsp Hon Mirin
1 tsp Water

Blend nectar, soy sauce, Hon Mirin and water together. Pour half of the blend in a different bowl, put aside as this will be utilized as sauce present with salmon. Set up together the salmon and the marinade blend let it marinate for something like 2 hours. Pre-heat the Air-fryer at 180°C. Air-flame broiled the salmon for 8 minutes, flip over midway and proceed for an extra 5 minutes. Treat the salmon with the marinade blend like clockwork. To set up the sauce, pour the rest of the sauce in a dish and let it stew for 1 minute. Present with salmon.

RECIPE 507: ALMOND PORK BITE

Serve: 10 | Total Time: 35 minutes

16 oz. sausage meat
1 whole egg, beaten
1/3 cup chopped onion
2 tbsp. almonds, chopped
1/2 tsp. pepper
2 tbsp. dried sage
1/3 cup sliced apples, sliced
1/2 tsp. salt

Preheat the PowerXL Air Fryer Grill by selecting grill mode. Adjust temperature to 350°F and Time to 5 minutes. Combine all the ingredients in a bowl. Pour into a Ziploc bag and marinate for 15 minutes. Form into cutlets. Arrange on the PowerXL Air Fryer Grill grilling plate. Transfer into the PowerXL Air Fryer Grill. Grill for 20 minutes. Serve and enjoy!

RECIPE 508: APPLE SLAW TOPPED ALASKAN COD FILET

Serve: 3 | Total Time: 25 minutes

¼ cup mayonnaise
½ red onion, diced
1 ½ pounds frozen Alaskan cod
1 box whole-wheat panko bread crumbs
1 granny smith apple, julienned
1 tbsp vegetable oil
1 tsp paprika
2 cups Napa cabbage, shredded
Salt and pepper to taste

Preheat the Air Fryer to 3900F. Place the grill pan accessory in the Air Fryer. Brush the fish with oil and dredge in the breadcrumbs. Place the fish on the grill pan and cook for 15 minutes. Make sure to flip the fish halfway through the cooking time. Meanwhile, prepare the slaw by mixing the remaining ingredients in a bowl. Serve the fish with the slaw.

RECIPE 509: APRICOTS WITH BRIOCHE

Serve: 8 | Total Time: 21 minutes

8 ripe apricots
2 tbsp butter
2 tbsp sugar
4 slice brioches, diced

2 tbsp Honey
2 cup vanilla ice cream

Toss the apricot halves with butter and sugar. Place brioche slices in the Ninja Foodi Smart XL grill. Cover the Ninja Foodi Grill's hood, select the Manual Mode, set the temperature to 350 degrees F and grill on the "Grill Mode" for 1 minute per side. Now grill the apricots in the same grill for 1 minute per side. Top these slices with apricot slices, honey, and a scoop of vanilla ice cream. Serve.

RECIPE 510: AROMATIC T-BONE STEAK WITH GARLIC

Serve: 3 | Total Time: 25 minutes

1-pound T-bone steak
4 garlic cloves, halved
1/4 cup all-purpose flour
2 tbsp olive oil
1/4 cup tamari sauce
2 tsp brown sugar,
4 tbsp tomato paste
1 tsp sriracha sauce,
2 tbsp white vinegar
1 tsp dried rosemary,
1/2 tsp dried basil
2 heaping tbsp cilantro, chopped

Rub the garlic halves all over the T-bone steak. Toss the steak with the flour. Drizzle the oil all over the steak and transfer it to the grill pan; grill the steak in the preheated Air Fryer at 400 degrees f for 10 minutes. Meanwhile, whisk the tamari sauce, sugar, tomato paste, sriracha, vinegar, rosemary, and basil. Cook an additional 5 minutes Serve garnished with fresh cilantro. Bon appétit!

RECIPE 511: ARTICHOKE TURKEY PIZZA

Serve: 2 | Total Time: 20 minutes

2 cups of chopped cooked turkey
1 ½ cup of mozzarella cheese
2 baked pizza crust
1 can of black olives
1 can of diced tomatoes with garlic, oregano, and basil

½ cup of shredded parmesan cheese
1 can of artichoke hearts

Place the pizza crusts on a working surface. Place turkey, olive, tomatoes mix, parmesan cheese, olives, and artichokes on them. Transfer the pizza crusts to the PowerXL Air Fryer Grill pan. Set the PowerXL Air Fryer Grill to the pizza function. Cook for 10 minutes at 450°F. Serve immediately.

RECIPE 512: ARTICHOKE WITH RED PEPPER PIZZA

Serve: 1 | Total Time: 30 minutes

1 tsp. of dried basil
1 can of artichoke hearts
1½ cup of mozzarella cheese
1 cup of red bell pepper
5 cloves of garlic
Cracked pepper
1 tbsp. of olive oil
1 pizza shell
1 tsp. of oregano
1 jar of sliced mushroom
Mix artichoke hearts, basil, bell pepper, garlic, and cracked pepper in a bowl. Add oregano, mushroom, and olive oil. Place the mixture on the pizza shell. Transfer the pizza shell to PowerXL Air Fryer Grill pan. Set the PowerXL Air Fryer Grill to the pizza function. Cook for about 20 minutes at temperature of 350°F. Serve immediately.

RECIPE 513: ASIAN PORK CHOPS

Serve: 4 | Total Time: 35 minutes

1/4 cup hoisin sauce
1 tsp. garlic powder
1 tsp. onion powder
1/4 cup soy sauce
1/4 cup apple cider vinegar
1 lb. pork rib

Take a mixing bowl and add all listed ingredients. Mix well. Add pork ribs and coat, let it chill for 2¬4 hours. Pre-heat Ninja Foodi by demanding the GRILL option and

situation it to MED and timer to 24 minutes. Let it pre-heat till you hear a beep. Arrange pork ribs over the grill grate, lock the lid and cook for 12 minutes, flip ribs and cook for 12 minutes more. Serve and enjoy!

RECIPE 514: ASPARAGUS STEAK TIPS

Serve: 2 | Total Time: 23 minutes

1 tsp olive oil
1 pound steak cubes
½ tsp salt
1/8 tsp cayenne pepper
½ tsp dried onion powder
½ tsp dried garlic powder
½ tsp black pepper, freshly ground

Select the "Grill" button on the Ninja Foodi Smart XL Grill and regulate the settings at Medium for 10 minutes. Mingle garlic powder, cayenne pepper, onion powder, salt, and black pepper in a bowl. Shift the steak cubes in a Ziploc bag along with the garlic powder mixture. Arrange the chicken in the Ninja Foodi when it displays "Add Food". Grill for about 10 minutes, tossing the steaks once in between. Dole out in a platter and serve warm.

RECIPE 515: AUTHENTIC KOREAN CHILI PORK

Serve: 2 | Total Time: 18 minutes

2 lbs. pork, cut into 1/8-inch slices
5 garlic cloves, minced
3 tbsp. green onion, minced
1 yellow onion, sliced
1/2 cup soy sauce
1/2 cup brown sugar
3 tbsp. Korean Red Chili Paste
2 tbsp. sesame seeds
3 tsp. black pepper
Red pepper flakes

Take a zip bag and add listed ingredients, shake well and let it chill for 6–8 hours. Pre-heat Ninja Foodi by demanding the GRILL option and situation it to MED and timer to 8 minutes. Let it pre-heat

till you hear a beep. Arrange sliced pork over grill grate, lock the lid and cook for 4 minutes. Flip pork and cook for 4 minutes more, serve warm and enjoy with some chopped lettuce.

RECIPE 516: AWESOME KOREAN PORK LETTUCE WRAPS

Serve: 8 | Total Time: 40 minutes

¼ cup of miso
¼ cup of soy sauce (Low Sodium)/ Coconut Aminos
3 tbsp of Korean red paste
1 tsp of ground sesame oil
1 tsp of ground black pepper
1 pork shoulder trimmed of excess fat

Take a small bowl and add miso, soy sauce, ¼ cup of water Korean red paste, black pepper, and sesame oil. Mix well until smooth Pour half of the sauce into your Ninja Foodi. Add pork and pour the rest of the sauce on top Press the GRILL button. Set the temperature to 360°F and adjust the time to 30 minutes. Press the START/STOP button to pre-heat the appliance for 8 minutes. Cook it when the unit is ready. Shred the pork and serve in lettuce wraps with cucumbers, radish, green onion, etc.

RECIPE 517: BABY BACK RIB RECIPE FROM KANSAS CITY

Serve: 2 | Total Time: 60 minutes

1/4 cup apple cider vinegar
1/4 cup molasses
1/4 tsp cayenne pepper
1 cup ketchup
1 tbsp brown sugar
1 tbsp liquid smoke seasoning, hickory
1 tbsp Worcestershire sauce
1 tsp dry mustard
1 pound pork ribs, small
2 cloves of garlic
Salt and pepper to taste

Bring all ingredients in a Ziploc bag and allow marinating in the fridge for at least 2 hours. Preheat the Air Fryer to 390F. Place the grill pan accessory in the Air Fryer. Grill meat for 25 minutes per batch. Flip the meat halfway through the cooking time. Pour the marinade in a saucepan and allow to simmer until the sauce thickens. Pour glaze over the meat before serving.

RECIPE 518: BACON CHEESEBURGER PIZZA

Serve: 2 | Total Time: 20 minutes

6 bacon strips
½ pound of ground beef
1 tsp. of pizza seasoning
2 cups of mozzarella cheese
2 baked-bread crush
20 slices of dill pickles
1 chopped small onion
2 cups of shredded cheddar cheese
8 ounces of pizza sauce

Cook the onion and beef for 5 minutes over medium heat. Drain the meat. Add bacon, seasonings, sauce, cheeses, and pickles. Place the bread crusts on a working surface. Place the ingredients on them. Transfer it to the PowerXL Air Fryer Grill pan. Set the PowerXL Air Fryer Grill to the pizza function. Cook for 10 minutes at 450°F.

RECIPE 519: BACON EGG MUFFINS WITH CHIVES

Serve: 10 | Total Time: 30 minutes

10 eggs, lightly beaten
10 bacon rashers, cut into small pieces
½ cup chopped chives
1 brown onion, chopped
1 cup grated cheddar cheese
Salt and black pepper
Preheat the PowerXL Air Fryer Grill to 360 F on Bake function. Spray a 10-hole muffin pan with cooking spray. In a bowl, add eggs, bacon, chives, onion, cheese, salt and pepper. Stir to combine. Pour into muffin pans and place inside the PowerXL Air Fryer Grill. Cook

for 12 minutes until nice and set. Serve and enjoy!

RECIPE 520: BACON 'N' BELL PEPPER PITA POCKETS

Serve: 4 | Total Time: 25 minutes

8 bacon slices, cut into thirds
1/3 cup spicy BBQ sauce
2 tbsp honey
1 red bell pepper, sliced
1 yellow bell pepper, sliced
2 pita pockets, cut in half
2 cups torn romaine lettuce
2 tbsp sliced scallions
2 tomatoes, sliced

Preheat Air Fryer to 350°F. In a bowl, combine BBQ sauce and honey. Lightly brush the pepper slices with the barbecue mix and then the bacon, but do not dip your brush back into the sauce. Place the peppers into the frying basket. Air Fry for 4 minutes, shake the basket and add the bacon. Grill until the bacon browns and peppers are tender, 2 minutes. To assemble the sandwiches, layer the bacon, peppers, romaine lettuce, and tomatoes in the pita halves. Add any remaining barbeque sauce and top with scallions to serve.

RECIPE 521: BALSAMIC ARTICHOKES

Serve: 4 | Total Time: 19 minutes

2 tsp of balsamic vinegar
Black pepper and salt
1/4 cup of olive oil
1 tsp of oregano
4 big trimmed artichokes
2 tbsp of lemon juice
2 cloves of garlic

Sprinkle the artichokes with pepper and salt. Brush oil over the artichokes and add lemon juice. Place the artichokes on the 360 Deluxe Air Fryer Oven. Set the 360 Deluxe Air Fryer Oven at Air Fryer/Grill, timer at 7 minutes at 3600F. Mix garlic, lemon juice, pepper, vinegar, oil in a bowl. Add oregano and salt. Mix well.

RECIPE 522: BALSAMIC-GLAZED PORK CHOPS

Serve: 4 | Total Time: 55 minutes

3/4 cup balsamic vinegar
11/2 tbsp sugar
1 tbsp butter
½ tbsp olive oil
¼ tbsp salt
4 pork rib chops

Place all ingredients in a bowl and allow the meat to marinate in the fridge for at least 2 hours. Preheat the Pro Breeze Air Fryer to 390°F. Place the grill pan accessory in the Air Fryer. Grill the pork chops for 20 minutes making sure to flip the meat every 10 minutes for even grilling. Meanwhile, pour the balsamic vinegar into a saucepan and allow simmering for at least 10 minutes until the sauce thickens. Brush the meat with the glaze before serving.

RECIPE 523: BALSAMIC MUSHROOM SLIDERS WITH PESTO

Serve: 4 | Total Time: 18 minutes

8 small Portobello mushrooms, trimmed with gills removed
2 tbsp canola oil
2 tbsp balsamic vinegar
8 slider buns
1 tomato, sliced
½ cup pesto
½ cup microgreens

Close the hood and insert the Grill Grate. Choose GRILL, raise the temperature to HIGH, and cook for 8 minutes. Select START/STOP to begin preheating. While the unit is preheating, brush the mushrooms with oil and balsamic vinegar. When the unit beeps to signify it has preheated, place the mushrooms, gill-side down, on the Grill Grate. Close the hood and GRILL for 8 minutes until the mushrooms are tender. When cooking is complete, remove the mushrooms from the grill, and layer on the buns with tomato, pesto, and microgreens.

RECIPE 524: BANANA SKEWERS

Serve: 2 | Total Time: 21 minutes

1 loaf (10 3/4 oz.) cake, cubed
2 large bananas, one-inch slices
1/4 cup butter, melted
2 tbsp brown sugar
1/2 tsp vanilla extract
1/8 tsp ground cinnamon
4 cups butter pecan ice cream
1/2 cup butterscotch ice cream topping
1/2 cup chopped pecans, toasted
Thread the cake and bananas over the skewers alternately. Whisk butter with cinnamon, vanilla, and brown sugar in a small bowl. Brush this mixture over the skewers liberally. Place the banana skewers in the Ninja Foodi Smart XL grill. Cover the Ninja Foodi Grill's hood, select the Manual Mode, set the temperature to 310 degrees F and grill on the "Grill Mode" for 3 minutes per side. Serve with ice cream, pecan, and butterscotch topping on top.

RECIPE 525: BARBEQUE AIR FRIED CHICKEN

Serve: 10 | Total Time: 30 minutes

2 lb. chicken
1 tsp. Liquid Smoke
2 cloves Fresh Garlic smashed
1/2 cup Apple Cider Vinegar
1 Tbsp. Kosher Salt
1 Tbsp. Freshly Ground Black Pepper
2 tsp. Garlic Powder
1.5 cups Barbecue Sauce
1/4 cup Light Brown Sugar + more for sprinkling

Combine all the ingredients. Add the meat and let aside for a few minutes to marinate. Preheat the PowerXL Air Fryer Grill by selecting Air fry mode. Adjust the temperature to 390°F, set Time to 5 minutes. Pour into the Air Fryer baking tray. Transfer to the PowerXL Air Fryer Grill. Air fry for 20 minutes, flip halfway done. Enjoy.

RECIPE 526: BARLEY PORRIDGE

Serve: 6 | Total Time: 8 hours

1½ cups pearl barley
3 cups unsweetened almond milk
3 cups water
2 tbsp maple syrup
2 tsp grated fresh orange zest
1 tsp ground cinnamon
1 tsp ground ginger
¼ tsp salt
¼ cup chopped walnuts

Place all items in the inner pot of the PowerXL Grill Air Fryer Combo and whisk to mix. Select "Slow Cook" mode by using the "Control Knob." To set the time for 8 hours, press the "Timer Button" and twist the "Control Knob." To begin cooking, close the PowerXL with the "Glass Lid" and hit the "Start Button." To end cooking, hit the "Cancel Button" when the cooking time is up. Remove the cover and serve immediately.

RECIPE 527: BASIL BELL PEPPER BITES

Serve: 4 | Total Time: 20 minutes

1 medium red bell pepper, small portions
1 medium yellow pepper, small portions
1 medium green bell pepper, small portions
3 tbsp balsamic vinegar
2 tbsp olive oil
1 tbsp garlic, minced
½ tsp dried basil
½ tsp dried parsley
Salt and black pepper to taste
½ cup garlic mayo to serve
In a bowl, mix peppers, oil, garlic, balsamic vinegar, basil, and parsley; season with salt and black pepper. Preheat your PowerXL Air Fryer Grill to 390 F on Air Fry function. Place the pepper mixture inside; cook for 10-15 minutes, tossing once or twice. Serve with garlic mayo and enjoy.

RECIPE 528: BBQ LAMB

Serve: 8 | Total Time: 55 minutes

4 lbs. boneless leg of lamb, 2-inch chunks
2-1/2 tbsps. herb salt
2 tbsps. olive oil

Preheat the Power XL Air Fryer Grill by selecting Air Fryer mode. Adjust the temperature to 390°F, set Time to 5 minutes. Season the meat with salt and olive oil. Arrange on the Air Fryer baking tray. Transfer to the Power XL Air Fryer Grill. Cook for 15 minutes in the air, flipping halfway through. Serve and enjoy.

RECIPE 529: BBQ PORK RIBS

Serve: 3 | Total Time: 45 minutes

1 lb. pork ribs, cut into smaller pieces
1 tsp. soy sauce
1 tsp. sesame oil
1 tsp. oregano
1 tbsp. Plus 1 tbsp. maple syrup
3 tbsp. barbecue sauce
Salt and black pepper to taste
2 cloves garlic, minced
1 tbsp. cayenne pepper

Combine all the ingredients in a bowl Add the pork chops and let aside for 5 hours to marinade. Preheat the PowerXL Air Fryer Grill by selecting Grill/ air fry mode Adjust temperature to 390°F and Time to 5 minutes Remove the pork chops and arrange them on the grilling plate Transfer into the PowerXL Air Fryer Grill Air fry for 15 minutes, flip, and brush with the remaining 1 tbsp. maple syrup. Air fry for additional 10 minutes. Serve and enjoy!

RECIPE 530: BEEF AND MANGO SKEWERS

Serve: 4 | Total Time: 15 minutes

350 g beef sirloin, cut into 2 cm thick cubes
2 tbsp balsamic vinegar
1 tbsp olive oil
1 tbsp honey

½ tsp dried marjoram
salt and pepper
1 mango

Combine the beef cubes, balsamic vinegar, olive oil, honey, marjoram, salt, and pepper in a medium mixing basin. Mix thoroughly, then use your hands to massage the marinade into the steak. Put aside. Now remove the peel from the mango and remove the stone. Cut the mango into 2 cm thick cubes. Now put the mango and beef cubes on the skewers. Grill the skewers in the frying basket for 4-7 minutes at 60 degrees or until the beef is cooked through.

RECIPE 531: BEEF BULGOGI WITH SCALLIONS AND SESAME

Serve: 4 | Total Time: 15 minutes

1/3 cup soy sauce
2 tbsp sesame oil
2½ tbsp brown sugar
3 garlic cloves, minced
½ tsp freshly ground black pepper
1-pound (454 g) rib-eye steak, thinly sliced
2 scallions, thinly sliced, for garnish
Toasted sesame seeds for garnish

Add sesame oil, soy sauce, brown sugar, garlic, and pepper to a small bowl. Pour the sauce over the meat pieces in a large shallow dish. Cover and chill for 1 hour. The Grill Grate closes the hood. Choose GRILL, MEDIUM temp, 5 min timer START/STOP to start preheating. When the machine beeps, lay the steak on the Grill Grate. 4 minutes no flipping. Check the steak after 4 minutes and cook for 1 minute further if required. Serve immediately with scallions and sesame seeds.

RECIPE 532: BEEF RECIPE TEXAS-RODEO STYLE

Serve: 6 | Total Time: 70 minutes

1/2 cup honey

1/2 cup ketchup
1/2 tsp dry mustard
1 clove of garlic, minced
1 tbsp chili powder
2 onion, chopped
3 pounds beef steak sliced
Salt and pepper to taste

Stick all ingredients in a Ziploc bag and allow marinating in the fridge for at least 2 hours. Preheat the Air Fryer to 390F. Place the grill pan accessory in the Air Fryer. Grill the beef for 15 minutes per batch making sure that you flip it every 8 minutes for even grilling. Meanwhile, pour the marinade on a saucepan and allow simmering over medium heat until the sauce thickens. Baste the beef with the sauce before serving.

RECIPE 533: BEEF STRIPS, CORN AND TOMATOES

Serve: 2 | Total Time: 15 minutes

½ lb. beef tenderloins, cut into strips.
1 cup corn kernels
1 cup cherry tomatoes, stems removed. and halved
2 tbsp. soy sauce
1 tbsp. garlic, minced.
2 tbsp. olive oil
salt and pepper, to taste

Attach the Air Fryer Grill Pan and preheat the Air Fryer to 350 degrees F. Season the beef strips with the olive oil, soy sauce, garlic, salt and pepper and place on the Air Fryer Grill Pan. Add the tomatoes and corn kernels to the Air Fryer Grill Pan. Cook for 8 minutes or until desired doneness of the meat. Serve and enjoy!

RECIPE 534: BEEF WELLINGTON

Serve: 4 | Total Time: 50 minutes

Beef fillet
Salt and pepper, to taste
Short crust pastry
1 medium egg, beaten
1 cup chicken liver pâté

Clean up the beef fillet and take out any visible fat. Season with salt and pepper. Then, seal the fillet with cling film and place in the fridge for an hour. Roll out the short crust pastry. Brush the edges with egg for sealing. Then, inside the outside egg line, apply a thin layer of homemade pâté until the white pastry is gone. Discard the plastic wrap and push the meat into the pâté. Seal the pastry around the filling. Score the top of the pastry, then place on the Air Fryer grill pan. Cook for 35 minutes at 320°F (160°C). Let it cool before slicing and serving.

RECIPE 535: BEEF WITH CAULIFLOWER AND GREEN PEAS

Serve: 4 | Total Time: 25 minutes

2 beef steaks, sliced into thin strips
2 garlic cloves, chopped
2 tsp maple syrup
1 tsp oyster sauce
1 tsp cayenne pepper
½ tsp olive oil
Juice of 1 lime
Salt and black pepper
1 cauliflower, cut into florets
2 carrots, cut into chunks
1 cup green peas

Preheat the PowerXL Air Fryer Grill to 400 F on Bake function. In a bowl, add beef, garlic, maple syrup, oyster sauce, cayenne, oil, lime juice, salt, and black pepper, and stir to combine. Place the beef along with the garlic and some of the juices into the baking pan. Top with the veggies. Insert in your PowerXL Air Fryer Grill.Cook at 400 F for 8 minutes, turning once halfway through. Serve and enjoy!

RECIPE 536: BELL PEPPERS WITH POTATO STUFFING

Serve: 4 | Total Time: 20 minutes

4 green bell peppers, top cut and deseeded
4 potatoes, boiled, peeled and mashed

2 onions, finely chopped
1 tsp lemon juice
2 tbsp coriander leaves, chopped
2 green chilies, finely chopped
Olive oil as needed
Salt to taste
¼ tsp Garam Masala
½ tsp chili powder
¼ tsp turmeric powder
1 tsp cumin seeds

Sauté the onion, chillies, and cumin seeds in the oil. Add the rest of the ingredients except the bell peppers and mix well. Preheat your Air Fryer to 390°Fahrenheit for 10-minutes. Brush your bell peppers with olive oil, inside and out and stuff each pepper with potato mixture. Place in Air Fryer basket and grill for 10-minutes. Check and grill for an additional 5-minutes.

RECIPE 537: BLACK BEAN FAJITAS

Serve: 2 | Total Time: 20 minutes

1 (15.5-oz) black beans
1 tbsp fajita seasoning
2 tbsp lime juice
2 flour tortillas
¼ cup salsa
2 scallions, thinly sliced
1 tbsp hot sauce

Preheat Air Fryer to 400°F. Using a fork, mash the beans until smooth. Stir in fajita seasoning and lime juice. Set aside. Place tortillas on a flat surface, spread half of the salsa on each tortilla, scatter with scallions, and top with the bean mixture. Drizzle with the hot sauce. For the burritos, fold in the sides of the tortilla, then fold up the bottom, and finally roll up. Grill for 10 minutes until crispy, turning once. Serve warm.

RECIPE 538: BOURBON-BBQ SAUCE MARINATED BEEF BBQ

Serve: 4 | Total Time: 70 minutes

1/4 cup bourbon
1/4 cup barbecue sauce
1 tbsp Worcestershire sauce

2 pounds beef steak, pounded
Salt and pepper to taste

Stick all ingredients in a Ziploc bag and allow marinating in the fridge for at least 2 hours. Preheat the Air Fryer to 390F. Place the grill pan accessory in the Air Fryer. Set on the grill pan and cook for 20 minutes per batch. Halfway through the cooking time, give a stir to cook evenly. Meanwhile, pour the marinade on a saucepan and allow to simmer until the sauce thickens. Serve beef with the bourbon sauce.

RECIPE 539: BREAKFAST GRILLED HAM AND CHEESE

Serve: 2 | Total Time: 15 minutes

1 tsp butter
4 slices bread
4 slices smoked country ham
4 slices Cheddar cheese
4 thick slices tomato

Spread ½ tsp of butter onto one side of 2 slices of bread. Each sandwich will have 1 slice of bread with butter and 1 slice without. Assemble each sandwich by layering 2 slices of ham, 2 slices of cheese, and 2 slices of tomato on the unbuttered pieces of bread. Top with the greased side of the remaining bread pieces. Place the sandwiches in the Air Fryer buttered-side down. Cook for 4 minutes Open the Air Fryer. Flip the grilled cheese sandwiches. Cook for an additional 4 minutes. Cool before serving. Cut each sandwich in half and enjoy.

RECIPE 540: BROCCOLI CHICKEN

Serve: 4 | Total Time: 22 minutes

1 lb. chicken breast, boneless and cut into bite-sized pieces
1 tbsp. soy sauce, low sodium
1 tbsp. olive oil
1/2 lb. broccoli, small florets
2 tsp. spicy sauce
1/2 onion, sliced
1 tsp. sesame seed oil

Salt to taste
Black pepper to taste
1/2 tsp. garlic powder
1 tbsp. fresh minced ginger
2 tsp. rice vinegar

Select the GRILL button on the Ninja Foodi Smart XL Grill and regulate Medium settings for 20 minutes. Mingle the chicken breasts with onion and broccoli in a bowl. Merge in the remaining ingredients and toss thoroughly. Arrange the chicken in the Ninja Foodi when it displays ADD FOOD. Grill for about 20 minutes, flipping once in between. Dole out on a platter and shower with a sauce prepared to serve.

RECIPE 541: BROCCOLI CHICKEN CASSEROLE

Serve: 4 | Total Time: 55 minutes

4 chicken breasts, skinless & boneless
1 cup Ritz crackers, crushed
1/2 tsp. paprika
10.5 oz. can cheddar cheese soup
10 oz. frozen broccoli florets
1 cup sharp cheddar cheese, shredded
1 cup milk
Black pepper
Kosher salt

Place the inner pot in the PowerXL grill Air Fryer combo base. Season chicken with pepper and salt and place into the inner pot. In a large bowl, mix together milk, cheddar cheese, paprika, cheddar cheese soup, half crackers, and broccoli and pour over chicken. Top with remaining crackers. Cover the inner pot with an air frying lid. Set the oven to bake mode at 350°F for 25 minutes. Press start. When the Timer reaches 0, then press the cancel button. Serve and enjoy.

RECIPE 542: BRUSSEL SPROUTS, MANGO, AVOCADO SALSA TACOS

Serve: 4 | Total Time: 40 minutes

4 taco shells

8 ounces brussels sprouts, diced
Half a mango, diced
Half of an avocado, diced
½ cup black beans, cooked
2 tbsp. onions, chopped
¼ cup cilantro, chopped
1 tbsp. jalapeno, chopped
Lime juice
Olive oil
1 tbsp. taco seasoning
Salt & Pepper

Preheat the PowerXL Air Fryer Grill at 230°C or 400°F. Mix the sprouts with taco seasoning, olive oil, and salt and pepper on the pan. Roast for 15 mins. Turn every 5 mins. To make the salsa, combine the mango, avocado, black beans, lime juice, cilantro, onion, jalapeno, salt, and pepper. Cook taco shells and fill them with sprouts and salsa.

RECIPE 543: BUTTERMILK BRINED TURKEY BREAST

Serve: 8 | Total Time: 45 minutes

3-1/2 pounds boneless, skinless turkey breast
3/4 cup brine from can of olives
1 fresh rosemary sprig
2 fresh thyme sprigs
1/2 cup buttermilk

Combine all the ingredients. Add the turkey and pour into a sealable bag. Leave to marinate for 12 hours in the refrigerator. Preheat the PowerXL Air Fryer Grill by selecting Air fry mode. Preheat the oven to 350°F and set the timer for 5 minutes. Arrange on the PowerXL grill baking tray. Transfer to the PowerXL Air Fryer Grill. Air fry for 20 minutes, flip halfway done. Enjoy.

RECIPE 544: BUTTERY PARMESAN BROCCOLI FLORETS

Serve: 2 | Total Time: 25 minutes

2 tbsp butter, melted
1 egg white
1 garlic clove, grated
¼ tsp salt

A pinch of black pepper
½ lb broccoli florets
¼ cup grated Parmesan cheese

Preheat the PowerXL Air Fryer Grill to 400 F on Air Fry function. Whisk together the butter, egg, garlic, salt, and black pepper in a mixing bowl. Toss in broccoli to coat well. Top with Parmesan cheese and; toss to coat. Arrange broccoli in a single layer in the PowerXL Air Fryer Grill without overcrowding. Cook in batches for 10 minutes. Remove to a serving plate and sprinkle with Parmesan cheese. Serve.

RECIPE 545: BUTTERY SCRAMBLE EGGS

Serve: 2 | Total Time: 11 minutes

2 slices bread
2 eggs
Salt and black pepper to taste
2 tbsp butter

Preheat the PowerXL Air Fryer Grill to 330 F on Bake function. Place a 3 X 3 cm heatproof bowl in the baking pan and brush with butter. Make a hole in the middle of the bread slices with a bread knife and place in the heatproof bowl in 2 batches. Break an egg into the center of each hole. Season with salt and pepper. Close the PowerXL Air Fryer Grill and cook for 4 minutes. Turn the bread with a spatula and cook for another 4 minutes. Serve and enjoy!

RECIPE 546: CADIENNE CHICKEN PASTA

Serve: 4 | Total Time: 25 minutes

2 chicken breasts; cut into thin strips
1/4 cup mushrooms, sliced.
1 green bell pepper; chopped
1/4 cup red bell pepper; chopped
1/4 cup onions, sliced.
1/4 cup parmesan cheese, shavings.
12 oz linguine, cooked.
2 tbsp. Cajun seasoning
1 tbsp. butter

Attach the Air Fryer Grill Pan and preheat the Air Fryer to 350 degrees F. Season the chicken with Cajun seasoning and place them on the Air Fryer Grill Pan. Cook for 10 minutes. Turn the chicken halfway through the cooking time. Add the butter, bell peppers, mushrooms and onions to the Air Fryer Grill Pan and cook for 5 minutes. Add the parmesan cheese and cook for 5 more minutes. Remove from the Air Fryer, pour over pasta and toss well to combine. Serve and enjoy!

RECIPE 547: CAESAR CHICKEN

Serve: 2 | Total Time: 80 minutes

2 chicken breasts, skinless and boneless
1/4 cup creamy Caesar dressing
1/4 tsp. dried parsley
2 tbsp. fresh basil, chopped
1/8 tsp. black pepper
1/8 tsp. salt

Place the inner pot in the PowerXL grill Air Fryer combo base. Add all ingredients into the inner pot and stir well. Cover the inner pot with a glass lid. Select slow cook mode then press the temperature button and set the timer for 6 hours. Press start. When the Timer reaches 0, then press the cancel button. Shred the chicken using a fork and serve.

RECIPE 548: CAESAR MARINATED GRILLED CHICKEN

Serve: 3 | Total Time: 34 minutes

¼ cup crouton
1 tsp lemon zest. Form into ovals, skewer and grill.
1/2 cup parmesan
1/4 cup breadcrumbs
1 lb ground chicken
2 tbsp Caesar dressing and more for drizzling
2-4 romaine leaves

In a shallow dish, mix well chicken, 2 tablespoons caesar dressing, parmesan, and breadcrumbs. Mix well with hands.

Form into 1-inch oval patties. Thread chicken pieces in skewers. Place on skewer rack in cuisinart Air Fryer oven. For 12 minutes, cook on 360°f. Halfway through cooking time, turnover skewers. If needed, cook in batches. Enjoy on a lettuce bed with croutons and additional dressing.

RECIPE 549: CAJUN SWEET-SOUR GRILLED PORK

Serve: 3 | Total Time: 22 minutes

1/4 cup brown sugar
1/4 cup cider vinegar
1 lb pork loin, sliced into 1-inch cubes
2 tbsp Cajun seasoning
3 tbsp brown sugar

In a shallow dish, mix well pork loin, 3 tbsp brown sugar, and Cajun seasoning. Toss well to coat. Marinate in the ref for 3 hours. In a medium bowl mix well, brown sugar and vinegar for basting. Thread pork pieces in skewers. Baste with sauce and place on skewer rack in Air Fryer. For 12 minutes, cook on 360F. Halfway through cooking time, turnover skewers and baste with sauce. If needed, cook in batches. Serve and enjoy.

RECIPE 550: CAPERS 'N OLIVES TOPPED FLANK STEAK

Serve: 4 | Total Time: 55 minutes

1 anchovy fillet, minced
1 clove of garlic, minced
1 cup pitted olives
1 tbsp capers, minced
1/3 cup olive oil
2 pounds flank steak, pounded
2 tbsp fresh oregano
2 tbsp garlic powder
2 tbsp onion powder
2 tbsp smoked paprika
Salt and pepper to taste

Preheat the Air Fryer to 390F. Place the grill pan accessory in the Air Fryer. Season the steak with salt and pepper. Rub the oregano,

paprika, onion powder, and garlic powder all over the steak. Set on the grill pan and cook for 45 minutes. Make sure to flip the meat every 10 minutes for even cooking. Meanwhile, mix together the olive oil, olives, capers, garlic, and anchovy fillets. Serve the steak with the tapenade.

RECIPE 551: CAPRESE GRILLED CHICKEN WITH BALSAMIC VINEGAR

Serve: 6 | Total Time: 20 minutes

6 grilled chicken breasts, boneless, skinless
6 large basil leaves
6 slices of tomato
6 slices of mozzarella cheese
1 tbsp butter
¼ cup balsamic vinegar
Prepare chicken in Air Fryer at 400°Fahrenheit for 15-minutes or until chicken is cooked. As chicken is cooking, pour balsamic vinegar into the pan and cook until reduced by half, for about 5-minutes. Add in the butter and stir with a flat whisk until well combined. Set aside. Top chicken with mozzarella cheese slices, basil leaves, and tomato slice each. Drizzle with balsamic reduction and serve warm.

RECIPE 552: CARAWAY, SICHUAN 'N CUMIN LAMB KEBABS

Serve: 3 | Total Time: 70 minutes

11/2 pounds lamb shoulder, bones removed and cut into pieces
1 tbsp Sichuan peppercorns
1 tsp sugar
2 tbsp cumin seeds, toasted
2 tsp caraway seeds, toasted
2 tsp crushed red pepper flakes
Salt and pepper to taste

Place all ingredients in bowl and allow the meat to marinate in the fridge for at least 2 hours. Preheat the Air Fryer to 390F. Place the grill pan accessory in the Air Fryer. Grill the meat for 15 minutes per batch. Flip the meat every 8 minutes for even grilling.

RECIPE 553: CATFISH FILLETS WITH PARSLEY

Serve: 2 | Total Time: 40 minutes

2 catfish fillets
3 tbsp breadcrumbs
1 tsp cayenne pepper
1 tsp dry fish seasoning, of choice
2 sprigs parsley, chopped
Salt to taste, optional

Preheat the PowerXL Air Fryer Grill to 400 F on Air Fry function. Meanwhile, pour all the dry ingredients, except the parsley, in a zipper bag. Pat dry and add the fish pieces. Close the bag and shake to coat the fish well. Do this with one fish piece at a time. Lightly spray the fish with olive oil. Arrange them in the fryer basket, one at a time, depending on the size of the fish. Cook for 10 minutes. Flip the fish and cook further for 10 minutes. For extra crispiness, cook for 3 more minutes. Garnish with parsley and serve as a lunch accompaniment.

RECIPE 554: CAULIFLOWER, OKRA, AND PEPPER CASSEROLE

Serve: 4 | Total Time: 20 minutes

1 head cauliflower, cut into florets
1 cup okra, chopped
1 yellow bell pepper, chopped
2 eggs, beaten
1/2 cup chopped onion
1 tbsp soy sauce
2 tbsp olive oil
Salt and ground black pepper, to taste

Spray baking pan with cooking spray. Put cauliflower inside food processor and pulse to rice the cauliflower. Pour the cauliflower rice in the baking pan and add the remaining ingredients. Stir to mix well. Place the pan on the bake position. Select Bake, set temperature to 380°F (193°C) and set time to 12 minutes. When cooking is complete, the eggs should be set. Remove the baking pan from the Air Fryer grill and serve immediately.

RECIPE 555: CHARRED ONIONS AND STEAK CUBE BBQ

Serve: 3 | Total Time: 48 minutes

1 cup red onions, cut into wedges
1 tbsp. dry mustard
1 tbsp. olive oil
1-lb. boneless beef sirloin, cut into cubes
Salt and pepper, to taste

Preheat the Air Fryer to 390°F. Place the grill rack in the Air Fryer. Toss all the listed ingredients in a bowl and mix until everything is coated with the seasonings. Place on the grill rack and put the rack in the oven. Select GRILL. Grill for 40 minutes. Halfway through the cooking time, give a stir to cook evenly. When done, transfer to a plate and enjoy.

RECIPE 556: CHEDDAR PIMIENTO STRIPS

Serve: 4 | Total Time: 35 minutes

8 oz shredded sharp cheddar cheese
1 (4-oz) jar chopped pimientos, including juice
¼ cup mayonnaise
¼ cup cream cheese
Salt and pepper to taste
1 tsp chopped parsley
8 slices sandwich bread
4 tbsp butter, melted

Salted pimientos and mayonnaise are mixed with cheddar cheese and cream cheese. Let chill covered in the fridge for 30 minutes. Preheat Air Fryer at 350°F. Spread pimiento mixture over 4 bread slices, then top with the remaining slices and press down just enough to not smoosh cheese out of sandwiches edges. Brush each sandwich with melted butter on top and bottom. Place sandwiches in the frying basket and Grill for 6 minutes, flipping once. Slice each sandwich into 16 sections and serve warm.

RECIPE 557: CHEESE STUFFED CHICKEN

Serve: 4 | Total Time: 35 minutes

1 tbsp creole seasoning
1 tbsp olive oil
1 tsp garlic powder
1 tsp onion powder
4 chicken breasts, butterflied and pounded
4 slices colby cheese
4 slices pepper jack cheese

Preheat the cuisinart Air Fryer oven to 390°f. Place the grill pan accessory in the Air Fryer. Create the dry rub by mixing in a bowl the creole seasoning, garlic powder, and onion powder. Season with salt and pepper if desired. Rub the seasoning on to the chicken. Place the chicken on a working surface and place a slice each of pepper jack and colby cheese. Fold the chicken and secure the edges with toothpicks. Brush chicken with olive oil.

RECIPE 558: CHEESY BBQ CHICKEN PIZZA

Serve: 1 | Total Time: 13 minutes

1 piece naan bread
¼ cup Barbecue sauce
¼ cup shredded Monterrey Jack cheese
¼ cup shredded Mozzarella cheese
½ chicken herby sausage, sliced
2 tbsp. red onion, thinly sliced
Chopped cilantro or parsley, for garnish
Cooking spray

Spritz the bottom of naan bread with cooking spray, then transfer to the air fry basket. Brush with the Barbecue sauce. Top with the sausage, cheeses, and finish with the red onion. Place the basket on the air fry position. Select Air Fry, set the temperature to 400°F (205°C), and set time to 8 minutes. When cooking is complete, the cheese should be melted. Remove the basket from the Air Fryer grill. Garnish with the chopped cilantro or parsley before slicing to serve.

RECIPE 559: CHEESY CREAMY BROCCOLI CASSEROLE

Serve: 4 | Total Time: 35 minutes

4 cups broccoli florets
¼ cup heavy whipping cream
1/2 cup sharp Cheddar cheese, shredded
¼ cup ranch dressing
Kosher salt and grind black pepper, to taste

Combine all ingredients in a large bowl. Toss to coat well broccoli well. Pour mixture into a baking pan. Place the pan on the bake position. Select Bake, set temperature to 375°F (190°C) and set time to 30 minutes. When cooking is complete, the broccoli should be tender. Remove the baking pan from the Air Fryer grill and serve immediately.

RECIPE 560: CHEESY RICE CROQUETTES

Serve: 4 | Total Time: 45 minutes

2 cups cooked rice
1 brown onion, chopped
2 garlic cloves, chopped
2 eggs, lightly beaten
½ cup grated Parmesan cheese
Salt and black pepper to taste
½ cup breadcrumbs
1 tsp dried mixed herbs

Preheat the PowerXL Air Fryer Grill to 400 F on Air Fry function. Combine rice, onion, garlic, eggs, Parmesan cheese, salt, and pepper. Shape into 10 croquettes. Spread the crumbs onto a plate and coat each croquette in the crumbs. Spray each croquette with oil. Arrange the croquettes in the PowerXL Air Fryer Grill. Cook for 16 minutes, turning once halfway through cooking. Serve with plum sauce.

RECIPE 561: CHICKEN CACCIATORE

Serve: 2 | Total Time: 85 minutes

1 3/4 lb. chicken thighs
1 cherry pepper
1 small onion, chopped
6 oz. cremini mushrooms
1 medium red pepper
14 oz. tomato paste
1 tbsp. capers
1 fresh rosemary sprig
1 garlic clove
1 cup chicken broth
Pepper
Salt

Place the inner pot in the PowerXL grill Air Fryer combo base. Whisk together tomato paste and broth in a bowl. Season chicken with pepper and salt. Place season chicken into the inner pot. Add remaining ingredients to the inner pot then pour tomato paste mixture over chicken. A glass lid should be used to cover the inner pot. Select slow cook mode then press the temperature button and set the timer for 5 hours. Press start. When the Timer reaches 0, then press the cancel button. Serve and enjoy.

RECIPE 562: CHICKEN PAILLARD

Serve: 8 | Total Time: 35 minutes

4 chicken breasts, skinless and boneless
1/2 cup olives, diced
1 small onion, sliced
1 fennel bulb, sliced
28 oz. can tomatoes, diced
1/4 cup fresh basil, chopped
1/4 cup fresh parsley, chopped
1/4 cup pine nuts
2 tbsp. olive oil
Pepper
Salt

Arrange chicken in baking dish and season with pepper and salt and drizzle with oil. In a bowl, mix together olives, tomatoes, pine nuts, onion, fennel, pepper, and salt. Pour olive mixture over chicken. Place the inner pot in the PowerXL grill Air Fryer combo base. Place the baking dish into the inner pot. Cover the inner pot with an air frying lid. Set the oven to bake mode at 450°F for 25

minutes. Press start. When the timer reaches 0, then press the cancel button. Serve and enjoy.

RECIPE 563: CHICKEN ROAST WITH PINEAPPLE SALSA

Serve: 2 | Total Time: 55 minutes

¼ cup extra virgin olive oil
¼ cup freshly chopped cilantro
1 avocado, diced
1-pound boneless chicken breasts
2 cups canned pineapples
2 tsp honey
Juice from 1 lime
Salt and pepper to taste
Preheat the cuisinart Air Fryer oven to 390°f. Place the grill pan accessory in the Air Fryer. Season the chicken breasts with lime juice, olive oil, honey, salt, and pepper. Place on the grill pan and cook for 45 minutes. Flip the chicken every 10 minutes to grill all sides evenly. Once the chicken is cooked, serve with pineapples, cilantro, and avocado.

RECIPE 564: CHICKEN SHAWARMA

Serve: 5 | Total Time: 85 minutes

1 1/4 lb. chicken thigh, skinless and boneless
1 tsp. garlic powder
1 tsp. cumin
2 tbsp. garlic, minced
1/2 cup Greek yogurt
1/4 cup chicken stock
1/4 tsp. ground coriander
1/4 tsp. cinnamon
1/2 tsp. curry powder
1/2 tsp. dried parsley
1 tsp. paprika
1/4 cup fresh lemon juice
1 1/2 tbsp. tahini
1 tbsp. olive oil
Pepper
Salt

Place the inner pot in the PowerXL grill Air Fryer combo base. Add all ingredients into the inner pot and mix well. Glass lid the inside pot. Select slow cook mode then press the temperature button and set the timer for 3 hours. Press start.

When the Timer reaches 0, then press the cancel button. Serve and enjoy.

RECIPE 565: CHICKEN WITH ARTICHOKE HEARTS

Serve: 2 | Total Time: 70 minutes

6 chicken thighs, skinless and boneless
3 tbsp. fresh lemon juice
10 oz. frozen artichoke hearts
14 oz. can tomatoes, diced
1/2 tsp. garlic powder
1 tsp. dried basil
1 tsp. dried oregano
15 olives, pitted
Pepper
Salt

Place the inner pot in the PowerXL grill Air Fryer combo base. Add all ingredients into the inner pot and mix well. Glass lid the inside pot. Select slow cook mode then press the temperature button and set the timer for 8 hours. Press start. When the Timer reaches 0, then press the cancel button. Serve and enjoy.

RECIPE 566: CHICKEN WITH CASHEW NUTS AND BELL PEPPER

Serve: 4 | Total Time: 30 minutes

1 lb chicken cubes
2 tbsp soy sauce
1 tbsp corn flour
2 ½ onion cubes
1 carrot, chopped
¼ cup cashew nuts, fried
1 bell pepper, cut
2 tbsp garlic, crushed
Salt and white pepper

Marinate the chicken cubes with ½ tbsp of white pepper, ½ tsp salt, 2 tbsp soya sauce, and add 1 tbsp corn flour. Set aside for 25 minutes. Preheat the PowerXL Air Fryer Grill to 380 F on Bake function. Transfer the marinated chicken. Add the garlic, the onion, the bell pepper, and the carrot; cook for 5-6 minutes. Roll it in the cashew nuts before serving.

RECIPE 567: CHILI CHICKEN SLIDER

Serve: 4 | Total Time: 28 minutes

1-1/2 cups chicken, minced
1/3 tsp. paprika
1/2 tbsp. chili sauce
3 cloves garlic, peeled and minced
1 tsp. ground black pepper, or to taste
1/2 tsp. fresh basil, minced
1-1/2 tbsp. coconut aminos
1/3 cup scallions, peeled and chopped
1/2 tsp. grated fresh ginger
1 tsp. salt
Preheat the PowerXL Air Fryer Grill by selecting grill mode. Adjust the temperature to 355°F, set Time to 5 minutes. Combine all the ingredients in a bowl. Form into patties. Arrange on the PowerXL grill grilling plate. Transfer to the PowerXL Air Fryer Grill. Air fry for 18 minutes, flip halfway done. Enjoy.

RECIPE 568: CHILI GARLIC CHICKEN WINGS

Serve: 4 | Total Time: 20 minutes

12 chicken wings
1 tsp. granulated garlic
1 tbsp. chili powder
1/2 tbsp. baking powder
1/2 tsp. sea salt

Add chicken wings into the large bowl and toss with remaining ingredients. Place the inner pot in the PowerXL grill Air Fryer combo base. Place grill plate in the inner pot. Cover. Select air fry mode then set the temperature to 410°F and Time for 20 minutes. Press start. Let the appliance preheat for 3 minutes. Open the lid then place chicken wings on the grill plate. Serve and enjoy.

RECIPE 569: CHILI-RUBBED FLANK STEAK

Serve: 2 | Total Time: 19 minutes

1 tbsp chili powder

1 tsp dried oregano
2 tsp ground cumin
1 tsp sea salt
¼ tsp freshly ground black pepper
2 (8-ounce) flank steaks

Reinstall the Grill Grate and hood. Select GRILL, HIGH temperature, and 8 minutes. Select START/STOP to begin preheating. Chili powder, oregano, cumin, salt, and pepper Use your hands to rub the spice mixture on all sides of the steaks. When the unit beeps to signify it has preheated, place the steaks on the Grill Grate. Gently press the steaks down to maximize grill marks. Cook for 4 minutes. After 4 minutes, flip the steaks, close the hood, and cook for 4 minutes more. Transfer the steaks to a chopping board. Allow for about 5 minutes at least of the resting time before slicing and serving.

RECIPE 570: CITRUSY CHICKEN BREASTS

Serve: 4 | Total Time: 32 minutes

4 boneless and skinless chicken breasts
1 tbsp. lemon pepper
1 tsp. table salt
1 1/2 tsp. granulated garlic

Select the GRILL button on the Ninja Foodi Smart XL Grill and regulate MED settings for 20 minutes. Dust the chicken breasts with salt, garlic, and lemon pepper. Arrange the chicken in the Ninja Foodi when it displays ADD FOOD. Grill for about 20 minutes, flipping once in between. Dole out on a platter and serve warm.

RECIPE 571: CLASSIC GRILLED CHEESE

Serve: 2 | Total Time: 15 minutes

1 cup of shredded cheddar cheese
½ cup of melted butter
4 slices of bread

Preheat your Air Fryer to 360 degrees Fahrenheit. Using two bowls, add the cheddar cheese to the first bowl and the melted butter to the second bowl. Brush the butter on each side of all the bread pieces. Add a ½ cup of cheese on the 2 pieces of bread, place the other slice of bread on top and put it inside your basket. Allow it to cook for 5 minutes or until it has golden brown color, and the cheese has completely melted. Thereafter, carefully remove it from your Air Fryer and allow it to cool. Serve and enjoy!

RECIPE 572: CLASSIC MAPLE-GLAZED CHICKEN

Serve: 4 | Total Time: 25 minutes

2 lbs. chicken wings, bone-in
1 tsp. black pepper, ground
1/4 cup teriyaki sauce
1 cup maple syrup
1/3 cup soy sauce
3 garlic cloves, minced
2 tsp. garlic powder
2 tsp. onion powder

Take a mixing bowl, add garlic, soy sauce, black pepper, maple syrup, garlic powder, onion powder, and teriyaki sauce, combine well. Add the chicken wings and combine well to coat. Position the grill grate and adjacent the cover. Pre-heat Ninja Foodi by demanding the GRILL option and situation it to MED and timer to 10 minutes. Let it pre-heat till you hear a beep. Arrange the chicken wings over the grill grate, lock the lid and cook for 5 minutes Flip the chicken and close the lid, cook for 5 minutes more Cook until it reaches 165°F. Serve warm and enjoy!

RECIPE 573: CLASSIC SPRING CHICKEN

Serve: 4 | Total Time: 40 minutes

Salt and pepper to taste
2 tsp dried rosemary, crushed
2 tsp oyster sauce

4 bell pepper, seeded and cut into chunks
1 pound spring chicken
1 tbsp olive oil
2 bay leaves

In a large bowl, add oyster sauce, rosemary, salt and pepper. Mix well. Rub the chicken with oyster mixture and then stuff its cavity with bay leaves. Meanwhile, preheat the Air Fryer to 355°F. Grease the Air Fryer grill pan and place potatoes on it. Cook for about 15 mins and remove the grill pan from the Air Fryer. Now, coat the bell pepper pieces with oil and line the grill pan with them. Arrange grill pan in the Air Fryer and transfer chicken pieces. Cook for 15 mins. Serve and enjoy!

RECIPE 574: COCONUT BATTERED FISH FILLETS

Serve: 2 | Total Time: 26 minutes

Salt and pepper to taste
½ tsp mustard powder
2 tsp of garlic powder
1/3 cup plain flour
1 cup coconut flour
Oil spray, for greasing
2 fish fillets, salmon (6 ounces each)

Select the grill function and place the grill grate in the Ninja Foodi Smart XL Grill. Remember to grease the grill grate with oil spray. Set the time to MAX for 8 minutes, buy selecting grill function. Select start to begin preheating. Meanwhile, mix salt, pepper, mustard powder, garlic powder, and coconut flour in a bowl. Season the fish with salt and black pepper and coat it with oil spray. Once the unit is preheated add the fish to the grill grate and grill at MAX for 10 minutes No needed to flip the fillets. Once it's done serve.

RECIPE 575: COCONUT FISH WITH A FINE NOTE

Serve: 4 | Total Time: 60 minutes

1.25 kg of Amur carp
2 small onions
150 coconut flakes
1 small piece of fresh ginger
1 stick of lemongrass
2 chili peppers
1 clove of garlic
Tamarind paste
0.5 tsp coriander powder
0.5 tsp turmeric powder
oil
pepper and salt

Peel and chop onions and garlic. Halve the lemongrass and the chili peppers and chop them just as finely. Cut the peeled ginger into fine strips and puree with coriander and turmeric in a blender. Afterwards, season with tamarind paste and salt and mix in the coconut flakes. Now use a baking paper and brush this with oil. Place the fish on top and distribute the coconut mixture on top. Seal the baking paper well and grill in the hot fryer at 180 degrees for a good 15 minutes.

RECIPE 576: COCONUT PORK CHOPS

Serve: 2 | Total Time: 20 minutes

4 pork chops
1 tbsp coconut oil
1 tbsp coconut butter
1 tbsp fresh parsley, chopped
3 garlic cloves, grated
Pepper
Salt

Preheat the Air Fryer to 350 F. In a prepared medium-sized bowl, mix together coconut butter, coconut oil, garlic, parsley, pepper, and salt. Rub coconut butter mixture over pork chops and place in the refrigerator for 1 hour. Place grill pan in the Air Fryer. Place marinated chops into the Air Fryer and cook for 7 minutes. Turn pork chops to another side and cook for 8 minutes. Serve and enjoy.

RECIPE 577: COD FILLET WITH HUMMUS

Serve: 2 | Total Time: 21 minutes

2 cod fillets
1 cup hummus
1 tbsp. lemon juice
1 tsp. garlic, minced.
1 tsp. chili flakes
salt and pepper, to taste
Attach the Air Fryer Grill Pan to the Air Fryer and preheat to 350 degrees F. Place the cod fillets on the Air Fryer Grill Pan and season with the lemon juice, salt and pepper. Spray the fillets with cooking spray and cook for 7 minutes. Mix the hummus, minced garlic and chili flakes in a bowl. Season with more pepper and dollop the hummus on the cod fillets. Cook for 4 minutes more. Serve and enjoy!

RECIPE 578: COD STEAKS AND PLUM SAUCE

Serve: 3 | Total Time: 40 minutes

1 tbsp. plum sauce
1/2 tsp. garlic powder
3 large cod steaks
Cooking spray
1/2 tsp. ginger powder
Black pepper and salt
1/4 tsp. turmeric powder

Drizzle the cod steaks with cooking spray. Add pepper, ginger powder, salt, turmeric powder, and garlic powder. Place the coated cod steaks in the PowerXL Air Fryer Grill. Set the function to Air Fryer/ Grill. Grill for about 20 minutes at 360°F. Flip while cooking for uniformity. Heat plum sauce over medium heat for 2 minutes at reheat function. Divide the cod steaks and serve immediately.

RECIPE 579: COD WITH CHORIZO POTATOES

Serve: 2 | Total Time: 20 minutes

2 cod fillets
1 cup Spanish chorizo; casings removed and diced
1 cup potatoes, diced.
1/2 cup onions, chopped.

1 tbsp. garlic, minced.
2 tbsp. butter
1 tsp. garlic powder
2 tsp. lemon juice
salt and pepper, to taste

Preheat the Air Fryer to temperature of 350 degrees F. Season the chorizos and potatoes with salt and pepper and place them in the Air Fryer Basket. Season the cod fillets with salt, pepper & garlic powder. Drizzle over the lemon juice and place them on the Air Fryer Grill Pan. Place the cod fillets on the Air Fryer Grill Pan and top with the butter and onions. Cook for 10 minutes. Serve and enjoy!

RECIPE 580: CREOLE FRIED TOMATOES

Serve: 3 | Total Time: 15 minutes

1 green tomato, sliced
¼ tbsp creole seasoning
Salt and black pepper to taste
¼ cup flour
½ cup buttermilk
Breadcrumbs as needed

Preheat your PowerXL Air Fryer Grill to 400 F on Air Fry function. Add flour to one bowl and buttermilk to another. Season the tomatoes with salt and pepper. Make a mix of creole seasoning and breadcrumbs. Cover tomato slices with flour, dip in buttermilk, and then into the breadcrumbs. Do the same for all the slices. Cook the tomato slices in your PowerXL Air Fryer Grill for 5 minutes. Serve and enjoy!

RECIPE 581: CRISPY BREAKFAST TACO WRAPS

Serve: 4 | Total Time: 30 minutes

1 tbsp water
4 pieces commercial vegan nuggets, chopped
1 small yellow onion, diced
1 small red bell pepper, chopped
2 cobs grilled corn kernels

4 large tortillas mixed greens for garnish

Preheat the Air Fryer to 400F. In a skillet heated over medium heat, water sauté the vegan nuggets together with the onions, bell peppers, and corn kernels. Set aside. Place filling inside the corn tortillas. Fold the tortillas and place inside the Air Fryer and cook for 15 minutes until the tortilla wraps are crispy. Serve with mix greens on top.

RECIPE 582: CRISPY CRUSTED CHICKEN

Serve: 4 | Total Time: 40 minutes

1 egg, lightly beaten
2 tbsp. butter, melted
4 chicken breasts, skinless and boneless
1 tsp. water
3 cups corn flakes, crushed
1 tsp. poultry seasoning
Pepper
Salt

Season chicken with poultry seasoning, pepper, and salt. In a medium-sized mixing bowl, combine and whisk together the egg and water until well combined. In a separate shallow bowl, mix together crushed cornflakes and melted butter. Dip chicken into the egg mixture then coats with crushed cornflakes. Place the inner pot in the PowerXL grill Air Fryer combo base. Place the coated chicken into the inner pot. Cover the inner pot with an air frying lid. Set the oven to bake mode at 400°F for 30 minutes. Press start. When the Timer reaches 0, then press the cancel button. Serve and enjoy.

RECIPE 583: CURRY PORK ROAST IN COCONUT SAUCE

Serve: 6 | Total Time: 85 minutes

1/2 tsp curry powder
1/2 tsp ground turmeric powder
1 can unsweetened coconut milk
1 tbsp sugar

2 tbsp fish sauce
2 tbsp soy sauce
3 pounds of pork shoulder
Salt and pepper to taste
Place all ingredients in a bowl and allow the meat to marinate in the fridge for at least 2 hours. Preheat the Air Fryer to 390F. Place the grill pan accessory in the Air Fryer. Grill the meat for 20 minutes making sure to flip the pork every 10 minutes for even grilling and cook in batches. Meanwhile, merge the marinade into a saucepan and allow to simmer for 10 minutes until the sauce thickens. Baste the pork with the sauce before serving.

RECIPE 584: EFFORTLESS PEPPERONI PIZZA

Serve: 2 | Total Time: 25 minutes

8 ounces fresh pizza dough
¼ cup tomato sauce
¼ cup mozzarella cheese, shredded
8 pepperonis, sliced
Flour, to dust

Preheat the PowerXL Air Fryer Grill to 360 F on Air Fry function. On a floured surface, place dough and dust with flour. Stretch with hands into an air-fryer fitting shape. Place the pizza in the oven/ pizza rack. Brush with sauce, leaving some space at the border. Scatter with mozzarella and top with pepperonis. Cook for 15 minutes or until crispy. Serve and enjoy!

RECIPE 585: EGGPLANT ROLLS WITH QUINOA

Serve: 3 | Total Time: 15 minutes

1 whole eggplant, sliced
Marinara sauce for dipping
½ cup cheese, grated
2 tbsp milk
1 whole egg, beaten
2 cups breadcrumbs

Preheat the PowerXL Air Fryer Grill to 400 F on Air Fry function. In a bowl, mix beaten egg and milk. In another bowl, mix crumbs and cheese until crumbly. Place eggplant slices in the egg mixture, followed by a dip in the crumb mixture. Place the eggplant slices in the crisper tray and cook for 5 minutes. Serve with marinara sauce.

RECIPE 586: ESPRESSO-GRILLED PORK TENDERLOIN

Serve: 4 | Total Time: 26 minutes

2 tsp espresso powder
1 tsp ground paprika
½ tsp dried marjoram
1 tbsp honey, lemon juice, brown sugar
1 (1-pound) pork tenderloin

Mix the brown sugar, espresso powder, paprika, and marjoram. Stir in the honey, lemon juice, and olive oil until well mixed. Spread the honey mixture over the pork and let stand for 10 minutes at room temperature. Roast the tenderloin in the Air Fryer basket until the pork registers at least 145°f on a meat thermometer. Slice the meat to serve.

RECIPE 587: FEISTY RUM AND PINEAPPLE SUNDAE

Serve: 4 | Total Time: 18 minutes

1/2 cup dark rum
1/2 cup packed brown sugar
1 tsp ground cinnamon, also for garnish
1 pineapple cored and sliced
Vanilla ice cream, for serving

Take a large-sized bowl and add rum, sugar, cinnamon Add pineapple slices, arrange them in the layer. Coat mixture then let them soak for 5 minutes, per side Pre-heat Ninja Foodi by pressing the "GRILL" option and setting it to "MAX" and timer to 8 minutes Let it pre-heat until you hear a beep Strain extra rum sauce from pineapple Transfer prepared fruit in grill grate in a single layer, press down fruit, and lock lid Grill

for 6-8 minutes without flipping, work in batches if needed Once done, remove and top each pineapple ring with a scoop of ice cream, sprinkle cinnamon, and serve. Enjoy!

RECIPE 588: FILET MIGNON

Serve: 2 | Total Time: 15 minutes

2 filet mignons
Salt and ground black pepper, as required

Season the filet mignons with salt and black pepper generously. Place the water tray in the bottom of Power XL Smokeless Electric Grill. Place about 2 cups of lukewarm water into the water tray. Place the drip pan over water tray and then arrange the heating element. Now, place the grilling pan over heating element. Plugin the Power XL Smokeless Electric Grill and press the 'Power' button to turn it on. Then press 'Fan' button. Set the temperature settings according to manufacturer's directions. Cover the grill with lid and let it preheat. After preheating, remove the lid and grease the grilling pan. Place the filet mignons over the grilling pan. Cover with the lid and cook for about 5 minutes per side. Serve immediately.

RECIPE 589: FISH WITH SEASONAL HERBS IN A PACKET

Serve: 1 | Total Time: 30 minutes

150 g fish fillet of choice
50 g peas
50 g cherry tomatoes
2 tbsp olive oil
20 ml dry white wine
chervil
1 clove of garlic peeled and pressed
1 sprig of thyme
Some slices of lemons
1 pinch of saffron threads
pepper and salt

Place the cleaned fish fillet with the washed tomatoes and peas as well as the lemon on top of a sheet of baking paper. Now drizzle with olive oil and refine the spices. Add a dash of white wine. Fold the paper up and tie it in a package with kitchen thread. Grill the fish at 120 degrees for 15 minutes. A baguette or boiled potatoes go well with it.

RECIPE 590: FRUITY LIME SALAD

Serve: 2 | Total Time: 15 minutes

1/2 pound strawberries washed, hulled, and halved
1 can (9 ounces) pineapple chunks, drained, juice reserved
2 peaches, pitted and sliced
6 tbsp honey, divided
1 tbsp freshly squeezed lime juice

Take a large bowl and add strawberries, pineapple, peaches, and 3 tbsp, honey, toss well. Pre-heat Ninja Foodi by pressing the "GRILL" option and setting it to "MAX" and timer to 4 minutes. Let it pre-heat until you hear a beep. Transfer fruits to Grill Grate, lock lid and cook for 4 minutes. Take a small-sized bowl and add the remaining 3 tbsp of honey, lime juice, 1 tbsp reserved pineapple juice. Once cooking is done, place fruits in a large-sized bowl and toss with honey mixture, serve and enjoy!

RECIPE 591: GARLIC CHICKEN KEBAB

Serve: 2 | Total Time: 10 minutes

1 lb. chicken fillet, cut into small pieces
1 tbsp garlic, minced
½ cup plain yogurt
1 tbsp olive oil
Juice of one lime
1 tsp turmeric powder
1 tsp red chili powder
1 tsp black pepper
1 tbsp chicken masala

Mix the yogurt and spices in a bowl. Add the oil and squeeze half a lime into it and stir. Coat the chicken pieces with mixture one at a time. Marinate the chicken pieces in the fridge for 2 hours. Preheat your Air Fryer to 356°Fahrenheit. Place the grill pan into the Air Fryer and put the chicken pieces into it. Cook chicken for 10-minutes.

RECIPE 592: GARLIC LAMB SHANK

Serve: 4 | Total Time: 39 minutes

17 oz. lamb shanks
2 tbsp. garlic, peeled and coarsely chopped
1 tsp. kosher salt
1/2 cup chicken stock
1 tbsp. dried parsley
1 tsp. dried rosemary
4 oz. chive stems, chopped
1 tsp. butter
1 tsp. nutmeg
1/2 tsp. ground black pepper

Make the cuts in the lamb shank and fill the cuts with the chopped garlic. Sprinkle the lamb shank with kosher salt, dried parsley, dried rosemary, nutmeg, and ground black pepper. Stir the spices on the lamb shank gently. Preheat the PowerXL Air Fryer Grill by selecting air fry mode. Adjust the temperature to 380°F, set Time to 5 minutes. Put the butter, chives, and chicken stock in the Air Fryer baking tray. Add the lamb shank and air fry the meat for 24 minutes. Serve and enjoy

RECIPE 593: GENEROUS HOT PEPPER WINGS

Serve: 4 | Total Time: 35 minutes

1/2 tsp. paprika
1 tbsp. ranch salad dressing
1 lb. chicken wings
1 tbsp. coconut oil
2 tbsp. butter, melted
1/2 cup hot pepper sauce

Take a mixing bowl and add oil, chicken, ranch dressing, paprika,

and mix well. Let it chill for 30–60 minutes. Take another bowl and add pepper sauce, butter. Pre-heat Ninja Foodi by demanding the GRILL option and situation it to MED and timer to 25 minutes. Let it pre-heat till you hear a beep. Arrange chicken wings over grill grate, lock lid, and let it cook until the timer runs out. Serve chicken warm with pepper sauce. Enjoy!

RECIPE 594: GINGER, GARLIC AND PORK DUMPLINGS

Serve: 8 | Total Time: 25 minutes

¼ tsp crushed red pepper
½ tsp sugar
1 tbsp chopped fresh ginger
1 tbsp chopped garlic
1 tsp canola oil
1 tsp toasted sesame oil
18 dumpling wrappers
2 tbsp rice vinegar
2 tsp soy sauce
4 cups bok choy, chopped
4 ounces ground pork

Heat oil in a skillet and sauté the ginger and garlic until fragrant. Stir in the ground pork and cook for 5 minutes. Stir in the bok choy and crushed red pepper. Season with salt and pepper to taste. Allow to cool. Place the meat mixture in the middle of the dumpling wrappers. Fold the wrappers to seal the meat mixture in. Place the bok choy in the grill pan. Cook the dumplings in the Air Fryer at 330°F for 15 minutes. Meanwhile, prepare the dipping sauce by combining the remaining Ingredients in a bowl.

RECIPE 595: GLAZED LAMB CHOPS

Serve: 4 | Total Time: 45 minutes

4 (4-ounce) lamb loin chops
1 tbsp. Dijon mustard
1 tsp. honey
1/2 tbsp. fresh lime juice
1/2 tsp. olive oil
Salt and ground black pepper, as required

Preheat the PowerXL Air Fryer Grill by selecting Air Fryer mode. Adjust the temperature to 390°F, set Time to 5 minutes. Combine all the ingredients in a bowl. Add the pork chops and toss to coat. Arrange on the Air Fryer baking tray. Transfer to the PowerXL Air Fryer Grill. Air fry for 15 minutes, flipping halfway through. Serve and enjoy.

RECIPE 596: GOLDEN SQUASH CROQUETTES

Serve: 4 | Total Time: 22 minutes

1/3 butternut squash, peeled and grated
1/3 cup all-purpose flour
2 eggs, whisked
4 cloves garlic, minced
11/2 tbsp olive oil
1 tsp fine sea salt
1/3 tsp ground black pepper, to taste
1/3 tsp dried sage
A pinch of ground allspice

Line the air fry basket with parchment paper. Set aside. In a mixing bowl, stir together all the ingredients until well combined. Make the squash croquettes: Use a small cookie scoop to drop tablespoonfuls of the squash mixture onto a lightly floured surface and shape into balls with your hands. Transfer them to the air fry basket. Place the basket on the air fry position. Select Air Fry, set temperature to 345ºF (174ºC), and set time to 17 minutes. When cooking is complete, the squash croquettes should be golden brown. Remove from the Air Fryer grill to a plate and serve warm.

RECIPE 597: GREEK CHICKEN BREASTS

Serve: 4 | Total Time: 30 minutes

4 chicken breasts
1 ½ tsp. dried oregano
1 tsp. paprika
6 garlic cloves, minced
6 tbsp. fresh parsley, minced

6 tbsp. olive oil
6 tbsp. fresh lemon juice
Pepper
Salt

Add all ingredients except chicken into the zip-lock bag and mix well. Add chicken into the bag, seal bag shakes well, and place in the refrigerator overnight. Select grill mode on the Ninja Foodi Smart XL Grill, then set the temperature to medium and set the timer to 12 minutes. Press start to begin preheating. Once the unit is preheated it will beep then place marinated chicken on grill grates and close the hood. Cook chicken for 12 minutes or until the internal temperature of chicken reaches 165 F. Serve and enjoy.

RECIPE 598: GREEK POTATOES

Serve: 4 | Total Time: 50 minutes

1 lb. potatoes, sliced into wedges
2 tbsp. olive oil
1 tsp. paprika
2 tsp. dried oregano
Salt and pepper to taste
¼ cup onion, diced
2 tbsp. lemon juice
1 tomato, diced
¼ cup black olives, sliced
½ cup feta cheese, crumbled

Add crisper plate to the Air Fryer basket inside the PowerXL Grill. Choose air fry setting. Set it to 390°F. Preheat for 3 minutes. While preheating, toss potatoes in oil. Sprinkle with paprika, oregano, salt, and pepper. Add potatoes to the crisper plate. Air fry for 18 minutes. Toss and cook for another 5 minutes. Add onion and cook for 5 minutes. Transfer to a bowl. Stir in the rest of the ingredients.

RECIPE 599: GREEK TOMATO OLIVE CHICKEN

Serve: 4 | Total Time: 28 minutes

4 chicken breast, boneless and halves

15 olives, pitted and halved
2 cups cherry tomatoes
3 tbsp. olive oil
3 tbsp. capers, rinsed and drained
Pepper
Salt

In a bowl, toss tomatoes, capers, olives, and olive oil. Set aside. Season chicken with pepper and salt. Place chicken in the baking dish and top with tomato mixture. Place the inner pot in the PowerXL grill Air Fryer combo base. Place the baking dish into the inner pot. Cover the inner pot with an air frying lid. Set the oven to bake mode at 475°F for 25 minutes. Press start. When the Timer reaches 0, then press the cancel button. Serve and enjoy.

RECIPE 600: GREEN BEANS WITH SESAME SEEDS

Serve: 4 | Total Time: 13 minutes

1 tbsp reduced-sodium soy sauce or tamari
1/2 tbsp Sriracha sauce
4 tsp toasted sesame oil, divided
12 oz (340 g) trimmed green beans
1/2 tbsp toasted sesame seeds

Whisk together the Sriracha sauce, soy sauce, and 1 teaspoon of sesame oil in a small bowl until smooth. Set aside. Toss the green beans with the remaining sesame oil in a large bowl until evenly coated. Place the green beans in the air fry basket in a single layer. Place the basket on the air fry position. Select Air Fry, set temperature to 375ºF (190ºC), and set time to 8 minutes. Stir the green beans halfway through the cooking time. When cooking is complete, the green beans should be lightly charred and tender. Remove from the Air Fryer grill to a platter. Pour the prepared sauce over the top of green beans and toss well. Serve sprinkled with the toasted sesame seeds.

RECIPE 601: GREEN BELL PEPPER WITH CALIFLOWER STUFFING

Serve: 4 | Total Time: 20 minutes

4 green bell peppers, top cut, deseeded
1 tsp lemon juice
2 tbsp coriander leaves, finely chopped
2 green chilies, finely chopped
2 cups cauliflower, cooked and mashed
2 onions, finely chopped
1 tsp cumin seeds
¼ tsp turmeric powder
¼ tsp chili powder
¼ tsp garam masala
Salt to taste
Olive oil as needed
In a pan heat the oil and sauté the chilies, onion, and cumin seeds. Add the rest of the ingredients except the bell peppers and mix well. Preheat your Air Fryer to 390°Fahrenheit for 10-minutes. Brush the green bell peppers with olive oil, inside and out and stuff each pepper with cauliflower mixture. Place them into Air Fryer and grill for 10-minutes.

RECIPE 602: GRILLED ASPARAGUS

Serve: 8 | Total Time: 10 minutes

3 lb. asparagus, with the woody parts cut off
3 tbsp. olive oil
3 tbsp. salt
Pepper to taste
Place the grill grate in your unit according to your manual. Select the GRILL function on HOT heat with a 4-minute timer. Close the hood and press "START/STOP" to start the preheating process. When it's preheated, open the hood and arrange the asparagus on the grill. Grill for 4 minutes with the hood closed. Test for doneness by piercing with a fork. If needed, cook for another couple of minutes.

RECIPE 603: GRILLED BBQ TURKEY

Serve: 6 | Total Time: 40 minutes

1–3 lbs. turkey breast, half and bone-in
1 cup Greek yogurt
1/2 cup lemon juice
1 tsp. rosemary, dried and crushed
1/3 cup canola oil
1/2 cup parsley, minced
1/2 green onion, chopped
4 garlic cloves, minced
4 tbsp. dill, minced
1 tsp. salt
1/2 tsp. pepper

Yield a mingling bowl, complement all the ingredients except the turkey. Add and coat the turkey evenly and refrigerate for 8 hours to marinate. Position the grill grate and adjacent the cover. Pre-heat Ninja Foodi by demanding the GRILL option and situation it to HIGH and timer to 30 minutes. Let it pre-heat till you hear a beep. Arrange the turkey over the grill grate, lock the lid and cook for 15 minutes more. Flip the turkey and cook for 15 minutes more. Take out your when it reaches 350°F. Serve warm and enjoy!

RECIPE 604: GRILLED BROCCOLI

Serve: 4 | Total Time: 15 minutes

4 cups of broccoli
2 tsp of garlic powder
1 tsp of pepper
½ tsp of salt
1/8 tsp of paprika
1/6 tsp of oregano
1 tbsp of olive oil
1 tbsp of coconut oil
1 big red pepper
½ tsp of onion powder
½ cup of sauce

Wash and cup broccoli in the pieces. Wash and chop the red pepper in the strings. Mix the red pepper with broccoli. Then add pepper, salt, paprika, oregano, coconut oil and onion powder to the bowl with vegetables. Mix everything well. Sprinkle the crying basket with oil. Preheat the Air Fryer to 350F. Cook broccoli for 5 minutes. Then shake well, cover with sauce and cook for 5

minutes again. Serve warm and you can decorate it with parsley or sprinkle with lemon.

RECIPE 605: GRILLED BUFFALO CHICKEN WINGS

Serve: 4 | Total Time: 60 minutes

500g chicken wings
2 tbsp melted butter
2 tbsp hot chili sauce depending on your taste
2 tbsp paprika powder
125 g of flour
1 tbsp canola oil
salt and pepper
Mix salt, pepper, paprika and flour together well. Rub the chicken legs with it and cover with the ingredients. Fry the chicken legs at 200 degrees until brown. Then set the temperature to 150 degrees and fry for another 10 minutes until the chicken legs are cooked. In the meantime, mix the hot sauce with the butter in a bowl and serve with the chicken thighs. A delicious, light summer dish that really comes into its own with a fine wine, a baguette and a fresh salad.

RECIPE 606: GRILLED CHEESE AND PRAWN SANDWICHES

Serve: 4 | Total Time: 15 minutes

1 ¼ cups shredded halloumi cheese
1 (6-oz) can prawns, minced
3 tbsp mayonnaise
2 tbsp minced green onion
4 bread slices
2 tbsp butter, softened
Preheat Air Fryer to 400°F. Mix together halloumi cheese, prawns, mayonnaise, and green onion. On a work surface, lay out the bread. Spread half of the mixture on one slice of bread, and then half on another slice of bread. Cover each slice with the remaining bread to make sandwiches. Spread butter on both sides of each sandwich. Place the sandwich into the Air Fryer and Bake until the bread is toasted and crisp while the cheese is melted. Remove from the Air Fryer, cut in half, and serve warm.

RECIPE 607: GRILLED CHEESE FISH

Serve: 4 | Total Time: 20 minutes

1 bunch basil
2 garlic cloves
1 tbsp olive oil
1 tbsp olive oil
1 tbsp parmesan cheese
Salt and pepper to taste
2 tbsp pine nuts
1 and 1/2 pounds white fish fillets

Pepper and salt the fish fillets after coating them with oil. Preheat your Air Fryer to temperature of 356°F. Carefully transfer the fillets to your Air Fryer cooking basket. Cook for about 8 mins. Take a small bowl and add basil, olive oil, pine nuts, garlic, parmesan cheese and blend using your hand. Serve this mixture with the fish!

RECIPE 608: GRILLED CHEESE SANDWICH

Serve: 1 | Total Time: 15 minutes

2 sprouted bread slices
1 tsp sunflower oil
2 Halloumi cheese slices
1 tsp mellow white miso
1 garlic clove, minced
2 tbsp kimchi
1 cup Iceberg lettuce, torn

Preheat Air Fryer to 390°F. Brush the outside of the bread with sunflower oil. Put the sliced cheese, buttered sides facing out inside and close the sandwich. Put the sandwich in the frying basket and Air Fry for 12 minutes, flipping once until golden and crispy on the outside. On a plate, open the sandwich and spread the miso and garlic clove over the inside of one slice. Top with kimchi and lettuce, close the sandwich, cut in half, and serve.

RECIPE 609: GRILLED CHICKEN

Serve: 2 | Total Time: 20 minutes

1/4 cup onions, sliced.

1/4 cup horseradish
6 asparagus stalks
2 salmon fillets
4 lemon slices
2 tbsp. olives, sliced.
1 tbsp. lemon juice
2 tbsp. dill
salt and pepper, to taste

Preheat the Air Fryer to temperature of 350 degrees F. Season the asparagus with salt and pepper and place them in the Air Fryer Basket. Attach the Air Fryer Grill Pan to the Air Fryer Basket and place the salmon fillets on the Air Fryer Grill Pan. Season the salmon fillets with the salt, pepper and lemon juice. Cook for 10 minutes with lemon slices on fish. Remove the salmon and asparagus from the Air Fryer. Top the salmon with the horseradish, olives and dill. Serve and enjoy!

RECIPE 610: GRILLED CHICKEN AND SAUCE

Serve: 2 | Total Time: 40 minutes

2 cups granny smith apples; peeled, cored and sliced
2 chicken breast fillets
1/4 cup mint leaves, chopped.
salt and pepper, to taste

Preheat the Air Fryer and to 350 degrees F. Place the apples in the Air Fryer Basket and attach the Air Fryer Grill Pan. Prepare the chicken on the Air Fryer Grill Pan. Spray the chicken with cooking spray and cook for 20 minutes. Remove the apples from the Air Fryer Basket. Flip the chicken and cook for another 10 minutes. Mash the apples with a fork and add to the chopped mint. Remove the chicken fillets from the Air Fryer and top over with the apple mint sauce. Serve and enjoy!

RECIPE 611: GRILLED CHICKEN BREASTS

Serve: 4 | Total Time: 19 minutes

½ tsp garlic powder

salt and black pepper to taste
1 tsp dried parsley
2 tbsp olive oil, divided
3 boneless, skinless chicken breasts

Preparing the ingredients. Combine the garlic powder, salt, pepper, and parsley. Using 1 tbsp of olive oil and half of the seasoning mix, rub each chicken breast with oil and seasonings. Place the chicken breast in the Air Fryer basket. Set the temperature of your AF to 370 °F. Set the timer and grill for 7 minutes. Using tongs, flip the chicken and brush the remaining olive oil and spices onto the chicken. Reset the timer and grill for 7 minutes more. Check that the chicken has reached an internal temperature of 165 °F. Add Cooking Time if needed. Before serving, let the chicken finish cooking.

RECIPE 612: GRILLED CHICKEN BREASTS WITH BROCCOLI

Serve: 4 | Total Time: 25 minutes

1 pound chicken breast, boneless and cut into bite-sized pieces
1 tbsp soy sauce, low sodium
1 tbsp olive oil
½ pound broccoli, cut into small florets
2 tsp hot sauce
½ onion, sliced
1 tsp sesame seed oil
Salt, to taste
Black pepper, to taste
½ tsp garlic powder
1 tbsp fresh minced ginger
2 tsp rice vinegar

Select the "Grill" button on the Ninja Foodi Smart XL Grill and regulate the settings at Medium for 20 minutes. Mingle the chicken breasts with onion and broccoli in a bowl. Throw in the remaining ingredients and toss thoroughly. Arrange the chicken in the Ninja Foodi when it displays "Add Food". Grill for about 20 minutes, flipping once in between. Dole out in a platter and shower with lemon juice to serve.

RECIPE 613: GRILLED COD FILLETS MIXED WITH GRAPES SALAD AND FENNEL

Serve: 3 | Total Time: 40 minutes

1 tbsp. olive oil
1/2 cup pecans
1 sliced fennel bulb.
3 black cod fillets
Black pepper and salt
1 cup grapes
Rub oil all over the fish fillets. Sprinkle with pepper and salt. Place the fish on the PowerXL Air Fryer Grill basket. Place the basket at position 6 in the PowerXL Air Fryer Grill. Set the PowerXL Air Fryer Grill to Air Fryer/Grill function at 1450F. Grill for about 10 minutes. Mix grapes, pecans, oil, and fennel in another bowl, sprinkle with pepper and salt. Place the mixture in the PowerXL Air Fryer Grill basket. Set the PowerXL Air Fryer Grill to the air fry function. Cook for about 5 minutes at 400°F. Serve cod with grape and fennel mix.

RECIPE 614: GRILLED COD WITH AVOCADO AND OLIVES SALAD

Serve: 4 | Total Time: 13 minutes

4 cod fillets
1/4 cup feta cheese, crumbled.
1/4 cup olives, sliced.
1/4 cup dill, chopped.
1-tsp. lemon juice
2 avocados, diced.
salt and pepper, to taste

Preheat the Air Fryer to temperature of 350 degrees F. Season the cod fillets with salt, pepper and lemon juice. Arrange all the cod fillets in the Air Fryer Basket, if required. Cook for 8 minutes or until the fish is cooked through. Remove from the Air Fryer and top with the feta cheese, olives, avocados and dill. Serve and enjoy!

RECIPE 615: GRILLED CUMIN HANGER STEAK

Serve: 2 | Total Time: 25 minutes

2 hanger steaks
1/4 cup mint leaves, chopped.
1/4 cup parmesan cheese, shavings.
1 cup green peas
2 tbsp. olive oil
1 tsp. ground cumin
1 tsp. paprika
salt and pepper, to taste

Rub the steaks with cumin and paprika. Add 1 tbsp olive oil, pepper, salt. Rest for 10 minutes. Attach the Air Fryer Grill Pan and preheat the Air Fryer to 350 degrees F. Arrange the steaks on the Air Fryer Grill Pan and cook for 5 minutes. Remove the steaks from the Air Fryer Grill Pan and place the green peas and mint leaves on the Air Fryer Grill Pan. Flip over the steaks and place them on top of the vegetables. Drizzle with remaining olive oil and top with the parmesan cheese shavings. Cook for 5 more minutes or until desired doneness of meat. Serve and enjoy!

RECIPE 616: GRILLED FISH AND CHEESE

Serve: 4 | Total Time: 20 minutes

1 bunch basil
2 garlic cloves
1 tbsp olive oil (for cooking)
1/4 cup olive oil (extra)
1 tbsp parmesan cheese
Salt and pepper to taste
2 tbsp peanuts
6 ounces white fish fillet

Pepper and salt the fish fillets after coating them with oil. Pre-heat your Air Fryer to 356°F in "Air Fry" mode. Carefully transfer the fillets to your Air Fryer cooking basket. Cook for about 8 mins. Take a small bowl and add basil, olive oil, pine nuts, garlic, parmesan cheese and blend using your hand. Serve this mixture with the fish!

RECIPE 617: GRILLED FISH FILLET WITH PESTO SAUCE

Serve: 2 | Total Time: 20 minutes

2 white fish fillets (8 oz each)
1 tbsp olive oil
Ground black pepper and salt to taste

Pesto sauce:
1 bunch fresh basil
1 tbsp pine nuts
2 garlic cloves
1 cup extra-virgin olive oil
1 tbsp grated Parmesan cheese
Ensure that your Air Fryer is preheated to 360 F. Grab each fish fillet and brush with the oil and season with salt and pepper. Transfer the coated fillet into the Air Fryer cooking basket and allow to cook for 8 minutes. While cooking the fish fillet, pick the basil leaves and combine them with pine nuts, garlic, olive oil, and the Parmesan cheese. Transfer the mixture into a food processor or mortar and pestle. Pulse or grind the mixture until you have a sauce. Salt to taste. Serve the cooked fish fillets drizzled with pesto sauce on a serving plate.

RECIPE 618: GRILLED FRUIT

Serve: 6 | Total Time: 5 minutes

4 peaches
1 pear
4 plums
2 tbsp melted butter
1 tbsp brown sugar
1 tsp curry powder

Wash the fruits thoroughly and remove the pits and seeds of fruits. Cut each fruit in half. Now place some foil on your workplace and arrange all the fruits on the foil. Drizzle the fruits with the butter and honey. Next, sprinkle curry powder on top. Trap the fruit in the foil. Make sure to leave some air space in the foil. Put the foil package in the basket of an Air Fryer and grill for 5 minutes at 350 degrees F. Serve.

RECIPE 619: GRILLED HALIBUT WITH SUN DRIED TOMATOES

Serve: 2 | Total Time: 15 minutes

2 halibut fillets, cut into cubes.
1/2 cup tomato sauce
1/4 cup pecorino cheese, shavings.
1/4 cup sun dried tomatoes, chopped.
1/4 cup butter; small pieces
2 tbsp. dill, chopped.
2 tsp. garlic, minced.
salt and pepper, to taste

Attach the Air Fryer Grill Pan and preheat the Air Fryer to 350 degrees F. Season the fillets with salt and pepper and place them on the Air Fryer Grill Pan. Dot the fish with the butter slices and cook for 5 minutes. Flip the fish and add the tomato sauce, minced garlic, sun dried tomatoes, and pecorino cheese. Top with some dill and cook for 5 more minutes. Serve and enjoy!

RECIPE 620: GRILLED HAWAIIAN CHICKEN

Serve: 2 | Total Time: 25 minutes

4 chicken breasts, cubed
2 garlic cloves, minced.
1/2 cup ketchup
1/2-tbsp. ginger, minced.
1/2 cup soy sauce
2 tbsp. sherry
1/2 cup pineapple juice
2 tbsp. apple cider vinegar
1/2 cup brown sugar

Preheat the Air Fryer to temperature of 360 degrees F. Take a bowl and, mix in ketchup, pineapple juice, sugar, cider vinegar, ginger. Heat the sauce in a frying pan over low heat. Cover chicken with the soy sauce and sherry; pour the hot sauce on top. Set aside for 15 minutes to marinate. Place the chicken in the Air Fryer cooking basket and cook for 15 minutes.

RECIPE 621: GRILLED HAWAIIAN CHICKEN BREASTS

Serve: 4 | Total Time: 25 minutes

4 chicken breasts
2 garlic cloves
1/2 cup ketchup, keto-friendly
1/2 teaspoon ginger
1/2 cup coconut aminos
2 tablespoons red wine vinegar
1/2 cup pineapple juice
2 tablespoons apple cider vinegar

Pre-heat your Instant Vortex Air Fryer to 360°F. Take a bowl and mix in ketchup, pineapple juice, cider vinegar, ginger. Take a fry pan and place it over low heat, add sauce and let it heat up. Cover chicken with the amino and vinegar pour hot sauce on top. Let the chicken sit for 15 mins to marinade. Transfer chicken to your instant vortex Air Fryer and bake for 15 mins. Serve and enjoy!

RECIPE 622: GRILLED HIGH RIB WITH SPICY SAUCE

Serve: 4 | Total Time: 30 minutes

1.2 kg high rib
2 tbsp ketchup
1 tbsp olive oil
½ tsp grated ginger
1 tbsp Dijon mustard
½ tsp ground turmeric
½ tsp salt

To ensure that the meat is particularly tender, take the high rib out of the refrigerator approx. 1 hour before the processing time. Afterwards, salt and brush with oil. Prepare the sauce with the remaining ingredients. Now bring the Air Fryer to 120 degrees and place the high rib on the grid. Depending on your wishes and taste, for example Cook for 7 to 8 minutes per side 9 to 10 minutes per side (medium rare) 11 to 12 minutes per side (pink) If you want, you can fry the high rib through it takes 13 to 14 minutes per side. Then let the high rib rest a little, cut into slices and enjoy with a delicious sauce.

RECIPE 623: GRILLED LEMONY SABA FISH

Serve: 1 | Total Time: 18 minutes

2 tbsp. lemon juice
2 tbsp. minced garlic
Black pepper and salt
2 tbsp. olive oil
4 saba fish fillet
3 chopped red chili pepper

Drizzle the fish with oil, sprinkle salt and pepper. Add chili, lemon juice, and garlic. Toss well. Place the fish on the PowerXL Air Fryer Grill basket at position 6. Set the PowerXL Air Fryer Grill to Air Fryer/Grill. Grill for about 8 minutes at 3600F. Flip while cooking. Serve immediately.

RECIPE 624: GRILLED MASALA LAMB CHOPS

Serve: 8 | Total Time: 90 minutes

2 kg Lamb chops
200g Natural yogurt
80ml Oil
1 tsp. Salt
1 tsp. Kashmiri chili powder
3/4 tsp. Paprika powder
1/2 tsp. turmeric powder
½ tsp. Chili flakes
1 tsp. Garlic powder
3/4 tsp. Ginger powder
1 tsp. Onion powder
1 tsp. Coriander powder
1 tsp. Cumin powder
4 tsp. Garam masala powder
½ tsp. ground black pepper

Add all the ingredients for two hours and marinate the chops. Place the grill grate in the Ninja Foodi. Choose the Grill and adjust the temperature to medium. Adjust the timer for twenty minutes. Press the start/stop button to start preheating. When ready, place four chops. Close the lid. After five minutes, flip the chop and close the lid. When done, remove and serve! Serve with green chutney. Sprinkle with fresh cilantro.

RECIPE 625: GRILLED ORANGE CHICKEN

Serve: 4 | Total Time: 25 minutes

2 tsp. ground coriander
1/2 tsp. garlic salt
1/4 tsp. ground black pepper
12 chicken wings
1 tbsp. canola oil
1/4 cup butter, melted
3 tbsp. honey
1/2 cup orange juice
1/3 cup Sriracha chili sauce
2 tbsp. lime juice
1/4 cup cilantro, chopped
Coat chicken with oil, season with spices, and let it chill for 2 hours Add other listed ingredients and keep them on the side. Cook for 3-4 minutes in a saucepan Pre-heat Ninja Foodi by demanding the GRILL option and situation it to MED and timer to 10 min. Let it pre-heat till you hear a beep. Arrange chicken over grill grate, cook for 5 minutes. Flip and let it cook for 5 minutes more. Serve with sauce on top, enjoy!

RECIPE 626: GRILLED PARSLEY AND THYME SALMON

Serve: 5 | Total Time: 20 minutes

5 parsley sprigs
5 salmon fillets
1 chopped yellow onion
3 tbsp. olive oil
3 sliced tomatoes
5 thyme sprigs
Black pepper and salt
1 lemon juice

Pour 1 tbsp. oil on the PowerXL Air Fryer Grill pan. Add the sliced tomatoes to the grill pan. Sprinkle pepper and salt on the tomatoes. Pour another 1 tbsp. of oil on the grill pan. Place onion, fish, parsley spring, lemon juice, thyme sprig on the tomatoes. Transfer the pan to the PowerXL Air Fryer Grill basket. Set the PowerXL Air Fryer Grill to Air Fryer/Grill. Set the Timer to 12 minutes and temperature at 360°F. Serve immediately.

RECIPE 627: GRILLED PEACHES

Serve: 3 | Total Time: 15 minutes

2 yellow peaches
Whipped Cream or Ice Cream
1/4 cup brown sugar
1/4 cup butter diced into tiny cubes
1/4 cup graham cracker crumbs

Peel peaches and cut them into wedges, removing the pits. Place a piece of parchment paper on top of the rack in the Air Fryer. Place peach wedges on parchment, skin side up (on the side). Air fry at 3500F for 5 minutes Combine the crumbs, brown sugar, and butter in a mixing bowl. Flip the peaches over to expose the peel. Spread the crumb mixture over the peaches, keeping the butter near to the peaches. Continue to air fry at 350°F for another 5 minutes. Spoon peaches onto plates with a big spoon. Top with whipped topping. Spoon any excess butter/topping combination from the parchment onto the whipped topping.

RECIPE 628: GRILLED PEARS WITH CINNAMON DRIZZLE

Serve: 3 | Total Time: 30 minutes

3 ripe pears
2 tbsp honey
1 tbsp cinnamon
1/4 cup pecans, chopped
coconut oil
sea salt

Peel and cut the pears into quarters. Toss pears with honey, cinnamon, and coconut oil. Place the pears in the Ninja Foodi Smart XL. Cover the Ninja Foodi Grill's hood, select the Manual Mode, set the temperature to 375 degrees F, and grill them on the "Grill Mode" for 7 minutes per side. Garnish with pecans and sea salt. Serve.

RECIPE 629: GRILLED PORK AND BELL PEPPER SALAD

Serve: 4 | Total Time: 25 minutes

1 cup sautéed button mushrooms, sliced
2 lb pork tenderloin, sliced

1 tsp olive oil
1 tsp dried marjoram
6 tomato wedges
6 green olives
6 cups mixed salad greens
1 red bell pepper, sliced
1/3 cup vinaigrette dressing

Preheat Air Fryer to 400°F. Combine the pork and olive oil, making sure the pork is well-coated. Season with marjoram. Lay the pork in the Air Fryer. 3-4 minutes each side until meat is cooked through. While the pork is cooking, toss the salad greens, red bell pepper, tomatoes, olives, and mushrooms into a bowl. Toss the salad with the pork pieces and the vinaigrette. Serve while the pork is still warm.

RECIPE 630: GRILLED PORK CHOPS WITH SWEET POTATOES

Serve: 4 | Total Time: 90 minutes

4 pork loin chops; 1-inch thick
1 large zucchini, diced.
1/4 cup fresh parsley, chopped.
2 cups sweet potatoes, cubed.
2 tbsp. garlic, minced.
3 tbsp. fresh oregano, chopped.
1 tbsp. lemon juice
4 tbsp. olive oil
salt and pepper, to taste

Marinate the pork chops with the lemon juice, olive oil, minced garlic, fresh oregano, salt and pepper. Cover with plastic wrap and chill overnight. Preheat the Air Fryer to temperature of 350 degrees F. Mix the sweet potatoes and zucchinis with the olive oil and the fresh parsley. Arrange the pork chops in the Air Fryer Basket and cook for 8 minutes. Add in the potatoes and zucchinis and cook for another 8 minutes. Top with the fresh parsley. Serve and enjoy!

RECIPE 631: GRILLED PORK IN CAJUN SAUCE

Serve: 3 | Total Time: 22 minutes

1-lb pork loin, sliced into 1-inch cubes
2 tbsp Cajun seasoning
3 tbsp brown sugar + ¼ cup
1/4 cup cider vinegar

In a plate, mix pork loin, Cajun seasoning, and three tbsp brown sugar. Stir well to coat. Marinate in the ref for three hours. In a medium bowl mix well, brown sugar and vinegar to baste. Thread pork pieces onto skewers. Baste with sauce and place on skewer rack in the oven. Cook on 360 degrees F for twelve mins. Halfway through cook time, turn skewers over and baste with sauce. If necessary, bake in batches.

RECIPE 632: GRILLED PORK SHOULDER

Serve: 2 | Total Time: 15 minutes

1/2 lb pork shoulder, cut into 1/2-inch slices
1/2 tsp Swerve
1/2 tbsp sesame oil
1/2 tbsp rice wine
1/2 tbsp soy sauce
1 tbsp green onion, sliced
1/2 tbsp sesame seeds
1/4 tsp cayenne pepper
1/2 tbsp garlic, minced
1/2 tbsp ginger, minced
1 tbsp gochujang
1/2 onion, sliced

In a prepared large bowl, mix together all ingredients and place in the refrigerator for 60 minutes. Place Air Fryer grill pan into the Air Fryer. Add pork mixture into the Air Fryer and cook at 400 F for 15 minutes. Turn halfway through. Serve and enjoy.

RECIPE 633: GRILLED SALMON WITH CAPERS AND DILL

Serve: 2 | Total Time: 8 minutes

1 tsp capers, chopped
2 sprigs dill, chopped
1 lemon zest
1 tbsp olive oil
4 slices lemon (optional)

11 oz salmon fillet

Dressing:
5 capers, chopped
1 sprig dill, chopped
2 tablespoons plain yogurt
Pinch of lemon zest
Salt and black pepper to taste

Preheat your Air Fryer to 400°Fahrenheit. Mix dill, capers, lemon zest, olive oil and salt in a bowl. Cover the salmon with this mixture. Cook salmon for 8-minutes. Combine the dressing ingredients in another bowl. When salmon is cooked, place on serving plate and drizzle dressing over it. Place lemon slices at the side of the plate and serve.

RECIPE 634: GRILLED SCALLION CHEESE SANDWICH

Serve: 1 | Total Time: 20 minutes

2 tsp butter (room temperature)
¾ cup grated cheddar cheese
2 slices of bread
1 tbsp grated parmesan cheese
2 scallions (thinly sliced)

Spread a teaspoon of butter on a slice of bread. Place it in the cooking basket with the buttered side facing down. Add scallions and cheddar cheese on top. Spread the rest of the butter in the other slice of bread. Place it on top of the sandwich and sprinkle with parmesan cheese. Cook for 10 minutes at 3560 F. Serve and Enjoy!

RECIPE 635: GRILLED SKIRT STEAK WITH SAUCE

Serve: 4 | Total Time: 55 minutes

1 lb skirt steak, cut into 4 pieces
⅛ tsp crushed red pepper flakes
2 tbsp adobo sauce
1 chipotle pepper in adobo sauce, minced
⅛ tsp pepper

In a bowl, mix the salt, pepper, minced chipotle pepper, red pepper flakes, and adobo sauce. Rub both sides of the steaks with the marinade. Let the steaks sit for at least 20 minutes at room temperature or refrigerate up to 12 hours. Arrange the steaks in the Air Fryer basket. Put the Air Fryer lid on and grill in batches in the preheated instant pot at 400°F for 10 minutes, or until the steaks are cooked to medium doneness. Serve in a serving dish, sliced.

RECIPE 636: GRILLED SOY SALMON FILLETS

Serve: 4 | Total Time: 15 minutes

4 salmon fillets
1/4 tsp ground black pepper
1/2 tsp cayenne pepper
1/2 tsp salt
1 tsp onion powder
1 tbsp fresh lemon juice
1/2 cup soy sauce
1/2 cup water
1 tbsp honey
2 tbsp extra-virgin olive oil

Firstly, pat the salmon fillets dry using kitchen towels. Season the salmon with black pepper, cayenne pepper, salt, and onion powder. To make the marinade, combine together the lemon juice, soy sauce, water, honey, and olive oil. Before serving, chill the salmon for at least 2 hours. Arrange the fish fillets on a grill basket in your XL Air Fryer oven. Air Frying. Bake at 330 degrees for 8 to 9 minutes, or until salmon fillets are easily flaked with a fork. Work with batches and serve warm.

RECIPE 637: GRILLED STUFFED LOBSTER

Serve: 3 | Total Time: 25 minutes

1 lobster
2 tbsp freshly chopped basil
1 medium-sized zucchini
1 lemon
2 tbsp butter
Olive oil
Salt, to taste

Boil the lobster for 5 minutes until nice and red. Place the knife in the groove between the lobster's eyes. Cut the lobster in half. Then remove the intestinal tract, liver and stomach. Cut the zucchini in long slices and coat them with a little olive oil. Mix chopped basil with butter. Season the mixture with salt, to taste. Preheat the Air Fryer to 360 F. Add lobster halves, brush with butter and cook for about 6-8 minutes. Remove the lobster from the grill pan and let it rest. Grill the zucchini slices for 4 to 5 minutes at 390 F. Place the lobster and the zucchini slices in a dish and sprinkle with a little lemon juice.

RECIPE 638: GRILLED TOFU SANDWICH

Serve: 1 | Total Time: 20 minutes

2 slices of bread
1 1-inch thick Tofu slice
1/4 cup red cabbage, shredded
1/4-tsp. vinegar
2-tsp. olive oil divided
Salt and pepper, to taste

Preheat your Air Fryer to temperature of 350 degrees F, add in the bread slices and toast for 3 minutes; set aside. Brush the tofu with 1-tsp. oil and place in the Air Fryer; grill for 5 minutes on each side. Combine the cabbage, remaining oil and vinegar and season with salt and pepper. Place the tofu on top of one bread slice, place the cabbage over and top with the other bread slice. Serve and enjoy.

RECIPE 639: GRILLED TOMATO SALSA

Serve: 8 | Total Time: 25 minutes

1 onion, sliced
1 jalapeño pepper, sliced in half
5 tomatoes, sliced
2 tbsp. oil
Salt and pepper to taste
1 cup cilantro, trimmed and sliced
1 tbsp. lime juice

1 tsp. lime zest
2 tbsp. ground cumin
3 cloves garlic, peeled and sliced

Coat onion, jalapeño pepper, and tomatoes with oil. Season with salt and pepper. Add grill grate to your PowerXL Grill. Press grill setting. Choose max temperature and set it to 10 minutes. Press start to preheat. Add vegetables to the grill. Cook for 5 minutes per side. Transfer to a plate and let cool. Add vegetable mixture to a food processor. Stir in the remaining ingredients. Pulse until smooth.

RECIPE 640: GRILLED TOMATOES

Serve: 3 | Total Time: 17 minutes

3 medium beefcake tomatoes
Salt and ground black pepper to taste
1 tsp oregano

With the tomatoes chopped into two halves, transfer them into the Air Fryer grill pan. Add sprinkles of salt, oregano, and pepper. Allow cooking for 8 minutes at 360 F. Reduce the heat to 320 F and allow to cook for an extra 5 minutes. This is to let the tomatoes to cook in the middle. Serve. The essence of chopping the tomatoes in half is to get equal sizes and ensure that each tomato has a bottom.

RECIPE 641: GRILLED TURKEY SKEWERS WITH SATAY SAUCE

Serve: 3 | Total Time: 30 minutes

12 ounces turkey breast, cut into chunks
½ cup soy sauce
½ cup peach juice
5 tbsp olive oil
3 garlic cloves, peeled and chopped
4 shallots, peeled and chopped
1 tbsp turmeric
2 tbsp caraway seeds
Cayenne pepper

Place the turkey breast in a bowl. In a prepared medium-sized mixing bowl combine the soy sauce, peach juice, olive oil, garlic, shallots, turmeric, caraway seeds, and cayenne pepper and mix well. Cover the turkey breast with the marinade, cover the bowl, and let rest in the refrigerator for at least two hours. Preheat the Air Fryer to 350ºF. Using a paper towel, blot the turkey dry after removing it from the marinade. Put the turkey on oven-safe skewers into the Air Fryer pan. Cook for 5-7 minutes. Serve with a spiced sauce that contains peanuts.

RECIPE 642: GRILLED VEGETABLES WITH LAMB

Serve: 3 | Total Time: 25 minutes

4 lamb chops
½ bunch fresh mint
4 tbsp olive oil
1 small parsnip
1 large carrot
1 fennel bulb
Salt and pepper, to taste
Fresh rosemary

Chop the mint and rosemary. 4 tbsp olive oil, salt, and pepper to season the marinade. Refrigerate the lamb chops for 3 hours. Cut the veggies into tiny cubes and soak them in water for a few minutes. Preheat the Air Fryer to temperature of 380 degrees F and cook the lamb chops for 2 minutes on each side. Remove the chops from the basket and place the veggies in the bottom. Place the lamb chops on top. Cook for another 6 minutes and then serve hot.

RECIPE 643: GRILLED VIENNA SAUSAGE WITH BROCCOLI

Serve: 4 | Total Time: 55 minutes

1-pound beef Vienna sausage
1/2 cup mayonnaise
1 tsp yellow mustard
1 tbsp fresh lemon juice
1 tsp garlic powder
1/4 tsp black pepper
1-pound broccoli

Start by preheating your Air Fryer to temperature of 380 degrees f. Spritz the grill pan with cooking oil. Cut the sausages into serving sized pieces. Cook the sausages for 15 minutes, shaking the basket occasionally to get all sides browned. Set aside. In the meantime, whisk the mayonnaise with mustard, lemon juice, garlic powder, and black pepper. Toss the broccoli with the mayo mixture. Turn up temperature to 400 degrees f. Cook broccoli for 6 minutes, turning halfway through the cooking time. Serve the sausage with the grilled broccoli on the side. Bon appétit!

RECIPE 644: GROUND PORK AND APPLE BURGERS

Serve: 2 | Total Time: 25 minutes

12 oz ground pork
1 apple, peeled and grated
1 cup breadcrumbs
2 eggs, beaten
½ tsp ground cumin
½ tsp ground cinnamon
Salt and black pepper to taste

Preheat the PowerXL Air Fryer Grill to 360 F on Air Fry function. In a bowl, add pork, apple, breadcrumbs, cumin, eggs, cinnamon, salt, and black pepper; mix with hands. Shape into 4 even-sized burger patties. Grease the PowerXL Air Fryer Grill with oil. Arrange the patties inside the crisper tray and cook for 14 minutes, turning once halfway through. Serve and enjoy!

RECIPE 645: FLAVORFUL AND JUICY GRILLED CHICKEN

Serve: 4 | Total Time: 30 minutes

4 chicken breasts
½ tsp. ground coriander
2 tbsp. olive oil
½ tsp. smoked paprika
1 tsp. ground cumin
1 tsp. garlic powder
¼ tsp. pepper
½ tsp. sea salt

Select grill mode on the Ninja Foodi Smart XL Grill, then set the temperature to medium and set the timer to 12 minutes. Press start to begin preheating. In a small bowl, mix oil, paprika, coriander, cumin, garlic powder, pepper, and salt and rub all over the chicken breasts. Once the unit is preheated it will beep then place chicken breasts on grill grates and close the hood. Cook chicken for 6 minutes then flip chicken and continue cooking for 6 minutes. Serve and enjoy.

RECIPE 646: FRUIT AND VEGETABLE SKEWERS

Serve: 4 | Total Time: 30 minutes

4 tbsp virgin olive oil
3 tbsp. lemon juice
1 garlic clove, minced
2 tbsp. chopped parsley
½ tsp. salt
½ tsp. black pepper
1 sliced zucchini
1 sliced yellow squash
½ red bell pepper
½ cup cherry tomatoes
½ cup pineapple chunks
4 wooden skewers

Combine olive oil, garlic, parsley, lemon juice, pepper, and salt in a mixing bowl. Pour into large resealable plastic bag. Add the zucchini, squash, bell pepper and tomatoes. Refrigerate for at least 1 hour after sealing the bag and shaking it to coat the veggies. Remove vegetables from marinade and thread onto skewers, along with pineapple, alternating each item. Place the skewers on the 4-inch grill. Bake on high power (350 degrees) for 8 mins. Flip the skewers over and cook for another 6-8 mins until the vegetables reach the desired cook level.

RECIPE 647: HAM AND PINEAPPLE SKEWERS

Serve: 2 | Total Time: 25 minutes

8 slices of ham
1/4 cup sour cream

2 tbsp. fresh parsley, chopped.
1 cup Greek yogurt
1/2 cup pineapple chunks
1 tsp. paprika
1 tsp. garlic, minced.
salt and pepper, to taste

To make the yogurt dip: Mix together the sour cream, Greek yogurt, minced garlic and fresh parsley. Set it aside with plenty of salt and pepper. Preheat the Air Fryer to temperature of 400 degrees F. Use the skewers from the Air Fryer Double Layer Rack and skewer the pineapples and ham slices alternately. Season with the paprika, salt and pepper. Place the rack in the Air Fryer Basket and cook for 10 minutes. Remove the skewers from the rack and drizzle over with the yogurt dip. Serve and enjoy!

RECIPE 648: HEALTHY FLAPJACKS

Serve: 4 | Total Time: 20 minutes

4 oz butter
10 oz gluten free oats
4 oz brown sugar
2 tbsp honey

Place the baking pan on top of the Air Fryer grill pan and ensure that it slots in place inside the Air Fryer. Dice the butter into quarters and transfer them onto the baking pan. Allow cooking for 2 minutes at 360 F or until you have the butter melted. Blend the gluten-free oats in the blender until they appear like breadcrumbs. Combine the brown sugar and the honey, and finally the oats. Mix well with a fork until you have a smooth mixture. Allow cooking for 10 minutes at 320 F. Raise the temperature to 360 F and allow cooking for an extra 5 minutes. Withdraw and serve.

RECIPE 649: HERBY TOMATO MEATLOAF

Serve: 4 | Total Time: 30 minutes

1 lb ground beef

2 eggs, lightly beaten
½ cup breadcrumbs
2 garlic cloves, crushed
1 onion, finely chopped
2 tbsp tomato puree
1 tsp mixed dried herbs

Preheat the PowerXL Air Fryer Grill to 380 F on Bake function. Line a loaf pan that fits in your fryer with baking paper. In a bowl, mix beef, eggs, breadcrumbs, garlic, onion, puree, and herbs. Gently press the mixture into the pan and slide in the PowerXL Air Fryer Grill. Cook for 25 minutes. If undercooked and slightly moist, cook for 5 more minutes. Wait 15 minutes before slicing it.Serve and enjoy!

RECIPE 650: HONEY GLAZED PINEAPPLE FRIES

Serve: 2 | Total Time: 25 minutes

4 oz. fresh pineapple
2 tsp cinnamon
2 tbsp honey

Chip the peeled pineapple into chunky chip sizes. Arrange the fries in the grill pan placed in your Air Fryer. Maintain a long neat row, without gaps. Allow cooking in the Air Fryer for 390 F for 3 minutes. Turn the fries over using thongs and allow cooking for another 3 minutes at 390 F. Withdraw the grill pan and sprinkle the pineapple fries with cinnamon, before glazing them with honey using a pastry brush. Serve immediately while warm.

RECIPE 651: HONEY-LUSCIOUS ASPARAGUS

Serve: 4 | Total Time: 25 minutes

2 pounds asparagus, trimmed
4 tbsp tarragon, minced
¼ cup honey
2 tbsp olive oil
1 tsp salt
½ tsp pepper

Add asparagus, oil, salt, honey, pepper, tarragon into a mixing bowl. Toss them well. Pre-heat Ninja Foodi by pressing the "GRILL" option and setting it to "MED." Set the timer to 8 minutes. Let it pre-heat until you hear a beep. Arrange asparagus over grill grate and lock lid. Cook for 4 minutes. Flip the asparagus and cook for 4 minutes more. Serve and enjoy!

RECIPE 652: HORSERADISH MAYO AND GORGONZOLA MUSHROOMS

Serve: 5 | Total Time: 25 minutes

½ cup of breadcrumbs
2 cloves garlic, pressed
2 tbsp. fresh coriander, chopped
1/3 tsp. kosher salt
½ tsp. crushed red pepper flakes
1 ½ tbsp. olive oil
2 medium-sized mushrooms, stems removed
½ cup Gorgonzola cheese, grated
¼ cup low-fat mayonnaise
1 tsp. horseradish, well-drained
1 tbsp. fresh parsley, finely chopped
Combine the breadcrumbs together with garlic, coriander, salt, red pepper, and olive oil. Take equal-sized amounts of the bread crumb mixture and use them to stuff the mushroom caps. Add the grated Gorgonzola on top of each. Put the mushrooms in the Air Fryer grill pan and transfer them to the fryer. Grill them at 380°F for 8–12 minutes, ensuring the stuffing is warm throughout. In the meantime, prepare the horseradish mayo. Mix together the mayonnaise, horseradish, and parsley. When the mushrooms are ready, serve with the mayo.

RECIPE 653: HOT PAPRIKA POTATO WEDGES

Serve: 6 | Total Time: 30 minutes

26 oz large waxy potatoes, cut into wedges
2 tbsp olive oil
2 tsp smoked paprika

2 tbsp sriracha hot chili sauce
½ cup Greek yogurt

Soak potatoes under cold water for 30 minutes; pat dry with a towel. Preheat the PowerXL Air Fryer Grill to 360 F on Air Fry function. Coat potatoes with oil and paprika. Cook them for 20 minutes, shaking once halfway through. Remove to a paper to let them dry.Season with salt and pepper. Serve with the yogurt and chili sauce on the side.

RECIPE 654: INDIAN MEATBALL WITH LAMB

Serve: 8 | Total Time: 24 minutes

1 lb. ground lamb
1 garlic clove, minced
1 egg
1 tbsp. butter
4 oz. chive stems, grated
1/4 tbsp. turmeric
1/3 tsp. cayenne pepper
1/4 tsp. bay leaf
1 tsp. ground coriander
1 tsp. salt
1 tsp. ground black pepper

Combine all of the listed above ingredients in a mixing bowl. Preheat the PowerXL Air Fryer by selecting the air fry mode. Adjust the temperature to 390°F and set Time to 5 minutes. Put the butter in the Air Fryer baking tray and melt it. Form the meatballs. Place them in the Air Fryer baking tray. Transfer to the PowerXL Air Fryer Grill. Cook the dish for 14 minutes. Stir the meatballs twice during the cooking.

RECIPE 655: ITALIAN CHICKEN MARSALA

Serve: 2 | Total Time: 35 minutes

4 chicken thighs
1 cup button mushrooms, sliced.
1/2 cup marsala wine
1/8 cup all-purpose flour
½ tsp. dried oregano
salt and pepper, to taste

Attach the Air Fryer Grill Pan and preheat the Air Fryer to 400

degrees F. Mix together the flour, salt, pepper and oregano. Coat the chicken in the flour mix and arrange them on the Air Fryer Grill Pan. Spray the chicken with some cooking spray and cook for 20 minutes. Add the mushrooms and marsala wine to the Air Fryer Grill Pan and cook for 10 more minutes. Serve and enjoy!

RECIPE 656: JUICY BONELESS BBQ RIBS

Serve: 3 | Total Time: 90 minutes

500 g beef sirloin
1 tbsp garlic powder
1 tbsp onion powder
50 ml smoky barbecue sauce
2 tbsp chili powder
1 tbsp yellow mustard
50 ml of melted apricot jam

Don't cut the loin lengthways. As a result, they may be opened like a book. Then tap until it is evenly thick. Now cut the loin halfway and leave a gap of 2.5 cm. So it resembles a piece of rib. Mix all the spices and distribute evenly over the meat. In the meantime, distribute the sauce with the mustard and the melted jam well. Use about 2 tbsp of the sauce to coat the loin. Set aside the legal sauce. Grill the BBQ ribs at 150 degrees for about 60-90 minutes.

RECIPE 657: KALE AND CHEESE SANDWICHES

Serve: 2 | Total Time: 25 minutes

1 ½ cups chopped kale
2 garlic cloves, sliced
2 tsp olive oil
2 slices Gruyère cheese
4 bread slices
1 dill pickle, sliced

Preheat Air Fryer to 400°F. Toss the kale, garlic, and some olive oil in a baking pan, then put the pan in the Air Fryer. Air Fry for 4-5 minutes until the kale is soft, making sure to stir at least once during cooking. Divide kale between two slices of bread and top with cheese and pickle slices, making 2 sandwiches. Spritz the outside of the bread slices with the remaining olive oil. Grill in the Air Fryer for 6-8 minutes, flipping once until the bread is browned and the cheese is melted. Serve warm.

RECIPE 658: LAMB GYRO

Serve: 4 | Total Time: 35 minutes

1-pound ground lamb
1/2 onion sliced
1/4 cup mint, minced
1/4 red onion, minced
1/8 tsp. rosemary
1/2 tsp. salt
1/2 tsp. black pepper
3/4 cup hummus
4 slices pita bread
1/2 cucumber, sliced into thin rounds
1 cup romaine lettuce, shredded
1 Roma tomato, diced
1/4 cup parsley, minced
2 cloves garlic, minced
12 mint leaves, minced

Preheat the PowerXL Air Fryer Grill by selecting broil mode. Adjust the temperature to temperature of 370°F, set Time to 5 minutes. Mix lamb with onions, mint, parsley, garlic, salt, rosemary, and pepper. Form into patties. Arrange in a lined Air Fryer baking tray. Transfer to the PowerXL Air Fryer Grill. Cook for 20 minutes in the air, flipping halfway through. Assemble the gyro with the remaining ingredients. Serve and enjoy.

RECIPE 659: LAMB MEATBALLS

Serve: 12 | Total Time: 30 minutes

1 lb. ground lamb
1/2 cup breadcrumbs
1 lemon, juiced and zested
1/4 cup milk
2 egg yolks
1 tsp. ground cumin
1 tsp. dried oregano
1/2 tsp. salt

1 tsp. ground coriander
1/2 tsp. black pepper
3 garlic cloves, minced
1/4 cup fresh parsley, chopped
1/2 cup crumbled feta cheese

Preheat the PowerXL Air Fryer Grill by selecting Broil mode. Adjust the temperature to 390°F, set Time to 5 minutes. Combine all the ingredients in a bowl. Form into 12 balls. Arrange on the Air Fryer baking tray. Transfer to the PowerXL Air Fryer Grill. Cook for 12 minutes. Serve and enjoy.

RECIPE 660: LEGS OF GOOSE WRAPPED IN BACON WITH PARSNIPS

Serve: 2 | Total Time: 60 minutes

2 goose legs
500 g parsnips
300 g thinly sliced pork belly
olive oil
1 pinch of whole caraway seeds
½ tsp paprika powder
½ tsp dried thyme
½ tsp peppercorns
½ coriander seeds
pepper and salt

Release the goose legs on the left and right of the bone and brush with olive oil. Clarified butter can also be used. Crush all the spices in a mortar and rub the goose legs with them. Remove the ends of the parsnips, peel and cut into 3 cm thick wedges and wrap with bacon. Then spread on the grill cup of the Air Fryer. Roast the goose legs at 160 degrees for 20 to 25 minutes, turn them once and cook for another 20 minutes. Check the cooking point. The parsnips wrapped in bacon can now be served with the goose legs and a salad.

RECIPE 661: LEG OF LAMB WITH SMOKED PAPRIKA

Serve: 6 | Total Time: 50 minutes

3 pounds lamb leg, bones removed
2 garlic cloves

1 tsp ground smoked paprika
2 tbsp dried oregano
1garlic clove, minced
2 tbsp olive oil
Salt and pepper to taste
Juice of 1 lemon

Preheat your Air Fryer machine to 134 degrees F. Prepare the seasoning: whisk together the minced garlic, olive oil, smoked paprika, salt, pepper, and oregano. Spread the mixture evenly over the lamb. Put the lamb into the bag, remove the air and cook for 10 hours. When the time is up, place the lamb under the preheated grill for 4-5 minutes just until it becomes crispy. Slice the cooked lamb and serve it sprinkled with lemon juice.

RECIPE 662: LEMON GRILLED CHICKEN

Serve: 2 | Total Time: 95 minutes

2 chicken breast fillets
4 lemon slices
2 tbsp. lemon juice
2 tbsp. fresh thyme, chopped.
2 tbsp. olive oil
salt and pepper, to taste

Marinate the chicken in the lemon juice, olive oil, thyme, salt and pepper for 3 hours. Attach the Air Fryer Grill Pan and preheat the Air Fryer to 350 degrees F. Place the chicken breasts on the Air Fryer Grill Pan and cook for 20 minutes. Flip the chicken and top with the lemon slices. Cook for 10 more minutes or until the chicken is cooked through. Serve and enjoy!

RECIPE 663: LEMON LAMB RACK

Serve: 4 | Total Time: 40 minutes

1/4 cup olive oil
3 tbsp. garlic, minced
1/3 cup dry white wine
1 tbsp. lemon zest, grated
2 tbsp. lemon juice
1-1/2 tsp. dried oregano, crushed
1 tsp. thyme leaves, minced
Salt and black pepper
4 lamb rack

1 lemon, sliced

Preheat the PowerXL Air Fryer Grill by selecting Air Fryer mode. Adjust the temperature to a heat of 370°F, set Time to 5 minutes. Whisk all the ingredients together in a bowl. Pour into Air Fryer baking tray. Add the lamb rack. Top with lemon. Transfer to the PowerXL Air Fryer Grill. Air fry for 30 minutes, flipping halfway through. Serve and enjoy.

RECIPE 664: LEMON PEPPER CHICKEN

Serve: 6 | Total Time: 41 minutes

6 chicken breast, boneless
2 lemon juice
½ onion, diced
2 tsp. garlic, minced
½ cup olive oil
1 tsp. pepper
1 tsp. salt

Add all ingredients except chicken into the zip-lock bag and mix well. Add chicken into the bag, seal bag shakes well, and place in the refrigerator overnight. Select grill mode on the Ninja Foodi Smart XL Grill, then set the temperature to medium and set the timer to 20 minutes. Press start to begin preheating. Once the unit is preheated it will beep then place marinated chicken on grill grates and close the hood. Cook chicken for 20 minutes. Flip chicken after every 5 minutes. Serve and enjoy.

RECIPE 665: LEMON PEPPER SHRIMP

Serve: 6 | Total Time: 22 minutes

10 large Shrimps
2 tbsp of Vegetable oil, avocado
1 tbsp of Lemon pepper seasoning

Coat the shrimp with vegetable oil and lemon pepper seasoning Rub it all well. Next, insert the grill grate in the Ninja Foodi Smart XL Grill and select the grill function. Remember to grease the grill grate

with oil spray. Set the time to MAX for 8 minutes, buy selecting grill function. Select start to begin preheating. Once the unit is preheated add the fish to the grill grate and close the hood Grill at MAX for 10 minutes. Flipping the shrimp is not necessary. Once done, serve.

RECIPE 666: MAPLE GLAZED SAUSAGES AND FIGS

Serve: 2 | Total Time: 50 minutes

2 tbsp. maple syrup
2 tbsp. balsamic vinegar
2 packages (12 ounces each) fully cooked chicken, cooked garlic sausages
8 fully ripe fresh figs, cut lengthwise
1/2 large sweet onion, minced
1-1/2 lb. Swiss chard, with sliced stems, minced leaves
2 tsp. olive oil
Salt and pepper

Preheat the PowerXL Air Fryer Grill to 232°C or 450°F, mix syrup with 1 tbsp. vinegar in a tiny bowl. Put sausages with figs on a one-layer foil-lined oven tray. Roast for 8–10 minutes by grazing the syrup mix throughout the cooking. Cook the onions in the PowerXL Air Fryer Grill in a bowl with wrapping for 9 minutes. Mix oil and seasoning with 1 tsp. of vinegar. Serve the chards with figs and sausages.

RECIPE 667: MARINATED BEEF BBQ

Serve: 4 | Total Time: 70 minutes

2 pounds beef steak, pounded
¼ cup bourbon
1 tbsp Worcestershire sauce
¼ cup barbecue sauce
Salt and pepper

Place all of the listed above ingredients in a medium-sized Ziploc bag and chill for 60 minutes. Preheat the oven to 390 degrees F. Place the beef steak on

the grill pan and cook for twenty mins per batch. Halfway through the cook time, give a stir to cook evenly. Meanwhile, pour the marinade over saucepan and simmer until sauce stars to thicken. Serve beef with the bourbon sauce.

RECIPE 668: MARSHMALLOW AND BANANA BOATS

Serve: 6 | Total Time: 25 minutes

4 ripe bananas
1 cup mini marshmallows
1/2 cup of chocolate chips
1/2 cup peanut butter chips
Slice a banana lengthwise, keeping its peel. Make sure you don't go all the way through the process. Use your hands to open banana peel like a book, revealing the inside of a banana. Divide marshmallow, chocolate chips, peanut butter among bananas, stuffing them inside. Pre-heat Ninja Foodi by pressing the "GRILL" option and setting it to "MEDIUM" and timer to 6 minutes. Let it pre-heat until you hear a beep. Transfer banana to Grill Grate and lock lid, cook for 4-6 minutes until chocolate melts and bananas are toasted. Serve and enjoy!

RECIPE 669: MAYONNAISE AND ROSEMARY GRILLED STEAK

Serve: 4 | Total Time: 20 minutes

1 cup mayonnaise
1 tbsp fresh rosemary, finely chopped
2 tbsp Worcestershire sauce
Sea salt, to taste
1/2 tsp ground black pepper
1 tsp smoked paprika
1 tsp garlic, minced
1 ½ pounds short loin steak

Combine the mayonnaise, rosemary, Worcestershire sauce, salt, pepper, paprika, and garlic; mix to combine well. Now, brush the mayonnaise mixture over both sides of the steak. Lower the steak onto the grill pan. Grill in the preheated Air Fryer at 390 degrees

F for 8 minutes. Turn the steaks over and grill an additional 7 minutes. Check for doneness with a meat thermometer. Serve warm and enjoy!

RECIPE 670: MEXICAN CHICKEN LASAGNA

Serve: 15 | Total Time: 25 minutes

1 1/2 lb. chicken breast, shredded
3/4 cup sour cream
2 cup cheese, shredded
4 tortillas
1 tsp. dry onion, minced
2 tsp. ground cumin
2 tbsp. chili powder
1 cup salsa

Mix together chicken, dried onion, cumin, chili powder, salsa, and sour cream. Spread half chicken mixture in a baking dish then place 2 tortillas on top. Sprinkle 1/2 cheese over the tortillas then repeat the layers. Place the inner pot in the PowerXL grill Air Fryer combo base. Place the baking dish into the inner pot. Cover the inner pot with an air frying lid. Set the oven to bake mode at 390°F for 15 minutes. Press start. When the Timer reaches 0, then press the cancel button. Serve and enjoy.

RECIPE 671: MEXICAN CORN DISH

Serve: 4 | Total Time: 23 minutes

2 tbsp lime juice
½ cup mayonnaise
½ cup sour cream
2 tsp garlic powder
2 tsp onion powder
1 and ¼ cups Cotija cheese, crumbled
Salt and pepper to taste
3 tbsp canola oil
6 ears corn

Set your Ninja Foodi Smart XL to grill mode, set temperature to MAX, and timer to 12 minutes. Let it preheat until you hear a beep. Brush the corn ears with oil, season with salt and pepper. Transfer to grill and cook for 6

minutes per side. Take a bowl and mix in the remaining ingredients; mix well. Cover corn mix and serve. Enjoy!

RECIPE 672: MORNING MINI CHEESEBURGER SLIDERS

Serve: 4 | Total Time: 15 minutes

1 lb. ground beef
6 slices cheddar cheese
6 dinner rolls
Salt and Black pepper

Adjust the Air Fryer to 390 °F. Form 6 beef patties (each about 2.5 oz.) and season with salt and black pepper. Add the burger patties to the cooking basket and cook them for 10 minutes. Remove the burger patties from the Air Fryer; place the cheese on top of the burgers and return to the Air Fryer and cook for another minute. Remove and put burgers on dinner rolls and serve warm.

RECIPE 673: MOZZARELLA AND SMOKED FISH TART

Serve: 5 | Total Time: 35 minutes

1 quiche pastry case
5 eggs, lightly beaten
4 tbsp heavy cream
¼ cup finely chopped green onions
¼ cup chopped parsley
1 tsp baking powder
Salt and black pepper
1 lb smoked fish
1 cup shredded mozzarella cheese

Preheat the PowerXL Air Fryer Grill to 360 F on Bake function. In a bowl, whisk eggs, cream, scallions, parsley, baking powder, salt, and black pepper. Add in fish and cheese, stir to combine. Line the crisper tray with baking paper. Pour the mixture into the pastry case and place it gently inside the PowerXL Air Fryer Grill. Cook for 25 minutes. Check past 15 minutes, so it's not overcooked.

RECIPE 674: MUSTARD AND VEGGIE

Serve: 4 | Total Time: 50 minutes

Vinaigrette
½ cup olive oil
½ cup avocado oil
¼ tsp pepper
1 tsp salt
2 tbsp honey
½ cup red wine vinegar
2 tbsp Dijon vinegar

Veggies
4 zucchinis, halved
4 sweet onion, quartered
4 red pepper, seeded and halved
2 bunch green onions, trimmed
4 yellow squash, cut in half

Take a small bowl and whisk in mustard, honey, vinegar, salt, and pepper. Add oil and mix well. Set your Ninja Foodi Smart XL Grill to GRILL mode and MED setting, set timer to 10 minutes. Transfer onion quarter to Grill Grate, cook for 5 minutes. Flip and cook for 5 minutes more. Grill remaining veggies in the same way, giving 7 minutes per side for zucchini and 1 minute for green onions. Serve with mustard vinaigrette on top. Enjoy!

RECIPE 675: MUSTARD FISH MANIA

Serve: 5 | Total Time: 23 minutes

1 cup soft bread crumbs
1 tsp whole-grain mustard
2 cans canned fish
2 celery stalks, chopped
1 egg, whisked
1/2 tsp sea salt
¼ tsp black peppercorns, cracked
1 tsp paprika

In a bowl of large size, thoroughly mix the fish, breadcrumbs, celery and other ingredients. Make four cakes shapes from them and refrigerate for 45-50 minutes. Place your Air Fryer on a flat kitchen surface; plug it and turn it on. Set temperature to 360 degrees F and let it preheat for 4-5 minutes. Take out the air-frying grill pan and gently coat it using a cooking oil or spray. Add the cakes to the pan and add the pan to the basket. Push the air-frying basket in the Air Fryer. Cook for 5 minutes. Slide out the basket; flip and cook for 3-4 minutes. Serve over mashed potatoes.

RECIPE 676: NUGGET AND VEGGIE TACO WRAPS

Serve: 4 | Total Time: 20 minutes

1 tbsp water
4 pieces commercial vegan nuggets, chopped
1 small yellow onion, diced
1 small red bell pepper, chopped
2 cobs grilled corn kernels
4 large corn tortillas
Mixed greens, for garnish

Preheat the Air Fryer to temperature of 400°F (204°C). Over a medium heat, sauté the nuggets in the water with the onion, corn kernels and bell pepper in a skillet, then remove from the heat. Fold the tortillas up after filling them with the nuggets and veggies. Air fried for 15 minutes after transferring to the interior of the fryer. Serve immediately, topped with mixed greens once crispy.

RECIPE 677: OREGANO CHICKEN LEGS WITH LEMON

Serve: 5 | Total Time: 50 minutes

5 quarters chicken legs
2 lemons, halved
5 tbsp garlic powder
5 tbsp dried basil
5 tbsp oregano, dried
½ cup olive oil
Salt and black pepper

Preheat the PowerXL Air Fryer Grill to 400 F on Roast function. In a big, deep bowl, place the chicken. Brush the chicken legs with a tbsp of olive oil. Sprinkle with the lemon juice and arrange in the oven. In another bowl, combine

basil, oregano, garlic powder, salt, and pepper. Sprinkle the seasoning mixture on the chicken. Cook in the oven for 50 minutes, shaking every 10-15 minutes. Serve and enjoy!

RECIPE 678: ORIGINAL GRILLED CHEESE SANDWICHES

Serve: 2 | Total Time: 15 minutes

¼ cup sliced roasted red peppers
¼ cup Alfredo sauce
4 bread slices
¼ cup mozzarella cheese
3 tbsp sliced red onions

Preheat Air Fryer to 400°F. Lay 2 bread slices on a flat surface, spread some Alfredo sauce on one side, and place them in frying the basket. Scatter with mozzarella cheese, roasted peppers, and red onion. Drizzle with the remaining Alfredo sauce and top with the remaining bread slices. Grill for 4 minutes, turn the sandwiches, and Grill for 3 more minutes until toasted. Serve warm.

RECIPE 679: OUTSTANDING RACK OF LAMB

Serve: 2 | Total Time: 15 minutes

2 racks of lamb
¼ cup of freshly chopped parsley
4 cloves of minced garlic
2 tbsp of olive oil
2 tbsp of honey
1 tsp of salt
1 tsp of black pepper

Preheat your Air Fryer to temperature of 390 degrees Fahrenheit. Using a blender or food processor, add the parsley, garlic cloves, olive oil, honey, salt, and black pepper and blend it until it gets totally grounded. Rub the grounded parsley-garlic on the lamb racks, without using them all as you will need them later. Put the grill pan accessory into your Air Fryer, and place the lamb racks on top. Cook it for 15 minutes at a 390 degrees Fahrenheit or until it

gets brown in color. Spread another layer of the puree on the lamb racks. Serve and enjoy!

RECIPE 680: OYSTER CHICKEN BREASTS

Serve: 2 | Total Time: 60 minutes

2 chicken breasts
1 tbsp minced ginger
2 rosemary sprigs
½ lemon, cut into wedges
1 tbsp soy sauce
½ tbsp olive oil
1 tbsp oyster sauce
3 tbsp brown sugar

Add the ginger, soy sauce, and olive oil to a bowl. Add the chicken and toss to coat well. Refrigerate for 30 minutes after covering the bowl. Preheat the Air Fryer to 370 F on Bake function. Cook for 6 minutes after transferring the marinated chicken to a baking tray. Meanwhile, mix the oyster sauce, rosemary, and brown sugar in a small bowl. Pour the sauce over the chicken. Arrange the lemon wedges in the dish. Return to oven for 13 minutes. Serve and enjoy!

RECIPE 681: PAPRIKA AND PICKLES FRITTERS

Serve: 2 | Total Time: 15 minutes

8 medium pickles
1 egg, beaten
½ cup breadcrumbs
1 tsp paprika
4 tbsp flour
1 tbsp olive oil
Salt, to taste

Preheat the PowerXL Air Fryer Grill to 400 F on Air Fry function. Cut the pickles lengthwise; pat them dry. In a medium-sized mixing bowl, combine the paprika, and salt together with the flour. In another bowl, combine the breadcrumbs and olive oil. Dredge in the flour first, dip them in the beaten egg, and then coat them with the crumbs. Arrange on a lined baking sheet and place in the PowerXL Air Fryer Grill. Cook for 10 minutes. Serve and enjoy!

RECIPE 682: PAPRIKA GRILLED SHRIMP

Serve: 24 | Total Time: 15 minutes

1-pound jumbo shrimps, peeled and deveined
2 tbsp brown sugar
1 tbsp paprika
1 tbsp garlic powder
2 tbsp olive oil
1 tsp garlic salt
½ tsp black pepper

Add listed ingredients into a mixing bowl. Mix them well. Let it chill and marinate for 30-60 minutes. Pre-heat Ninja Foodi by pressing the "GRILL" option and setting it to "MED." Set the timer to 6 minutes. Let it pre-heat until you hear a beep. Arrange prepared shrimps over the grill grate. Lock lid and cook for 3 minutes. Then turn and cook for another 3 minutes. Serve and enjoy!

RECIPE 683: PEPPERONI GRILLED CHEESE

Serve: 3 | Total Time: 18 minutes

6 pieces of bread
6 pieces mozzarella cheese
1 package pepperoni, sliced
3 tbsp butter
1 tbsp garlic powder
1 tbsp Italian seasoning

In a mixing bowl, mix butter, garlic, parsley, and Italian seasoning. Spread the butter mixture on one side of the bread slice. Add a piece of cheese and 12 slices of pepperoni slices on top. Place another cheese piece on top and another slice of a buttered piece of bread. Repeat the process with the remaining bread slices. Set the temperature at 360oF and cook the bread for 8 minutes flipping the sandwich halfway through the cooking process. Serve and enjoy.

RECIPE 684: PERFECT FILLET OF BEEF

Serve: 2 | Total Time: 30 minutes

1 Beef
2 Garlic cloves
3 Rosemary
7 mushrooms
2 spring onions
Oil for frying
Salt and pepper

Unpack the beef fillet and pat it dry, then seal it with the rosemary and peeled garlic in a vacuum bag. Place the bag in the Air Fryer bath at 53 - 54 ° C. The meat stays here for 2 hours. Clean the mushrooms and spring onions and cut them into pieces. When the meat comes out of the bath, you can start preparing the side dish so that it still has a bite and is not completely overcooked. Take the meat out of the bag and grill on the grill using the flip-flip. Turn every 20 - 30 seconds until a nice crust has formed. Fry the mushrooms and spring onions for about 5 - 10 minutes in the hot pan and season with just a little pepper and salt.

RECIPE 685: PINEAPPLE AND VEGGIE SOUVLAKI

Serve: 4 | Total Time: 35 minutes

1 (15-oz) can pineapple rings in pineapple juice
1 red bell pepper, stemmed and seeded
1/3 cup butter
2 tbsp apple cider vinegar
2 tbsp hot sauce
1 tbsp allspice
1 tsp ground nutmeg
16 oz feta cheese
1 red onion, peeled
8 mushrooms, quartered

Preheat Air Fryer to 400°F. Whisk the butter, pineapple juice, apple vinegar, hot sauce, allspice, and nutmeg until smooth. Set aside. Slice feta cheese into 16 cubes, then the bell pepper into 16 chunks, and finally red onion into 8 wedges, separating each wedge

into 2 pieces. Cut pineapple ring into quarters. Place veggie cubes and feta into the butter bowl and toss to coat. Thread the veggies, tofu, and pineapple onto 8 skewers, alternating 16 pieces on each skewer. Grill for 15 minutes until golden brown and cooked. Serve warm.

RECIPE 686: PINEAPPLE FISH FILLET

Serve: 2 | Total Time: 24 minutes

1 tsp of Chili powder as needed
1/ 2 cup cilantro leaves, chopped
1 tbsp lime juice
Salt and black pepper to taste
½ tbsp canola oil
2 fillet salmon, 6-8 ounces
2 tbsp of pineapple juice, fresh squeezed
1 cup grilled pineapple slices

Take a blender and pulse cilantro with canola oil. Add salt and black pepper. The lime juice, chile powder, and pineapple juice are then added. Now rub the fillet with the blended mixture. Pre-heat your Ninja Foodi Smart XL Grill to MAX set a timer to 15 minutes. Once preheating done, grill the fillets and grill for 8 minutes. Once done serve it with grilled pineapple.

RECIPE 687: PIZZA MARGHERITA WITH SPINACH

Serve: 4 | Total Time: 50 minutes

½ cup pizza sauce
1 tsp dried oregano
1 tsp garlic powder
1 pizza dough
1 cup baby spinach
½ cup mozzarella cheese

Preheat Air Fryer to 400°F. Whisk pizza sauce, oregano, and garlic in a bowl. Set aside. Form 4 balls with the pizza dough and roll out each into a 6-inch round pizza. Lay one crust in the basket, spread ¼ of the sauce, then scatter with ¼ of spinach, and finally top with mozzarella cheese. Grill for 8 minutes until golden brown and the crust is crispy. Repeat the process with the remaining crusts. Serve immediately.

RECIPE 688: PORK AND FRUIT KEBABS

Serve: 4 | Total Time: 25 minutes

1/3 cup apricot jam
2 tbsp freshly squeezed lemon juice
2 tsp olive oil
½ tsp dried tarragon
1 lbs pork tenderloin, 1-inch cubes
4 plums, pitted and quartered
4 small apricots, pitted and halved

Mix jam, lemon juice, olive oil, and tarragon. Stir in the meat. 10 minutes at room temperature. Alternating the items, thread the pork, plums, and apricots onto 4 metal skewers that fit into the Air Fryer. Brush with any remaining jam mixture. Discard any remaining marinade. In the Air Fryer, grill the kebabs for 9 to 12 minutes, or until the pork thermometer reads 145°F and the fruit is soft. Serve immediately.

RECIPE 689: PORK AND MIXED GREENS SALAD

Serve: 4 | Total Time: 25 minutes

2 lbs pork tenderloin, 1-inch slices
1 tsp olive oil
1 tsp dried marjoram
1/8 tsp freshly ground black pepper
6 cups mixed salad greens
1 red bell pepper, sliced
1 (8-ounce) package button mushrooms, sliced
1/3 cup low-sodium low-fat vinaigrette dressing

In a medium bowl, mix the pork slices and olive oil. Toss to coat. Sprinkle with the marjoram and pepper and rub these into the pork. Grill the pork in the Air Fryer for 4-6 minutes each batch, or until it registers 145°F on a meat thermometer. Meanwhile, in a

serving bowl, mix the salad greens, red bell pepper, and mushrooms. Toss gently. When the pork is cooked, add the slices to the salad. Drizzle with the vinaigrette and toss gently. Serve immediately.

RECIPE 690: PORK BALLS

Serve: 10 | Total Time: 45 minutes

10 ounces pork meat, minced
1 egg
1 tbsp light soy sauce
2 tsp sugar
2 tsp oyster sauce
½ tsp five-spice powder
1 tsp sesame oil
1 tbsp cornstarch
½ cup cornstarch, for coating

Combine minced pork meat with all seasonings and egg. Use a fork to mix them well. Use a tbsp to scope and shape into a ball. Lightly coat the meat ball with corn starch. Repeat step till all are done. Let coated meat balls rest and air dry for 15 minutes. Place meat balls on its non-stick grill pan or lined the basket with greased baking paper. Air fry at 392°F (200°C) for 20 minutes. When halfway air-frying, open the Air Fryer, drizzle some oil on the half done meat balls and flip them over to continue air-fry till crisped and golden browned.

RECIPE 691: PORK BURGERS WITH RED CABBAGE SALAD

Serve: 4 | Total Time: 29 minutes

½ cup greek yogurt
2 tbsp low-sodium mustard, paprika
1 tbsp lemon juice
¼ cup red cabbage, carrots
1-pound lean ground pork

Combine the yogurt, 1 tbsp mustard, lemon juice, cabbage, and carrots; mix and refrigerate. Mix the pork, remaining 1 tbsp mustard, and paprika. Form into 8 small patties. In the Air Fryer basket, place the sliders. Grill the

sliders until they reach 165°F on a meat thermometer. Assemble the burgers by putting some lettuce leaves on the bottom of a bun. A tomato slice, the patties, and the cabbage mixture go on top. Serve immediately with the bun top.

RECIPE 692: PORK CHOPS IN CREAM

Serve: 4 | Total Time: 25 minutes

4 pork chops, center-cut
2 tbsp flour
2 tbsp sour cream
Salt and black pepper
½ cup breadcrumbs

Preheat the PowerXL Air Fryer Grill to 400 F on Air Fry function. Coat the chops with flour. Drizzle the cream over and rub gently to coat well. Spread the breadcrumbs onto a bowl, and coat each pork chop with crumbs. Spray the chops with oil and arrange them in the basket of your PowerXL Air Fryer Grill. Cook for 14 minutes, turning once halfway through. Serve with salad, slaw or potatoes.

RECIPE 693: PORK RATATOUILLE

Serve: 4 | Total Time: 40 minutes

4 pork sausages

For Ratatouille:
pepper, chopped
15 oz. tomatoes, chopped
2 zucchinis, chopped
1 red chili, chopped
1 eggplant, chopped
2 sprigs fresh thyme
1 medium red onion, chopped
1 tbsp. balsamic vinegar
2 garlic cloves, minced

Preheat the PowerXL Air Fryer Grill by selecting pizza/bake mode. Adjust temperature to 392°F and Time to 10 minutes. Combine zucchini, eggplant, onions, and oil in the cooking tray. Transfer to the PowerXL Air Fryer Grill, bake for 20 minutes. Remove and add the remaining Ratatouille Ingredients.

Transfer to the PowerXL Air Fryer Grill and cook for an additional 20 minutes. Remove and season with salt and pepper. Add the sausage to the Pizza tray. Cook for 15 minutes, flipping halfway. Serve and enjoy.

RECIPE 694: PORK RIND NACHOS

Serve: 2 | Total Time: 10 minutes

1-ounce of pork rinds
4 ounces of shredded cooked chicken
1/2 cup of shredded Monterey jack cheese
1/4 cup of sliced pickled jalapeños
1/4 cup of guacamole
1/4 cup of full-Fat: sour cream

Put pork rinds in a 6 "round baking pan. Fill with grilled chicken and Monterey cheese jack. Place the pan in the basket with the Air Fryer. Set the temperature to 370° F and set the timer for 5 minutes or until the cheese has been melted. Eat right away with jalapeños, guacamole, and sour cream. Enjoy!

RECIPE 695: POTATO AND VEGETABLE STRUDEL

Serve: 4 | Total Time: 35 minutes

50 g broccoli
50 g carrots
50 g peas
250 g potatoes cooked floury
100 g cream cheese with herbs
Fresh herbs
1 egg
pepper and salt
2 strudel sheets (finished product)
Milk for brushing

Cut the broccoli up to mouth size and dice the peeled carrots, cook the vegetables and peas in boiling salted water until al dente. Meanwhile, wash and cut the herbs coarsely. Mix well the already cooked potatoes with the egg, the herbs, pepper and salt and the cream cheese. Now spread out the strudel leaves and place them on the grill cup, brush with the potato mixture and spread the vegetables evenly over the top. Then make a solid roll out of it and brush it with the milk. Bake at 180 degrees in the Air Fryer for about 30 minutes until golden yellow.

RECIPE 696: POTATOES WITH COTTAGE CHEESE

Serve: 3 | Total Time: 50 minutes

4 medium potatoes, cubed, skin shells reserved
1 bunch asparagus, trimmed
¼ cup fresh cream
¼ cup cottage cheese, cubed
1 tbsp wholegrain mustard

Preheat the PowerXL Air Fryer Grill to 400 F on Air Fry function. Place the potatoes in the crisper tray and cook for 25 minutes. Boil salted water in a pot over medium heat. Add asparagus and cook for 3 minutes until tender. In a bowl, mix cooked potatoes, cottage cheese, cream, asparagus, and mustard. Toss well and season with salt and black pepper. Transfer the mixture to the potato skin shells and serve.

RECIPE 697: PROSCIUTTO-WRAPPED ASPARAGUS

Serve: 6 | Total Time: 22 minutes

12 spears asparagus, trimmed
2 tsp. olive oil
Salt and ground black pepper, to taste
12 prosciutto slices

Drizzle the asparagus spears with oil and ten, sprinkle with salt and black pepper. Wrap one prosciutto slice around each asparagus spear from top to bottom. Turn the "Temperature Knob" of the PowerXL Air Fryer Grill to line the temperature to 300°F. Turn the "Function Knob" to settle on "Air Fry." Turn the "timer Knob" to line the time for 10 minutes. After preheating, arrange the asparagus spears into the greased air fry basket. Insert the air fry basket at position 2 of the Air Fryer Grill. Flip the asparagus spears once halfway through. When the cooking time is over, transfer the asparagus spears onto a platter. Serve hot.

RECIPE 698: QUICK TUNA TACOS

Serve: 4 | Total Time: 20 minutes

2 cups torn romaine lettuce
1 lb fresh tuna steak, cubed
1 tbsp grated fresh ginger
2 garlic cloves, minced
½ tsp toasted sesame oil
4 tortillas
¼ cup mild salsa
1 red bell pepper, sliced

Preheat Air Fryer to 390°F. Combine the tuna, ginger, garlic, and sesame oil in a bowl and allow to marinate for 10 minutes. Lay the marinated tuna in the fryer and Grill for 4-7 minutes. Serve right away with tortillas, mild salsa, lettuce, and bell pepper for delicious tacos.

RECIPE 699: SPICY HONEY MUSTARD CHICKEN

Serve: 4 | Total Time: 30 minutes

1/3 cup tomato sauce
2 tbsp yellow mustard
2 tbsp apple cider vinegar
1 tbsp honey
2 garlic cloves, minced
1 Fresno pepper, minced
1 tsp onion powder
4 chicken breasts

Preheat Air Fryer to 370°F. Mix the tomato sauce, mustard, apple cider vinegar, honey, garlic, Fresno pepper, and onion powder in a bowl, then use a brush to rub the mix over the chicken breasts. Put the chicken in the Air Fryer and Grill for 10 minutes. Remove it, turn it, and rub with more sauce. Cook further for about 5 minutes. Remove the basket and flip the chicken. Add more sauce, return to the fryer, and cook for 3-5 more minutes or until the chicken is cooked through. Serve warm.

RECIPE 700: QUINOA GREEN PIZZA

Serve: 2 | Total Time: 25 minutes

¾ cup quinoa flour
½ tsp dried basil
½ tsp dried oregano
1 tbsp apple cider vinegar
1/3 cup ricotta cheese
2/3 cup chopped broccoli
½ tsp garlic powder

Preheat the Air Fryer to 350°F. Whisk quinoa flour, basil, oregano, apple cider vinegar, and ½ cup of water until smooth. Set aside. Cut 2 pieces of parchment paper. Place the quinoa mixture on one paper, top with another piece, and flatten to create a crust. Discard the top piece of paper. Bake for 5 minutes, turn and discard the other piece of paper. Spread the ricotta cheese over the crust, scatter with broccoli, and sprinkle with garlic. Grill at a heat of 400°F for 5 minutes until golden brown. Serve warm.

RECIPE 701: RANCH CHICKEN

Serve: 2 | Total Time: 4 hours

3 chicken breasts, skinless and boneless
1 1/2 tbsp. dry ranch seasoning
1 1/2 tbsp. taco seasoning
1/4 cup water
2 garlic cloves, minced

Place the inner pot in the PowerXL grill Air Fryer combo base. Add chicken to the inner pot. In a small bowl, whisk together the remaining ingredients and pour over the chicken. Cover the inner pot with a glass lid. Select slow cook mode then press the temperature button and set the timer for 4 hours. Press start. When the Timer reaches 0, then press the cancel button. Shred the chicken using a fork and serve.

RECIPE 702: ROAST BEEF

Serve: 4 | Total Time: 50 minutes

2.5 pounds beef, for roasting
1 tsp oil
Pepper, to season

Preheat Air Fryer at 320°F (160°C) for approximately 5 minutes. The roast should be mixed with the oil in a mixing dish while the Air Fryer is preheating, so that it is evenly covered with oil. Rub in your seasoning afterwards. Place the seasoned roast in the Air Fryer and cook until done. Set it to 30 minutes and cook at 320°F (160°C). Once done, turn roast over and cook again for another 15 minutes. Serve with onions and potatoes.

RECIPE 703: ROASTED HAMBURGERS

Serve: 6 | Total Time: 25 minutes

1–1/2 tsp. kosher salt
2 lb. ground beef
1 tbsp. Worcestershire sauce
1/2 tsp. freshly ground black pepper
6 toasted hamburger buns
Hamburger toppings

Preheat the PowerXL Air Fryer Grill to 230°C or 450°F, and line a rimmed baking sheet with aluminum foil with some salt to absorb drippings. Season 1–2 inch lumps of meat by hand and split up meat into 6 parts to shape into 3"x1" disks. Place burgers an inch apart on a wire rack and roast for 10–16 minutes at 135°C or 250°F for medium-rare meat.

RECIPE 704: ROASTED PEPPER CHICKEN

Serve: 4 | Total Time: 4 hours

2 lb. chicken breasts, skinless and boneless
3 tbsp. red wine vinegar
1 onion, diced
1/2 cup olives

10 oz. roasted red peppers, drained and chopped
1/2 cup feta cheese, crumbled
1 tsp. dried thyme
1 tsp. dried oregano
1 tbsp. garlic, minced
1 tbsp. olive oil
1/4 tsp. pepper
1/2 tsp. kosher salt

Place the inner pot in the PowerXL grill Air Fryer combo base. Add all ingredients into the inner pot and mix well. A glass lid should be used to cover the inner pot. Select slow cook mode then press the temperature button and set the timer for 4 hours. Press start. When the Timer reaches 0, then press the cancel button. Serve and enjoy.

RECIPE 705: ROASTED PUMPKIN SEEDS

Serve: 4 | Total Time: 30 minutes

1 cup pumpkin seeds, pulp removed, rinsed
1 tbsp butter, melted
1 tbsp brown sugar
1 tsp orange zest
½ tsp cardamom
½ tsp salt

Preheat the PowerXL Air Fryer Grill to 400 F on Bake function. In a bowl, whisk melted butter, sugar, zest, cardamom, and salt. Toss the seeds in the basin. Transfer the seeds to the PowerXL Air Fryer Grill. Cook for 15 minutes, shaking the basket every 10-12 minutes. Cook until lightly browned. Serve and enjoy!

RECIPE 706: SAFFRON SPICED RACK OF LAMB

Serve: 4 | Total Time: 70 minutes

½ tsp crumbled saffron threads
1 cup plain greek yogurt
1 tsp lemon zest
2 cloves of garlic, minced
2 racks of lamb, rib bones frenched
2 tbsp olive oil
Salt and pepper to taste

Preheat the Air Fryer to 3900f. Place the grill pan accessory in the Air Fryer. Season the lamb meat to taste with salt and pepper. Set aside. In a bowl, combine the rest of ingredients. Brush the mixture onto the lamb. Place on the grill pan and cook for 1 hour and 10 minutes.

RECIPE 707: SALMON ASPARAGUS AND HORSERADISH

Serve: 2 | Total Time: 15 minutes

1/4 cup onions, sliced.
1/4 cup horseradish
6 asparagus stalks
2 salmon fillets
4 lemon slices
2 tbsp. olives, sliced.
1 tbsp. lemon juice
2 tbsp. dill
salt and pepper, to taste

Preheat the Air Fryer to temperature of 350 degrees F. Season the asparagus with salt and pepper and place them in the Air Fryer Basket. Attach the Air Fryer Grill Pan to the Air Fryer Basket and place the salmon fillets on the Air Fryer Grill Pan. Season the salmon fillets with the salt, pepper and lemon juice. Cook for 10 minutes with lemon slices on fish. Remove the salmon and asparagus from the Air Fryer. Top the salmon with the horseradish, olives and dill. Serve and enjoy!

RECIPE 708: SALMON IN PUFF PASTRY CROISSANTS

Serve: 6 | Total Time: 35 minutes

200 g smoked salmon
1 package of puff pastry
100 g creme fraîche
1 bunch of fresh dill
Lemon juice
4 egg yolks
2 eggs for brushing
pepper and salt

Mix the chopped salmon with the chopped dill, lemon juice, pepper and salt. Now whisk the eggs,

these will be used for brushing afterwards. Spread out the puff pastry and cut lengthways into 3 equal strips and cut out triangles. Brush with the beaten eggs and place the salmon mixture on the wide ends. Then shape the triangles into croissants and roll them up and again brush the outside with the whisked eggs. Then place on the greased grill plate and bake at 160 degrees for about 20 minutes.

RECIPE 709: SALMON WITH CREAM CHEESE

Serve: 2 | Total Time: 24 minutes

4 salmon fillets, 6 ounces each
6 ounces cream cheese
2 tbsp mayonnaise
2 tsp of parsley, chopped
2 tsp of lemon juice
Salt and black pepper
Oil spray, for greasing

Season the salmon fillet with salt, black pepper, and oil spray before cutting it into little pieces. Select the grill function and place the grill grate in the Ninja Foodi Smart XL Grill. Remember to grease the grill grate with oil spray. Set the time to MAX for 8 minutes, buy selecting grill function. Select start to begin preheating. Once beeps sound add salmon to the grill and grill it at MAX for 8 minutes. Meanwhile, take a bowl and combine parsley, lemon zest, salt, mayonnaise, cream cheese in a bowl. Serve the cooked fillet with creamy sauce and enjoy.

RECIPE 710: SALMON WITH HERBS

Serve: 2 | Total Time: 28 minutes

2 lemons, juice only
1/3 cup fresh mint, chopped
¼ cup fresh parsley, chopped
1 tbsp Dijon mustard
1 garlic clove
Salt and black pepper, to taste
1 pound center-cut salmon, skinned

Combine all the listed ingredients excluding fish in a blender and process. Add a few tbsp of water if needed. Once the smooth paste is formed, marinate fish in it for 30 minutes. Next, insert the grill grate in the Ninja Foodi Smart XL Grill and select the grill function. Remember to grease the grill grate with oil spray. Set the time to MAX for 8 minutes, buy selecting grill function. Select start to begin preheating. Once done with the preheating adds fillets to the grill and close the hood. GRILL at MAX, for 12 minutes. Flipping is not necessary. Once cooked, serve the fish.

RECIPE 711: SALMON WITH PESTO AND ROASTED TOMATOES

Serve: 4 | Total Time: 15 minutes

4 salmon steaks
4 tbsp pesto
1 pound pasta
8 large prawns
9 oz cherry tomatoes
1 medium lemon
Olive oil
Fresh thyme

Season the pasta water with salt and bring to a boil. Add the pasta when the water boils. Meanwhile, take an ovenproof dish and coat with one tbsp of pesto. Place the sliced salmon in the dish and top with the remaining pesto. Toss in two tbsp of extra virgin olive oil to the pan. After halving the tomatoes, toss them with the fish. Place the prawns on top of the salmon, sprinkle with lemon juice, and air fry for 8 minutes at 390°F. Drain the pasta and combine it with the salmon and prawns in a serving dish. Enjoy.

RECIPE 712: SALT-AND-PEPPER BEEF ROAST

Serve: 12 | Total Time: 45 minutes

4–6lb. boned beef cross rib roast
1/4 cup coarse salt
1/4 cup sugar

2 tbsp. coarse-ground pepper
1/2 cup prepared horseradish

Mix salt with sugar in a bowl. Pat the mixture on the beef, and marinate for 3–4 hours. Mix 1.5 tsp. salt, pepper, and horseradish. Put the beef on a rack in a 9"x13" pan and rub the horseradish mixture. Roast in 176°C or 350°F in the PowerXL Air Fryer Grill. Check if the internal temperature is 120–125°C. Rest for 20 minutes, and then slice the meat thinly across the grain.

RECIPE 713: SAUCY CHICKEN WITH LEEKS

Serve: 10 | Total Time: 28 minutes

6 chicken legs, boneless and skinless
2 leeks sliced
1/2 tsp. smoked cayenne pepper
2 tbsp. olive oil
2 large-sized tomatoes, chopped
1/2 tsp. dried oregano
3 cloves garlic, minced
A dash ground nutmeg

Combine all the ingredients. Place the meat in the marinade and let it sit for a few minutes. Preheat the PowerXL Air Fryer Grill by selecting Air fry mode. Adjust the temperature to 390|F, set Time to 5 minutes. Arrange the leeks on the PowerXL grill baking tray. Add the chicken on top. Transfer to the PowerXL Air Fryer Grill. Air fry for 18 minutes, flip halfway done. Enjoy.

RECIPE 714: SEASONED CHICKEN BREASTS

Serve: 4 | Total Time: 15 minutes

4 (4-ounce) boneless, skinless chicken breasts
1 tsp olive oil
1 tsp jerk seasoning

After brushing each chicken breast with olive oil, smear it with jerk seasoning. Place the water tray in the bottom of Power XL Smokeless Electric Grill. Place about 2 cups of lukewarm water into the water tray. Place the drip pan over water tray and then arrange the heating element. Now, place the grilling pan over heating element. Plugin the Power XL Smokeless Electric Grill and press the 'Power' button to turn it on. Then press 'Fan' button. Set the temperature settings according to manufacturer's directions. Cover the grill with lid and let it preheat. After preheating, remove the lid and grease the grilling pan. Place the chicken breasts over the grilling pan. Cover with the lid and cook for about 3-5 minutes per side. Serve hot.

RECIPE 715: SEASONED GARLIC CARROTS

Serve: 4 | Total Time: 20 minutes

Salt and pepper to taste
2 tsp garlic powder
2 tbsp olive oil
1-pound carrots, diced

Take a bowl and toss the carrot cubes generously in oil. Season the cube further with salt, pepper, and garlic powder. Make sure that they are coated evenly. Spread the carrots in the Air Crisp Basket. Set your Ninja Foodi Smart XL Grill to 390 degrees F in AIR CRISP mode and set the timer to 30 minutes. Cook for 10 minutes, stir once. Serve and enjoy!

RECIPE 716: SIMPLE CUBAN SANDWICHES

Serve: 4 | Total Time: 28 minutes

slices ciabatta bread, about ¼-inch thick
Cooking spray
1 tbsp. brown mustard
Toppings:
6 to 8 ounces thinly sliced leftover roast pork
4 ounces thinly sliced deli turkey
⅓ cup bread and butter pickle slices
2 to 3 ounces Pepper Jack cheese slices

On a clean work surface, spray one side of each slice of bread with cooking spray. Spread the other side of each slice of bread evenly with brown mustard. 4 of the bread pieces should be topped with turkey, roast pork, pickle slices, and cheese, followed by the remaining bread slices. Transfer to the air fry basket. Place the basket on the air fry position. Select Air Fry, set the temperature to 390°F (199°C), and set time to 8 minutes. Remove the basket from the Air Fryer grill after the cooking is finished. Cool for 5 minutes and serve warm.

RECIPE 717: SIRLOIN ROAST BEEF

Serve: 6 | Total Time: 35 minutes

3.3 lb. Sirloin Beef
2 tbsp. vegetable oil
6 ounces red wine
14 ounces beef consommé

Preheat the PowerXL Air Fryer Grill to 200°C or 400°F. Season the sirloin and cook it at medium heat in oil for 5 minutes, turning regularly. Roast it in the PowerXL Air Fryer Grill for 15 minutes to make it medium-rare. Flip it halfway. Remove it when the internal temperature is 145°F, and cover with foil. Make a gravy with the fat residue on the pan and some wine. Add beef consommé to the sauce and simmer for 5 minutes. Strain when completed and pour on the roast.

RECIPE 718: SLOW ROASTED BEEF SHORT RIBS

Serve: 6 | Total Time: 30 minutes

5 lb. beef short ribs
1/3 cup brown sugar
1 tsp. garlic powder
1 tsp. onion powder
1/4 tsp. marjoram
1/2 tsp. kosher salt
1/4 tsp. thyme
1 pinch cayenne pepper

Pat the ribs dry. Rub the ingredients on each rib, put them in a sealed plastic bag, and freeze overnight. Preheat the PowerXL Air Fryer Grill to 150°C or 300°F, and put ribs on a rack in a roasting pan. Roast for around 3 hours.

RECIPE 719: SMOKED SHRIMP

Serve: 1 | Total Time: 24 minutes

10 large shrimps
1 tsp smoked paprika
1 tsp thyme, dry
Salt, pinch
¼ tsp garlic powder
¼ onion powder
½ tsp cayenne pepper
¼ tsp of lemon zest

Select the grill function and place the grill grate in the Ninja Foodi Smart XL Grill. Remember to grease the grill grate with oil spray. Set the time to MAX for 8 minutes, buy selecting grill function. Select start to begin preheating. Mix the entire rub and spices in a bowl and then coat the shrimp with the spice rub. Spray the shrimp with oil spray and transfer it to the grill grate. Let it grill at MAX for 9 minutes. Flipping is not necessary. Once it's done, serve.

RECIPE 720: SOY CHORIZO AND SPRING ONION TOAST

Serve: 2 | Total Time: 12 minutes

1 cup soy chorizo, chopped
1 large spring onion, finely sliced
3 white bread slices
½ cup sweet corn
1 egg white, whisked
1 tbsp black sesame seeds
Preheat the PowerXL Air Fryer Grill to 370 F on Air Fry function. In a bowl, place the chopped soy chorizo, corn, spring onion, and black sesame seeds. Add the whisked egg and mix the ingredients. Spread the mixture over the bread slices. Place in the crisper tray and sprinkle oil. Cook

until golden, about 8-10 minutes. Serve with ketchup or chili sauce.

RECIPE 721: SOY SALMON FILLETS

Serve: 4 | Total Time: 18 minutes

4 salmon fillets
1/4 tsp ground black pepper
1/2 tsp cayenne pepper
1/2 tsp salt
1 tsp onion powder
1 tbsp fresh lemon juice
1/2 cup soy sauce
1/2 cup water
1 tbsp honey
2 tbsp extra-virgin olive oil

Firstly, pat the salmon fillets dry using kitchen towels. Season the salmon with black pepper, cayenne pepper, salt, and onion powder. To make the marinade, combine together the lemon juice, soy sauce, water, honey, and olive oil. Marinate the salmon for at least 2 hours in your refrigerator. Arrange the fish fillets on a grill basket in your Breville Air Fryer oven. Bake at 330 degrees for 8 to 9 minutes, or until salmon fillets are easily flaked with a fork. Work with batches and serve warm.

RECIPE 722: SPAGHETTI SQUASH BURRITO BOWLS

Serve: 2 | Total Time: 45 minutes

1 small spaghetti squash
Zucchini, diced
¼ onion, diced
Bell peppers, diced
¾ cup black beans, cooked
½ cup corn kernels
½ cup salsa
2 ounces cheese (optional)
Olive oil
½ tsp dried oregano
¼ tsp ground cumin
Salt & pepper

Preheat the PowerXL Air Fryer Grill at 230°C or 425°F on bake setting. Microwave the squash for 4 minutes and then cut it in half. Scoop out the seeds. Rub the squash with oil, salt, and pepper

and bake for 45 minutes. Make the filling by stir-frying bell pepper, zucchini, oregano, corn, salt, and pepper for 10 minutes. Add the salsa and black beans. Scrape squash flesh to make spaghetti and toss in the vegetables. Bake them at 176°C or 350°F for 10 minutes and then broil for 1–2 minutes.

RECIPE 723: SPICY AIR FRYER SALMON

Serve: 6 | Total Time: 25 minutes

¾ tsp ground cumin
2 tbsp. grill seasoning (i.e., Montreal Steak Flavor)
1/2 tsp ground coriander
1 tbsp. brown sugar
2 lbs. salmon fillets, skin is on
¼ tsp cayenne pepper

Pre-heat your Air Fryer to 330 °F (165 ° C) for 2 mins in the fish environment. In a mixing bowl, add steak seasoning, cumin, cayenne pepper, brown sugar, and coriander. Season each piece of salmon with about 2 tbsps. of the spice mix (or more, if desired). Arrange the salmon in a single layer in the basket of an Air Fryer. Cook fish in an Air Fryer for around 18 mins, in chunks if possible until it flakes comfortably by using a fork. Place the cooked salmon on a tray and keep it warm in an oven set to the minimum temperature. Repeat with the rest of the salmon fillets. Serve right away.

RECIPE 724: SPICY CHICKEN DRUMSTICKS WITH GRILL MARINADE

Serve: 4 | Total Time: 35 minutes

5 chicken drumsticks
½ tbsp mustard
1 peeled crushed clove of garlic
1 tsp brown sugar
1 tbsp olive oil
1 tsp chili powder
pepper and salt

Mix the grill marinade made of mustard, garlic, brown sugar, chili powder, pepper and salt with the oil and marinate the chicken legs in it for 30 minutes. Put the legs in the basket of the Air Fryer and fry for 10 to 12 minutes at 200 degrees. Switch on the temperature depending on the size. Serve the hot chicken legs with a baguette and fresh salad.

RECIPE 725: SPICY GRILLED STEAK

Serve: 4 | Total Time: 16 minutes

2 tbsp low-sodium salsa
1 tbsp minced chipotle pepper
1 tbsp apple cider vinegar
1 tsp ground cumin
1/8 tsp freshly ground black pepper
1/8 tsp red pepper flakes
¾ pound sirloin tip steak, 4 pieces and pounded to about 1/3 inch thick

Mix salsa, chipotle pepper, cider vinegar, cumin, black pepper, and red pepper flakes in a small bowl. Rub it onto the outside and inside of each steak. 15 minutes at room temperature. Grill the steaks in the Air Fryer for 6–9 minutes each side, or until a meat thermometer reads 145°F. To keep warm, transfer the steaks to a clean platter. Rep with the other steaks. Serve thinly sliced steaks against the grain.

RECIPE 726: SPICY GRILLED TOMATOES

Serve: 2 | Total Time: 25 minutes

2 medium tomatoes, sliced
Herbs you like
Ground pepper and salt to taste
1 tbsp olive oil or cooking spray

Tomatoes should be washed and dried with paper kitchen towels. They should be half-cut. Place the halves with the cut side up. Drizzle the tops with olive oil or cooking spray. Freshly ground pepper and dried or fresh herbs are used to season. Set your Air Fryer to 320°F (without preheating) and cook for 20 minutes with tomato halves. Preparation time depends on the size of the tomatoes, the quantity of halves, and your personal preferences. Tip: you can serve grilled tomatoes piping hot, room temperature or chilled.

RECIPE 727: STEAK AND VEGETABLE KEBABS

Serve: 4 | Total Time: 22 minutes

2 tbsp balsamic vinegar
2 tsp olive oil
½ tsp dried marjoram
1/8 tsp freshly ground black pepper
¾ pound round steak, cut into 1-inch pieces
1 red bell pepper, sliced
16 button mushrooms
1 cup cherry tomatoes

Combine the balsamic vinegar, olive oil, marjoram, and black pepper in a medium mixing basin. Add the steak and stir to coat. Allow for a 10-minute resting period at room temperature. Alternating items, thread the beef, red bell pepper, mushrooms, and tomatoes onto 8 bamboo or metal skewers that fit in the Air Fryer. In the Air Fryer, grill for 5 to 7 minutes, or until the beef is browned and a meat thermometer that registers at 145°F. Serve immediately.

RECIPE 728: STROGANOFF SHORT STEAK

Serve: 2 | Total Time: 91 minutes

1-lb. beef steak, sliced.
1/2 cup sour cream
1/4 cup cream
1/4 cup onions, sliced.
1/2 cup button mushrooms, sliced.
4 tbsp. olive oil
1 tbsp. garlic, minced.
2 tbsp. soy sauce
salt and pepper, to taste

Marinate the steak slices with the combined soy sauce, two-tbsp. of olive oil, garlic and pepper for 2 hours in the fridge. Attach the Air Fryer Grill Pan and preheat to 350 degrees F. Arrange the steak slices on the Air Fryer Grill Pan and cook for 8 minutes or until desired doneness of meat. To prepare the stroganoff sauce, sauté the onions and mushrooms in the remaining 2 tbsp olive oil for 5–8 minutes until tender. Add the sour cream and cream and season with salt and pepper. Remove from the heat and set aside. Serve and enjoy!

RECIPE 729: STUFFED PORTABELLA MUSHROOM

Serve: 2 | Total Time: 35 minutes

2 large portabella mushrooms
Breadcrumbs
Nutritional yeast (gives a cheesy, savory flavor)
1 cup tofu ricotta
½ cup canned marinara sauce
1 cup spinach
½ tsp. garlic powder
1 tsp. dry basil & 1 tsp. dry thyme
Salt & pepper

Make ricotta with tofu, lemon juice, nutritional yeast, salt, and pepper. Mix the tofu ricotta, spinach, thyme, basil, marinara sauce, and seasoning. Brush marinara sauce on each mushroom and stuff the filling. Top it with breadcrumbs, nutritional yeast, and some olive oil. Bake for 15 minutes at 230°C or 450°F in your PowerXL Air Fryer Grill.

RECIPE 730: STUFFED TOMATOES

Serve: 2 | Total Time: 20 minutes

2 cups brown rice, cooked
1 pound grilled chicken breasts, cut into pieces
4 large red tomatoes
4 tbsp fresh basil
2 tbsp olive oil
Black pepper, to taste
Sea salt
2 tbsp lemon juice
1 tsp red chili powder

Combine rice, chicken, basil, oil, salt, pepper, lemon juice and chili powder in a bowl. Wash and center core the tomatoes and fill the cavity with the bowl mixture. Oil the Air Fryer pan and place the tomatoes according to capacity. Bake tomatoes in the Air Fryer for 20 minutes. Serve and enjoy.

RECIPE 731: SUPER CHEESE SANDWICHES

Serve: 8 | Total Time: 16 minutes

8 ounces Brie
8 slices oat nut bread
1 large ripe pear, cored and cut into ½ -inch-thick slices
2 tbsp. butter, melted

Make the sandwiches: Spread each of 4 slices of bread with ¼ of the Brie. Top the Brie with the pear slices and the remaining 4 bread slices. Brush the melted butter lightly on both sides of each sandwich. Arrange the sandwiches in the air fry basket. Place the basket on the bake position. Select Bake, set the temperature to 360°F (182°C), and set the time to 6 minutes. When cooking is complete, the cheese should be melted. Remove the basket from the Air Fryer grill and serve warm.

RECIPE 732: SWEET AND SOUR PORK

Serve: 4 | Total Time: 37 minutes

2 pounds pork cut into chunks
2 large Eggs
1 tsp. olive oil
1 cup cornstarch
Salt and ground black pepper to taste
1/4 tsp. Chinese spice
Oil Mister

Preheat the PowerXL Air Fryer Grill by selecting grill mode. Adjust temperature to 350°F and Time to 5 minutes. In a medium-sized mixing dish, whisk together the egg and olive oil. Add breadcrumbs to another bowl. Dip the beef schnitzel in the egg mixture. Then coat with the breadcrumb mixture. Arrange on the PowerXL grilling plate. Transfer into the PowerXL Air Fryer Grill. Grill for 12 minutes, flipping halfway. Serve and enjoy!

RECIPE 733: SWEET AND SPICY SWORDFISH KEBABS

Serve: 4 | Total Time: 30 minutes

½ cup canned pineapple chunks, drained, juice reserved
1 lb swordfish steaks, cubed
½ cup large red grapes
1 tbsp honey
2 tsp grated fresh ginger
1 tsp olive oil
Pinch cayenne pepper

Preheat Air Fryer to 370°F. Poke 8 bamboo skewers through the swordfish, pineapple, and grapes. Mix the honey, 1 tbsp of pineapple juice, ginger, olive oil, and cayenne in a bowl, then use a brush to rub the mix on the kebabs. Allow the marinate to sit on the kebab for 10 minutes. Grill the kebabs for 8-12 minutes until the fish is cooked through and the fruit is soft and glazed. Brush the kebabs again with the mix, then toss the rest of the marinade. Serve warm and enjoy!

RECIPE 734: SWEET PLANTAINS

Serve: 2 | Total Time: 18 minutes

1 tbsp melted butter
1 tbsp brown sugar
⅛ tsp ground cinnamon

Each plantain was cut in half and then sliced horizontally 2. Evenly coat the plantain pieces with melted butter. Place the grill plate in the PowerXL Grill Air Fryer Combo's inner pot. Select "Grill" mode by rotating the "Control Knob." To set the time for 8 minutes, press the "Timer Button" and spin the "Control Knob." To begin preheating, close the PowerXL with the "Air Frying Lid"

and push the "Start Button." Open the lid and put the plantain slices on the grill plate when the machine says "Add Food." To begin cooking, close the lid and push the "Start Button." Flip the plantain slices after 4 minutes. To end cooking, hit the "Cancel Button" when the cooking time is up. Remove the plantain slices from the pot and place them on a platter. Serve with a sprinkling of brown sugar and cinnamon.

RECIPE 735: TACO BEEF AND GREEN CHILE CASSEROLE

Serve: 4 | Total Time: 25 minutes

1 pound (454 g) 85% lean ground beef
1 tbsp taco seasoning
1 (7-ounce / 198-g) can diced mild green chiles
1/2 cup milk
2 large eggs
1 cup shredded Mexican cheese blend
2 tbsp all-purpose flour
1/2 tsp kosher salt
Cooking spray

Spritz a baking pan with cooking spray. Toss the ground beef with taco seasoning in a large bowl to mix well. Pour the seasoned ground beef in the prepared baking pan. Combing the remaining ingredients in a medium bowl. Whisk to mix well, then pour the mixture over the ground beef. Place the pan on the bake position. Select Bake, set temperature to 350°F (180°C) and set time to 15 minutes. When cooking is complete, a toothpick inserted in the center should come out clean. Remove the casserole from the Air Fryer grill and allow to cool for 5 minutes, then slice to serve.

RECIPE 736: TASTY CARIBBEAN CHICKEN

Serve: 8 | Total Time: 20 minutes

3 lb. chicken thigh, skinless and boneless

3 tbsp. coconut oil, melted
1/2 tsp. ground nutmeg
1/2 tsp. ground ginger
1 tbsp. cayenne
1 tbsp. cinnamon
1 tbsp. coriander powder
Pepper
Salt

Assemble all components except chicken. Rub bowl mixture all over the chicken. Place the inner pot in the PowerXL grill Air Fryer combo base. Place grill plate in the inner pot. Cover. Select air fry mode then set the temperature to 390°F and Time for 10 minutes. Press start. Let the appliance preheat for 3 minutes. Open the lid then place chicken on the grill plate. Serve and enjoy.

RECIPE 737: TENDER AND JUICY CHICKEN

Serve: 6 | Total Time: 50 minutes

2 lb. chicken thighs, skinless and boneless
8 garlic cloves, sliced
2 tbsp. olive oil
2 tbsp. fresh parsley, chopped
1 fresh lemon juice
Pepper
Salt

Place chicken on a baking dish and season with pepper and salt. Sprinkle parsley and garlic over the chicken and drizzle oil and lemon juice on top of the chicken. Place the inner pot in the PowerXL grill Air Fryer combo base. Place the baking dish in the inner pot. Cover the inner pot with an air frying lid. Set the oven to bake mode at 450°F for 40 minutes. Press start. When the Timer reaches 0, then press the cancel button. Serve and enjoy.

RECIPE 738: TERIYAKI GLAZED SALMON

Serve: 2 | Total Time: 18 minutes

Teriyaki sauce:
118 ml soy sauce

50g of sugar
1g grated ginger
1 clove garlic, crushed
60 ml of orange juice

Salmon:
2 salmon fillets (5 oz)
20 ml of vegetable oil
Salt and white pepper, to taste

Put all the ingredients of the teriyaki sauce in a small pot. Boil the sauce, reduce by half, then let it cool. Preheat the Air Fryer set the temperature to 180°C. Cover the salmon with oil and season with salt and white pepper. Place the salmon in the preheated air and adjust to 8 minutes. Remove the salmon from the fryer when finished. Let stand for 5 minutes, then glaze with teriyaki sauce. Serve on a bed of white rice or grilled vegetables.

RECIPE 739: TERIYAKI SALMON

Serve: 4 | Total Time: 75 minutes

4 salmon fillets (6 ounces each), uncooked
1 cup teriyaki marinade
Oil spray, for greasing

Marinate the fish fillets in the teriyaki sauce for 1 hour in the refrigerator. Meanwhile, insert the grill grate in the Ninja Foodi Smart XL Grill and select the grill function. Remember to grease the grill grate with oil spray. Set the time to MAX for 10 minutes, by selecting the grill function. Select start to begin preheating. Once the timer beeps add fillets to the grill grate and cook for 6 minutes at MAX. If the desired doneness is not achieved let it grill for 2 more minutes. Then serve and enjoy hot.

RECIPE 740: TEX MEX CHICKEN

Serve: 6 | Total Time: 30 minutes

1 cup tomatoes, chopped finely
2 pounds chicken breasts
1 cup coconut cream
½ tsp salt

2 tbsp Mexican seasoning
2 tbsp olive oil
1 cup green chilies

Select the "Grill" button on the Ninja Foodi Smart XL Grill and regulate the settings at Medium for 20 minutes. Mingle chicken breasts with all other ingredients in a bowl. Arrange the chicken in the Ninja Foodi when it displays "Add Food". Grill for about 20 minutes, flipping once in between. Dole out in a platter and serve warm.

RECIPE 741: THYME MEATLESS PATTIES

Serve: 3 | Total Time: 25 minutes

½ cup oat flour
1 tsp allspice
½ tsp ground thyme
1 tsp maple syrup
½ tsp liquid smoke
1 tsp balsamic vinegar

Preheat Air Fryer to 400°F. Mix the oat flour, allspice, thyme, maple syrup, liquid smoke, balsamic vinegar, and 2 tbsp of water in a bowl. Make 6 patties out of the mixture. Place them onto a parchment paper and flatten them to ½-inch thick. Grease the patties with cooking spray. Grill for 12 minutes until crispy, turning once. Serve warm.

RECIPE 742: TOASTED VEGETABLES WITH RICE AND EGGS

Serve: 4 | Total Time: 18 minutes

2 tsp melted butter
1 cup chopped mushrooms
1 cup cooked rice
1 cup peas
1 carrot, chopped
1 red onion, chopped
1 garlic clove, minced
Salt and black pepper, to taste
2 hard-boiled eggs, grated
1 tbsp soy sauce

Coat a baking dish with melted butter. Stir together the mushrooms, carrot, peas, garlic, onion, cooked rice, salt, and pepper in a large bowl until well mixed. Fill the baking dish with the batter. Place the baking dish in the toast position. Select Toast, set temperature to 380 °F (193 °C), and set time to 12 minutes. When cooking is complete, remove from the Air Fryer grill. Divide the mixture among four plates. Serve warm with a sprinkle of grated eggs and a drizzle of soy sauce.

RECIPE 743: TOMATO SHORT RIBS

Serve: 2 | Total Time: 35 minutes

9 ounces short ribs
1 cup tomato sauce
1/2 cup mushrooms, sliced.
2 tbsp. fresh basil, chopped.
2 tbsp. garlic, minced.
salt and pepper, to taste

Attach the Air Fryer Grill Pan and preheat the Air Fryer to 350 degrees F. Season the short ribs with salt and pepper and spray with cooking spray. Arrange the ribs on the Air Fryer Grill Pan with the mushrooms. Mix together the tomato sauce, fresh basil and garlic and pour onto the Air Fryer Grill Pan. Cook for 30 minutes or until the ribs are cooked through. Halfway through the cooking time, flip the ribs over to allow even cooking. Serve and enjoy!

RECIPE 744: TUNA AND FRUIT KEBABS

Serve: 4 | Total Time: 27 minutes

1-pound tuna steaks, cut into 1-inch cubes
½ cup canned pineapple chunks, drained, juice reserved
½ cup large red grapes
1 tbsp. honey
tsp. grated fresh ginger
1 tsp. olive oil
Pinch cayenne pepper

Thread the tuna, pineapple, and grapes on 8 bamboo or 4 metal skewers that fit in the Air Fryer. In a small bowl, whisk the honey, 1

tbsp. of reserved pineapple juice, ginger, olive oil, and cayenne. Brush this mixture over the kebabs. Let them stand for 10 minutes. Grill the kebabs for 8 to 12 minutes at 370°F, or until the tuna reaches an internal temperature of at least 145°F on a meat thermometer, and the fruit is tender and glazed, brushing once with the remaining sauce. Discard any remaining marinade. Serve immediately.

RECIPE 745: TUNA WRAPS

Serve: 4 | Total Time: 17 minutes

1 lb fresh tuna steak, cut into 1-inch cubes
1 tbsp grated fresh ginger
garlic cloves, minced
½ tsp toasted sesame oil
low-sodium whole-wheat tortillas
¼ cup low-fat mayonnaise
cups shredded romaine lettuce
1 red bell pepper, thinly sliced

In a medium bowl, mix the tuna, ginger, garlic, and sesame oil. Let it stand for 10 minutes. Grill the tuna in the Air Fryer for 4 to 7 minutes at 390°F, or until done to your liking and lightly browned. Make wraps with tuna, tortillas, mayonnaise, lettuce, and bell pepper. Serve immediately.

RECIPE 746: TURKEY MEATBALLS

Serve: 8 | Total Time: 25 minutes

½ cup fresh parsley, chopped
1 pound extra-lean ground turkey
1 cup cooked black beans, mashed roughly
Olive oil, as required
1 yellow bell pepper, finely chopped
Salt and black pepper, to taste
1 red bell pepper, finely chopped

Select the "Grill" button on the Ninja Foodi Smart XL Grill and regulate the settings at Medium for 10 minutes. Mingle all the ingredients in a bowl and toss well. Form equal-sized 24 balls out of

this mixture. Arrange the meatballs in the Ninja Foodi when it displays "Add Food". Grill for about 10 minutes, flipping once in between. Dole out in a platter and serve warm.

RECIPE 747: TURKEY SPRING ROLLS

Serve: 4 | Total Time: 20 minutes

1 lb turkey breast, grilled, cut into chunks
1 celery stalk, julienned
1 carrot, grated
1 tsp fresh ginger, minced
1 tsp sugar
1 tsp chicken stock powder
1 egg
1 tsp corn starch
6 spring roll wrappers

Preheat the Air Fryer to 360°F. Mix the turkey, celery, carrot, ginger, sugar, and chicken stock powder in a large bowl. Combine thoroughly and set aside. In another bowl, beat the egg, and stir in the cornstarch. On a clean surface, spoon the turkey filling into each spring roll, roll up and seal the seams with the egg-cornstarch mixture. Put each roll in the greased frying basket and Air Fry for 7-8 minutes, flipping once until golden brown. Serve hot.

RECIPE 748: TWO-CHEESE GRILLED SANDWICHES

Serve: 2 | Total Time: 30 minutes

4 sourdough bread slices
2 cheddar cheese slices
2 Swiss cheese slices
1 tbsp butter
2 dill pickles, sliced

Preheat Air Fryer to 360°F. Smear both sides of the sourdough bread with butter and place them in the frying basket. Toast the bread for 6 minutes, flipping once. Divide the cheddar cheese between 2 of the bread slices. Cover the remaining 2 bread slices with Swiss cheese slices. Bake for 10 more minutes until the cheeses have melted and lightly bubbled and the bread has golden brown. Set the cheddar-covered bread slices on a serving plate, cover with pickles, and top each with the Swiss-covered slices. Serve and enjoy!

RECIPE 749: VEGGIES AND HALLOUMI CHEESE

Serve: 2 | Total Time: 15 minutes

1 large eggplant, peeled, cut into chunks
6 oz block of firm halloumi cheese, cubed
2 zucchinis, cut into even chunks
1 large carrot, cut into chunks
2 tsp olive oil
1 tsp dried mixed herbs
Salt and black pepper

Preheat the PowerXL Air Fryer Grill to 380 F on Bake function. To a bowl, add halloumi, zucchini, carrot, eggplant, olive oil, herbs, salt and pepper. Arrange halloumi and veggies on the baking pan. Cook for 14 minutes, shaking once

or twice. When ready, make sure the veggies are tender, and the halloumi is golden. Sprinkle with olive oil and scatter with fresh arugula leaves.

RECIPE 750: WHOLE CHICKEN WITH PRUNES AND CAPERS

Serve: 6 | Total Time: 55 minutes

1 whole chicken, 3 lb
½ cup pitted prunes
3 minced cloves of garlic
2 tbsp capers
2 bay leaves
2 tbsp red wine vinegar
2 tbsp olive oil
1 tbsp dried oregano
¼ cup packed brown sugar
1 tbsp chopped and fresh parsley
Salt and black pepper to taste

In a big and deep bowl, mix the prunes, olives, capers, garlic, olive oil, bay leaves, oregano, vinegar, salt, and pepper. Spread the mixture on the bottom of a baking tray, and place the chicken. Preheat the PowerXL Air Fryer Grill to 360

F on Roast function. Sprinkle a little bit of brown sugar on top of the chicken; cook for 55 minutes. Serve and enjoy!

RECIPE 751: ZUCCHINI FETA PAWS

Serve: 4 | Total Time: 15 minutes

2 zucchini
2 Show oregano
olive oil
150 g feta cheese
pepper and salt
Take the feta cheese out of the package and let it drain well, then cut into small sticks and then pluck the oregano and chop it into small pieces. Remove the washed zucchini from the stalk, cut in half and make incisions lengthways in the peel. The feta cheese is placed in it and seasoned with salt, pepper and oregano, as well as drizzled with olives. Place on the baking pan of the hot Air Fryer and grill at 160 degrees for about 25 minutes.

CHAPTER 3: 250 RECIPES FOR BAKE

RECIPE 752: ALMOND NUGGETS

Serve: 4 | Total Time: 23 minutes

1 egg white
1 tbsp freshly squeezed lemon juice
½ tsp dried basil
½ tsp ground paprika
1 lb low-sodium boneless, skinless chicken breasts, 1 ½-inch cubes
½ cup ground almonds
2 slices low-sodium whole-wheat bread, crumbled

With a fork, whisk together the egg white, lemon juice, basil, and paprika in a small basin until frothy. Add the chicken and stir to coat. On a plate, mix the almonds and bread crumbs. Toss the chicken cubes in the almond and bread crumb mixture until coated. Bake the nuggets in the Air Fryer, in two

batches, at 400ºF (204ºC) for 10 to 13 minutes, or until the chicken reaches an internal temperature of 165ºF (74ºC) on a meat thermometer. Serve immediately.

RECIPE 753: ALMOND ORANGE BUTTER CAKE

Serve: 6 | Total Time: 20 minutes

1/3 cup almonds, chopped
3 tbsp orange marmalade
1 stick butter
½ tsp allspice, ground
½ tsp anise seed, ground
½ tsp baking powder
1 tsp baking soda
6 oz almond flour
2 tbsp Truvia for baking
2 eggs plus 1 egg yok, beaten
Olive oil cooking spray for pans

Lightly grease cake pan with olive oil cooking spray. Mix the butter and Truvia until nice and smooth. Fold in the eggs, almonds, marmalade; beat again until well mixed. Add flour, baking soda, baking powder, allspice, star anise and ground cinnamon. Bake in the preheated air-fryer at 310˚Fahrenheit for 20-minutes.

RECIPE 754: ALMOND PECAN COOKIES

Serve: 16 | Total Time: 30 minutes

1/2 cup butter
1 tsp vanilla
2 tsp gelatin
2/3 cup Swerve
1 cup pecans
1/3 cup coconut flour
1 cup almond flour

Fit the Air Fryer oven with the rack in position. Add butter, vanilla, gelatin, swerve, coconut flour, and almond flour into the food processor and process until crumbs form. Add pecans and process until chopped. Make cookies from prepared mixture and place onto a parchment-lined baking pan. Set to bake at 350 F for 25 minutes. After 5 minutes place the baking pan in the preheated oven. Serve and enjoy.

RECIPE 755: ALMOND-PUMPKIN PORRIDGE

Serve: 4 | Total Time: 10 minutes

1 cup pumpkin seeds
2/3 cup chopped pecans
1/3 cup quick-cooking oats
¼ cup pumpkin purée
¼ cup diced pitted dates
1 tsp chia seeds
1 tsp sesame seeds
1 tsp dried berries
2 tbsp butter
2 tsp pumpkin pie spice
¼ cup honey
1 tbsp dark brown sugar
¼ cup almond flour
Salt to taste

Preheat Air Fryer at 350°F. Combine the pumpkin seeds, pecans, oats, pumpkin purée, dates, chia seeds, sesame seeds, dried berries, butter, pumpkin pie spice, honey, sugar, almond flour, and salt in a bowl. Press mixture into a greased cake pan. Place cake pan in the frying basket and Bake for 5 minutes, stirring once. Let cool completely for 10 minutes before crumbling.

RECIPE 756: ALMOND ORANGE CAKE

Serve: 6 | Total Time: 20 minutes

1/3 cup almonds, chopped
3 tbsp orange marmalade
1 stick butter
½ tsp allspice, ground
½ tsp anise seed, ground
½ tsp baking powder

1 tsp baking soda
6-ounces almond flour
2 tbsp Truvia for baking
2 eggs plus 1 egg yok, beaten
Olive oil cooking spray for pans

Lightly grease cake pan with olive oil cooking spray. Mix the butter and Truvia until nice and smooth. Fold in the eggs, almonds, marmalade; beat again until well mixed. Add flour, baking soda, baking powder, allspice, star anise and ground cinnamon. Bake in the preheated air-fryer at 310°Fahrenheit for 20-minutes.

RECIPE 757: APRICOT-CHEESE MINI PIES

Serve: 6 | Total Time: 35 minutes

2 refrigerated piecrusts
1/3 cup apricot preserves
1 tsp cornstarch
½ cup vanilla yogurt
1 oz cream cheese
1 tsp sugar
Rainbow sprinkles

Preheat Air Fryer to 370°F. Lay out pie crusts on a flat surface. Cut each sheet of pie crust with a knife into three rectangles for a total of 6 rectangles. Mix apricot preserves and cornstarch in a small bowl. Cover the top half of one rectangle with 1 tbsp of the preserve mixture. Repeat for all rectangles. Fold the bottom of the crust over the preserve-covered top. Crimp and seal all edges with a fork. Lightly coat each tart with cooking oil, then place into the Air Fryer without stacking. Bake for 10 minutes. Meanwhile, prepare the frosting by mixing yogurt, cream cheese, and sugar. When tarts are done, let cool completely in the Air Fryer. Frost the tarts and top with sprinkles. Serve.

RECIPE 758: APRICOT CRUMBLE WITH BLACKBERRIES

Serve: 4 | Total Time: 50 minutes

2 ½ cups fresh apricots, de-stoned and cubed
1 cup fresh blackberries
½ cup sugar
2 tbsp lemon Juice
1 cup flour
5 tbsp butter

Preheat Instant Vortex on Bake function to 360 F. Add the apricot cubes to a bowl and mix with lemon juice, 2 tbsp sugar, and blackberries. Scoop the mixture into a greased dish and spread it evenly. In another bowl, mix flour and remaining sugar. Add 1 tbsp of cold water and butter and keep mixing until you have a crumbly mixture. Pour over the fruit mixture and cook for 20 minutes.

RECIPE 759: AROMATIC MUSHROOM OMELET

Serve: 4 | Total Time: 30 minutes

6 eggs
2 tbsp milk
½ yellow onion, diced
½ cup diced mushrooms
2 tbsp chopped parsley
1 tsp dried oregano
1 tbsp chopped chives
½ tbsp chopped dill
½ cup grated Gruyère cheese

Preheat Air Fryer to 350°F. Beat eggs in a medium bowl, then add the rest of the ingredients, except for the parsley. Stir until completely combined. Pour the mixture into a greased pan and bake in the Air Fryer for 18-20 minutes until the eggs are set. Top with parsley and serve.

RECIPE 760: ASPARAGUS STRATA

Serve: 4 | Total Time: 30 minutes

6 asparagus spears, 2-inch pieces
2 slices whole-wheat bread, ½-inch cubes
4 eggs
3 tbsp whole milk
½ cup grated Havarti
2 tbsp chopped flat-leaf parsley
Salt and black pepper, to taste

1 tbsp water
Non-stick cooking spray

Place the asparagus spears and 1 tbsp. water in a baking pan and place in the basket. Select BAKE. Bake for 5 minutes at 325°F until crisp and tender. Drain the asparagus. Spray the pan with non-stick cooking spray. Place the bread cubes and asparagus in the pan and set them aside. Whisk the eggs and milk in a large mixing dish. Add the cheese, parsley, salt, and pepper. Pour into the baking pan. Select BAKE. Set temperature to 360°F, set time to 14 minutes or until the eggs are set, and the top starts to brown. When the cooking time is complete, transfer to a platter and serve hot.

RECIPE 761: AVOCADO AND SPINACH MELTS

Serve: 4 | Total Time: 15 minutes

4 tbsp cheddar cheese, grated
2 brioche buns, halved
2 tbsp Dijon mustard
8 baby spinach leaves
4 tomato slices
½ peeled avocado, sliced
8 basil leaves

Preheat Air Fryer to 390°F. Set the bun halves in the frying basket and Air Fry for 2 minutes until golden, then set them on a clean surface. Smear 1 ½ tsp of mustard on each bun piece, then put 2 spinach leaves, 1 tomato slice, ¼ of the avocado, 2 basil leaves and 1 tbsp of cheese on the top. Bake the sandwiches in the Air Fryer for 3-4 minutes. Make sure the cheese is melted. Serve hot.

RECIPE 762: BAKED ALMOND CHICKEN

Serve: 3 | Total Time: 25 minutes

2 lbs chicken breast tenderloins
3 organic eggs
1 cup almond meal
1 tbsp chili powder
2 tbsp Italian seasoning

2 tbsp onion powder
1/3 tbsp garlic powder
1 tsp cayenne pepper
Salt, to taste
Black pepper, to taste

Preheat the Air Fryer to temperature of 400 degrees F. Take a dish and grease it with oil spray. On a flat plate, combine chili powder, almond meal, onion powder, cayenne pepper, Italian seasoning, garlic powder, pepper, salt, and pepper. Whisk eggs in a small separate bowl. Dip the pieces of chicken in the eggs, then in the dry mix. Arrange the chicken in the dish and cook for about 25-30 minutes. Serve.

RECIPE 763: BAKED APPLE

Serve: 2 | Total Time: 40 minutes

1 medium apple or pear
¼ tsp cinnamon
2 tbsp raisins
2 tbsp chopped walnuts
¼ tsp nutmeg
1½ tsp light margarine, melted
¼ cup water
Ensure that your Air Fryer is preheated to 350 F. Cut the pear or apple in half, around the middle, to gain access to scrape out some of the flesh. Place the pear or apple at the base of the Air Fryer, or in the frying pan of the Air Fryer (if available). Get a clean small bowl, and in it, combine the cinnamon, raisins, walnuts, nutmeg, and margarine. Fill the pears or apples with the mixture. Add some water into the pan, and bake the halves for 20 minutes.

RECIPE 764: BAKED BACON EGG CUPS

Serve: 2 | Total Time: 12 minutes

2 eggs
1 tbsp chives, fresh, chopped
½ tsp paprika
½ tsp cayenne pepper
3 oz cheddar cheese, shredded
½ tsp butter
¼ tsp salt

4 oz bacon, cut into tiny pieces

Slice bacon into tiny pieces and sprinkle it with cayenne pepper, salt, and paprika. Mix the chopped bacon. Spread butter in bottom of ramekin dishes and beat the eggs there. Add the chives and shredded cheese. Add the chopped bacon over egg mixture in ramekin dishes. Place all of the ramekins in the basket of your Air Fryer. Preheat your Air Fryer to 360°Fahrenheit. Place the Air Fryer basket in your Air Fryer and cook for 12-minutes.

RECIPE 765: BAKED CHEESE CRISPS

Serve: 4 | Total Time: 20 minutes

1/2 cup Parmesan cheese, shredded
1 cup Cheddar cheese, shredded
1 tsp Italian seasoning
1/2 cup marinara sauce

Begin by preheating your Air Fryer and set it to 350 degrees F. Place a piece of parchment paper in the cooking basket. Mix the cheese with the Italian seasoning. Add around one tbsp of the cheese mixture (per crisp to the basket, making sure they are not touching—Bake for 6 minutes, or until the top is browned to your preference. Work in batches, transferring them to a large baking sheet to cool somewhat. Toss with the marinara sauce before serving. Greetings and best wishes!

RECIPE 766: BAKED CHEESE 'N PEPPERONI CALZONE

Serve: 4 | Total Time: 35 minutes

1 cup chopped pepperoni
1 loaf frozen bread dough, thawed
1 to 2 tbsp 2% milk
1 tbsp grated Parmesan cheese
1/2 cup pasta sauce with meat
1/2 tsp Italian seasoning, optional
1/4 cup shredded part-skim mozzarella cheese

In a bowl mix well mozzarella cheese, pizza sauce, and pepperoni. On a lightly floured surface, divide dough into four portions. Set each into a 6-in. circle; top each with a scant 1/3 cup pepperoni mixture. Fold dough over filling; pinch edges to seal. Lightly grease baking pan of Air Fryer with cooking spray. Place dough in a single layer and if needed, cook in batches. For 25 minutes, cook on 330F preheated Air Fryer or until dough is lightly browned. Serve and enjoy.

RECIPE 767: BAKED CHICKEN WINGS

Serve: 4 | Total Time: 42 minutes

2 lbs chicken wings
1 tsp baking powder
1 tsp salt
1 tbsp butter
1/3 cup hot wing sauce

Preheat the Air Fryer to 4000F for 5 minutes. Dry the chicken wings with paper towel and sprinkle with baking powder and salt. Place the chicken wings on the crisper tray. Make sure to leave enough space for the air to circulate. Select the Air Fry setting and adjust the cooking time to 30 minutes. Meanwhile, you have to melt the 1 tbsp of butter in a medium pot. Add the hot wing sauce. Stir for 5 minutes. Serve the air fried wings with the hot sauce.

RECIPE 768: BAKED EGGS FOR BREAKFAST

Serve: 5 | Total Time: 15 minutes

5 oz. Ham, sliced into pieces
1 cup pound baby spinach
5 organic eggs, refrigerated
6 tbsp full cream milk
2 tbsp olive oil
Salt and pepper, to taste
Butter, for greasing

First, preheat the Air Fryer to temperature of 350 degrees F. Now, butter a ramekin and set aside. Heat the olive oil in a desired pan and cook baby spinach until wilted. Divide this cooked spinach over the five ramekins. Divide the ham equally over the five ramekins. Crack one egg into each ramekin. Add milk to each ramekin. Sprinkle salt and pepper at the end. Bake for about 15 minutes in the Air Fryer. Serve and enjoy.

RECIPE 769: BAKED EGGS IN AVOCADO NESTS

Serve: 2 | Total Time: 25 minutes

1 large avocado, halved
2 eggs
4 grape tomato, halved
2 tsp chives, chopped
A pinch of salt and black pepper

Cut avocado in half length-wise. Remove the pit and widen the hole in each half by scraping out the avocado flesh with the help of the spoon.
Place avocado halves in a small oven proof baking dish cut side up. Beat an egg into each half of avocado. Season with salt and pepper.
Cook for about 10-15 minutes in 370°F into the Air Fryer.
Top with grape tomato halves and chives. Enjoy!

RECIPE 770: BAKED EGGS WITH CHEESE

Serve: 6 | Total Time: 25 minutes

Cooking spray
12 eggs
2/3 cup cheese, shredded
Salt and pepper

Spray a muffin pan with cooking spray. Crack an egg in each cup and make sure that you don't break the yolk. Sprinkle some shredded cheese on each cup. Place the muffin pan on the pizza rack on shelf position 5 of the Emeril Lagasse Air Fryer 360 and select the bake setting. Preheat the oven to temperature of 350 degrees

Fahrenheit set the timer for 20 minutes. Press the start button to start. Check if the eggs are fully cooked by running the tip of a knife on one egg. Add more time if not cooked through. Serve immediately when seasoned with salt and pepper.

RECIPE 771: BAKED EGGS AND SAUSAGE MUFFINS

Serve: 2 | Total Time: 20 minutes

3 eggs
¼ cup cream
2 sausages, boiled
Chopped fresh herbs
Sea salt to taste
4 tbsp cheese, grated
1 piece of bread, sliced lengthwise

Preheat your Air Fryer to 360°Fahrenheit. Scramble the eggs in a bowl with the milk and salt and pepper to taste. Cooking spray should be used to grease three muffin tins. Fill each with an equal quantity of the egg mixture. Arrange sliced sausages and bread slices into muffin cups, sinking into egg mixture. Sprinkle the tops with cheese, and salt to taste. Cook the muffins for 20-minutes. Season with fresh herbs and serve warm.

RECIPE 772: BAKED EGGS WITH SPINACH AND BASIL

Serve: 2 | Total Time: 22 minutes

2 tbsps olive oil
4 eggs, whisked
5 ounces (142 g) fresh spinach, chopped
1 medium-sized tomato, chopped
1 tsp fresh lemon juice
½ tsp ground black pepper
½ tsp coarse salt
½ cup chopped fresh basil leaves, for garnish

Olive oil should be used to grease a baking pan. Stir together the remaining ingredients except the basil leaves in the greased baking pan until well incorporated. Select Bake. Set temperature to 280°F

(137ºC) and set time to 10 minutes. Press Start to begin preheating. Place the pan in the oven after it has been warmed. When cooking is complete, the eggs should be completely set and the vegetables should be tender. Remove from oven and scatter the basil leaves on top.

RECIPE 773: BAKED EGGPLANT AND ZUCCHINI

Serve: 4 | Total Time: 45 minutes

1 medium eggplant, sliced
3 medium zucchinis, sliced
3 oz. Parmesan cheese, grated
4 tbsp. parsley, chopped
4 tbsp. basil, chopped
1 tbsp. olive oil
4 garlic cloves, minced
1 cup cherry tomatoes, halved
1/4 tsp pepper
1/4 tsp salt

In a mixing bowl, add cherry tomatoes, eggplant, zucchini, olive oil, garlic, cheese, basil, pepper, and salt toss well until combined. Transfer the eggplant mixture into the greased baking dish. Place the inner pot in the Air Fryer combo base. Place baking dish into the inner pot. Cover the inner pot with an air frying lid. Select bake mode, then set the temperature to 350 °F and time for 35 minutes. Click start. When the countdown approaches zero, press the cancel button. Garnish with chopped parsley and serve.

RECIPE 774: BAKED PEARS WITH CHOCOLATE

Serve: 4 | Total Time: 35 minutes

4 firm ripe pears, peeled, and sliced
2 tbsp Truvia for baking
½ tsp ground star anise
1 tsp pure vanilla extract
1 tsp orange extract
½ stick butter, cold
½ cup chocolate chips for garnish

Grease the baking dish with olive oil cooking spray; lay pear slices on the bottom of pan. In a bowl, mix Truvia, star anise, vanilla and orange extract. Sprinkle this mixture over the fruit layer. Cut in the butter and scatter it evenly over the top. Air-fry at 380°Fahrenheit for 35-minutes. Serve sprinkle with chocolate chips for garnish.

RECIPE 775: BAKED SHRIMP BITES

Serve: 4 | Total Time: 25 minutes

1 cup shrimps; peeled, deveined and chopped
8 ounces ready-made puff pastry; cut into 15 squares
1/2-tbsp. lemon juice
2-tbsp. olives, chopped
1-tbsp. dill, finely chopped
pepper, to taste

Mix the shrimps with the dill, lemon juice, olives and pepper. Place a full-tsp. of the shrimp mixture onto each pastry square. Fold each pastry square over into a triangle. Prepare the edges by moistening them with water and pressing them together firmly with a fork. Preheat the Air Fryer to temperature of 400 degrees F. Arrange the shrimp bites in the Air Fryer Basket and use the Air Fryer Double Layer Rack if needed. Spray the shrimp bites with cooking spray and cook for 10 minutes. Serve and enjoy!

RECIPE 776: BAKED STUFFED PEPPERS

Serve: 4 | Total Time: 15 minutes

4 cored pears, halved
½ cup chopped cashews
½ cup dried cranberries
¼ cup agave nectar
½ stick butter, softened
½ tsp ground cinnamon
½ cup apple juice

Preheat the Air Fryer to 350°F. Combine the cashews, cranberries, agave nectar, butter, and cinnamon

and mix well. Stuff this mixture into the pears, heaping it up on top. Set the pears in a baking pan and pour the apple juice into the bottom of the pan. Put the pan in the fryer and Bake for 10-12 minutes or until the pears are tender. Let cool before serving.

RECIPE 777: BAKED SWEET POTATO WITH YOGURT CHIVES SAUCE

Serve: 3 | Total Time: 65 minutes

2 large sweet potatoes
1 cup plain whole-milk yogurt
2 tbsp honey
2 tbsp chives, chopped
¼ tsp kosher salt

On the COSORI Air Fryer Toaster Oven, choose the Air Fry feature, set the timer to 1 hour and the temperature to 350°F, and then push Start/Cancel to warm. Place the sweet potatoes on the wire rack and place it in the preheated Air Fryer toaster oven in the middle position. Press the Start/Cancel button. In a small dish, combine the yogurt, honey, chives, and kosher salt; set aside until the sweet potatoes are entirely roasted. After 5 minutes, remove the sweet potatoes from the oven and cool. Serve with a dollop of chive yogurt sauce and an incision in the centre of the potatoes.

RECIPE 778: BAKED TOMATO

Serve: 2 | Total Time: 40 minutes

2 eggs
2 large fresh tomatoes
1 tsp fresh parsley
Pepper
Salt

Cut off the top of a tomato and spoon out the tomato innards. Break the egg in each tomato. Place the inner pot in the Air Fryer combo base. Place tomato into the inner pot. Cover the inner pot with an air frying lid. Select bake mode, then set the temperature to 350 °F and time for 15 minutes. Click start. When the countdown approaches zero, press the cancel button. Season tomato with parsley, pepper, and salt. Serve and enjoy.

RECIPE 779: BAKED ZUCCHINI EGGPLANT

Serve: 6 | Total Time: 40 minutes

3 medium zucchinis, sliced
1 medium eggplant, sliced
1 tbsp olive oil
4 garlic cloves, minced
1/4 tsp pepper
3 oz parmesan cheese, grated
1/4 cup parsley, chopped
1/4 cup basil, chopped
1 cup cherry tomatoes, halved
1/4 tsp salt

Spray baking dish with cooking spray. In a bowl, add cherry tomatoes, eggplant, zucchini, olive oil, garlic, cheese, basil, pepper, and salt toss well until combined. Transfer eggplant mixture into the baking dish. Select bake mode and set the Omni to 350° F for 35 minutes once the oven beeps, place the baking dish into the oven. Garnish with parsley and serve.

RECIPE 780: BALSAMIC LONDON BROIL

Serve: 4 | Total Time: 25 minutes

2 ½ lb top round London broil steak
¼ cup coconut aminos
1 tbsp balsamic vinegar
1 tbsp olive oil
1 tbsp mustard
2 tsp maple syrup
2 garlic cloves, minced
1 tsp dried oregano
Salt and pepper to taste
¼ tsp smoked paprika
2 tbsp red onions, chopped

Whisk coconut aminos, mustard, vinegar, olive oil, maple oregano, syrup, oregano garlic, red onions, salt, pepper, and paprika in a small bowl. Put the steak in a shallow container and pour the marinade over the steak. Cover and let sit for 20 minutes. Preheat Air Fryer to 400°F. Transfer the steak to the frying basket and bake for 5 minutes. Flip the steak and bake for another 4 to 6 minutes. Allow sitting for 5 minutes before slicing. Serve warm and enjoy.

RECIPE 781: BANANA AND WALNUT CAKE

Serve: 6 | Total Time: 35 minutes

1 pound (454 g) bananas, mashed
8 ounces (227 g) flour
6 ounces (170 g) sugar
3.5 ounces (99 g) walnuts, chopped
2.5 ounces (71 g) butter, melted
2 eggs, lightly beaten
¼ tsp baking soda

Preheat the Air Fryer to 355ºF (179ºC). In a bowl, combine the sugar, butter, egg, flour, and baking soda with a whisk. Stir in the bananas and walnuts. Pour the mixture to a baking dish that has been buttered. Put the dish in the Air Fryer and bake for 10 minutes. Reduce the temperature to 330ºF (166ºC) and bake for another 15 minutes. Serve hot.

RECIPE 782: BANANA MUFFINS WITH CHOCOLATE CHIPS

Serve: 8 | Total Time: 25 minutes

1 cup flour
½ tsp baking soda
1/3 cup brown sugar
¼ tsp salt
1/3 cup mashed banana
½ tsp vanilla extract
1 egg
1 tbsp vegetable oil
¼ cup chocolate chips
1 tbsp powdered sugar

Preheat Air Fryer at 375ºF. Combine dry ingredients in a bowl. In another bowl, mix wet ingredients. Pour wet ingredients into dry ingredients and gently toss to combine. Fold in chocolate chips. Do not overmix. Spoon mixture into 8 greased silicone cupcake liners, place them in the frying basket, and Bake for 6-8 minutes. Let cool onto a cooling rack. Serve right away sprinkled with powdered sugar.

RECIPE 783: BASIL FETA CROSTINI

Serve: 4 | Total Time: 10 minutes

1 baguette, sliced
¼ cup olive oil
2 garlic cloves, minced
4 oz feta cheese
2 tbsp basil, minced

Preheat Air Fryer to 380°F. Combine together the olive oil and garlic in a bowl. Brush it over one side of each slice of bread. Put the bread in a single layer in the frying basket and Bake for 5 minutes. In a small bowl, mix together the feta cheese and basil. Remove the toast from the Air Fryer, then spread a thin layer of the goat cheese mixture over the top of each piece. Serve.

RECIPE 784: BASMATI RISOTTO

Serve: 2 | Total Time: 40 minutes

1 onion, diced
1 small carrot, diced
2 cups vegetable broth, boiling
½ cup grated Cheddar cheese
1 clove garlic, minced
¾ cup long-grain basmati rice
1 tbsp olive oil
1 tbsp unsalted butter

Preheat the Air Fryer to temperature 390ºF (199ºC). Grease a baking tin with oil and stir in the butter, garlic, carrot, and onion. Put the tin in the Air Fryer and bake for 4 minutes. Pour in the rice and bake for a further 4 minutes, stirring three times throughout the baking time. Reduce the temperature to 320 degrees Fahrenheit (160 degrees Celsius). Add the vegetable broth and give the dish a gentle stir. Bake for 22 minutes, uncovered in the Air Fryer. Pour in the cheese, stir once more and serve.

RECIPE 785: BATTERED CHICKEN THIGHS

Serve: 4 | Total Time: 18 minutes

1 ½ lbs. chicken thighs
2 cups buttermilk
1 tbsp baking powder
2 tsp black pepper
2 cups almond flour
2 tsp sea salt
1 tsp cayenne pepper
1 tbsp paprika
1 tbsp garlic powder

Place chicken thighs into a bowl. In another bowl, mix buttermilk, salt, pepper, cayenne and black pepper. Pour mixture over chicken thighs. Use foil to cover the bowl, then place in the fridge for 4-hours. Preheat your Air Fryer to 400°Fahrenheit. Mix flour, baking powder, paprika and garlic powder I a shallow bowl. Line baking dish with parchment paper. Dip chicken thighs in flour mixture and bake for 10-minutes. Flip chicken thighs over and bake on the other side for an additional 8-minutes.

RECIPE 786: BEANS AND EGGS

Serve: 6 | Total Time: 27 minutes

Cooking spray
12 eggs
Salt and pepper

Spray a muffin pan with cooking spray. Crack an egg in each cup and make sure that you don't break the yolk. Place the muffin pan on the pizza rack on position 5 of the Emeril Lagasse Air Fryer 360 and select the bake setting. Preheat the oven to 350 degrees Fahrenheit. To begin, set a timer for 20 minutes. Press the start button to start. Check if the eggs are fully cooked by running the tip of a knife on one egg. Serve immediately after seasoning with salt and pepper.

RECIPE 787: BEEF CASSEROLE

Serve: 4 | Total Time: 40 minutes

1 pound ground beef
1 green bell pepper, seeded and chopped
1 onion, chopped
3 cloves of garlic, minced
6 cups eggs, beaten
3 tbsp olive oil
Salt and pepper

Preheat the Air Fryer for about 5 minutes. In an ovenproof dish, mix the ground beef, the garlic, the olive oil, the onion, and the bell pepper. Season with salt and pepper. Toss in the beaten eggs until fully combined. Place the dish with the beef and egg mixture in the Air Fryer. Cook for 30 mins at 325 degrees F.

RECIPE 788: BEEF ENCHILADA DIP

Serve: 8 | Total Time: 15 minutes

2 lbs. ground beef
½ onion, chopped fine
2 cloves garlic, chopped fine
2 cups enchilada sauce
2 cups Monterrey Jack cheese, grated
2 tbsp. sour cream

Place rack in position. Heat a large skillet over med-high heat. Cook until the steak begins to brown, about 5 minutes. Drain off fat. Stir in onion and garlic and cook until tender, about 3 minutes. Stir in enchilada sauce and transfer mixture to a small casserole dish and top with cheese. Set oven to convection bake on 325°F for 10 minutes. After 5 minutes, add casserole to the oven and bake 3-5 minutes until cheese is melted and mixture is heated through. Serve warm topped with sour cream.

RECIPE 789: BEEFY BELL PEPPER 'N EGG SCRAMBLE

Serve: 4 | Total Time: 40 minutes

1 green bell pepper, seeded and chopped
1 onion, chopped
1-pound ground beef
2 cloves of garlic, minced
3 tbsp olive oil
6 cups eggs, beaten
Salt and pepper to taste

Preheat the Air Fryer for 5 minutes with baking pan insert. In a baking dish mix the ground beef, onion, garlic, olive oil, and bell pepper. Season with salt and pepper to taste. Pour in the beaten eggs and give a good stir. Place the dish with the beef and egg mixture in the Air Fryer. Bake for 30 minutes at 330F.

RECIPE 790: BERBERE BEEF STEAKS

Serve: 4 | Total Time: 45 minutes

1 chipotle pepper in adobo sauce, minced
1 lb skirt steak
2 tbsp chipotle sauce
¼ tsp Berbere seasoning
Salt and pepper to taste

Cut the steak into 4 equal pieces, then place them on a plate. Mix together chipotle pepper, adobo sauce, salt, pepper, and Berbere seasoning in a bowl. Then coat both sides of the steak. Chill for 2 hours. Preheat Air Fryer to 390°F. Place the steaks in the frying basket and Bake for 5 minutes on each side for well-done meat. Allow the steaks to rest for 5 more minutes. To serve, slice against the grain.

RECIPE 791: BERRY-GLAZED TURKEY BREAST

Serve: 4 | Total Time: 75 minutes

1 (4 lb) bone-in, skin-on turkey breast
1 tbsp olive oil
Salt and pepper to taste
1 cup raspberries
1cup chopped strawberries
2 tbsp balsamic vinegar

2 tbsp butter, melted
1 tbsp honey mustard
1 tsp dried rosemary

Preheat the Air Fryer to 350°F. Lay the turkey breast skin-side up in the frying basket, brush with the oil, and sprinkle with salt and pepper. Bake for 55-65 minutes, flipping twice. Meanwhile, mix the berries, vinegar, melted butter, rosemary and honey mustard in a blender and blend until smooth. Turn the turkey skin-side up inside the fryer and brush with half of the berry mix. Bake for 5 more minutes. Put the remaining berry mix in a small saucepan and simmer for 3-4 minutes while the turkey cooks. Serve with the remaining glaze.

RECIPE 792: BLACK AND WHITE BROWNIES

Serve: 5 | Total Time: 20 minutes

1 egg
1/3 cup brown sugar
2 tbsp white sugar
2 tbsp coconut oil, melted
1 tsp vanilla
¼ cup cocoa powder
½ cup all-purpose flour
1/4 cup white chocolate chips

First, spray a non-stick baking dish with flour. Take a bowl and beat the egg in it. Then add both sugars. Beat in the oil and vanilla. Next, add the remaining ingredients and make brownie dough. Spoon the brownie batter into the pan. Bake for 20 minutes in the Air Fryer at 350 degrees. Let it cool for 30 minutes before slicing.

RECIPE 793: BLACK BEAN AND TOMATO CHILI

Serve: 6 | Total Time: 38 minutes

1 tbsp olive oil
1 medium onion, diced
3 garlic cloves, minced
1 cup vegetable broth
3 cans black beans, drained and rinsed

2 cans diced tomatoes
2 chipotle peppers, chopped
2 tsp cumin
2 tsp chili powder
1 tsp dried oregano
½ tsp salt

3 minutes over medium heat, sauté the garlic and onions in the olive oil. Add the remaining ingredients, stirring constantly and scraping the bottom to prevent sticking. Take a dish and place the mixture inside. Put a sheet of aluminum foil on top. Press "Power Button" turn the dial to select "bake". Push "Temp" to set the temperature at 400°F. Press "Timer" to set the cooking time to 20 minutes. When ready, plate up and serve immediately.

RECIPE 794: BLACK BEAN STUFFED POTATO BOATS

Serve: 4 | Total Time: 55 minutes

4 russets potatoes
1 cup chipotle mayonnaise
1 cup canned black beans
2 tomatoes, chopped
1 scallion, chopped
1/3 cup chopped cilantro
1 poblano chile, minced
1 avocado, diced

Preheat Air Fryer to 390°F. Clean the potatoes, poke with a fork, and spray with oil. Put in the Air Fryer and Bake for 30 minutes or until softened. Cook the beans in a pan over medium heat until they are hot. Put the potatoes on a plate and cut them across the top. Open them with a fork so you can stuff them. Top each potato with chipotle mayonnaise, beans, tomatoes, scallions, cilantro, poblano chile, and avocado. Serve immediately.

RECIPE 795: BLACK FOREST HAND PIES

Serve: 6 | Total Time: 18 minutes

3 tbsp chocolate chips
2 tbsp hot fudge sauce
2 tbsp chopped dried cherries
1 sheet of puff pastry, 16 inches

1 egg white, beaten
2 tbsp sugar
½ tsp cinnamon

Combine first four ingredients in a bowl. Now roll out the puff pastry on a flat floured space. Cut it into 6 squares and divide the bowl mixture onto the center of the puff pastry. Fold the pastry to make triangles. Press the edges of pastry and brush the sides of triangles with egg whites. Sprinkle cinnamon and sugar on top. Bake for 18 minutes at temperature of 340°F or until golden brown. Let it cool and then serve.

RECIPE 796: BLACK OLIVE AND SHRIMP SALAD

Serve: 4 | Total Time: 15 minutes

1 lb cleaned shrimp, deveined
½ cup olive oil
4 garlic cloves, minced
1 tbsp balsamic vinegar
¼ tsp cayenne pepper
¼ tsp dried basil
¼ tsp salt
¼ tsp onion powder
1 tomato, diced
¼ cup black olives

Preheat Air Fryer to 380°F. Place the olive oil, garlic, balsamic, cayenne, basil, onion powder and salt in a bowl and stir to combine. Divide the tomatoes and black olives between 4 small ramekins. Top with shrimp and pour a quarter of the oil mixture over the shrimp. Bake for 6-8 minutes until the shrimp are cooked through. Serve.

RECIPE 797: BLUEBERRY PANCAKES

Serve: 4 | Total Time: 25 minutes

½ tsp vanilla extract
2 tbsp honey
½ cup blueberries
½ cup sugar
2 cups plus
2 tbsp flour
3 eggs, beaten
1 cup milk

1 tsp baking powder
pinch of salt

Preheat the Air Fryer to 390F. Combine all of the dry ingredients. Whisk in the wet ingredients until the mixture is smooth. Fold in the blueberries, making sure not to color the dough. You can do that by coating the blueberries with some flour before adding them to the dough. Grease a baking dish. Drop the batter onto the dish, ensuring that the pancakes have some space between them. Do it in two batches if you have too much batter. Bake for about 10 minutes. Serve and enjoy.

RECIPE 798: BREAKFAST BLUEBERRY COBBLER

Serve: 4 | Total Time: 20 minutes

¾ tsp baking powder
⅓ cup whole-wheat pastry flour
Dash sea salt
⅓ cup unsweetened nondairy milk
2 tbsps maple syrup
½ tsp vanilla
Cooking spray
½ cup blueberries
¼ cup granola
Nondairy yogurt, for topping (optional)

Spritz a baking pan with cooking spray. Firstly, combine the baking powder, flour, and salt. Add the milk, maple syrup, and vanilla and whisk to combine. Scrape the mixture into the prepared pan. Scatter the blueberries and granola on top. Bake it for about 15 minutes at a temperature of 350ºF (177ºC) in the Air Fryer, or until the top starts to be brown and a knife inserted in the middle comes out clean. Let the cobbler cool for 5 minutes and serve with a drizzle of nondairy yogurt.

RECIPE 799: BREAKFAST CASSEROLE

Serve: 4 | Total Time: 40 minutes

3 tbsp brown sugar

1/2 cup of flour
1/2 tsp cinnamon powder
4 tbsp margarine
2 tbsp white sugar
2 eggs
2-1/2 tbsp white flour
1 tsp baking powder
1 tsp baking soda
2 tbsp sugar
4 tbsp margarine
1/2 cup of milk
1-1/3 cup of blueberries
1 tbsp lemon zest

Preheat the 360 Deluxe Air Fryer Oven by selecting the pizza/bake mode. Adjust the temperature to 300°F. In a bowl, mix the casserole ingredients, then pour it into the 360 Deluxe Air Fryer Oven baking pan. In a separate bowl, mix white sugar with flour, margarine, white sugar, and cinnamon. Mix until a crumbly mixture is achieved, spread over the blueberry's mixture. Transfer to the 360 Deluxe Air Fryer Oven and bake for 30 minutes.

RECIPE 800: BREAKFAST POCKET PIES

Serve: 2 | Total Time: 23 minutes

4-5 eggs
½ cup sausage crumble, cooked
½ cup bacon, cooked
1 box puff pastry sheets
½ cup cheddar cheese

On a stove, scramble the eggs. Slowly add the meat to the eggs as you cook them. Set aside. Spread out the puff pastry on a chopping board, cutting them into uniform rectangles. Portion the egg-and-meat mixture onto one half of the pastry, topping with cheddar cheese. Place the other pastry rectangle on top of it and seal with a fork. Bake it in your Air Fryer for about 8-10 minutes at 370°F (≈187°C), checking every 2-3 minutes for desired cooking. Serve.

RECIPE 801: BROCCOLI AND CHEESE EGG RAMEKINS

Serve: 4 | Total Time: 40 minutes

1 lb. broccoli
4 eggs, beaten
1 cup cheddar cheese, shredded
1 cup heavy cream
½ tsp ground nutmeg
1 tsp ginger powder
Salt and black pepper to taste

In boiling water, steam the broccoli for 5 minutes. Drain and place in a bowl to cool. Mix in the eggs, heavy cream, nutmeg, ginger, salt, and pepper. Divide the mixture between greased ramekins and sprinkle the cheddar cheese on top. Place it in a baking tray and cook in your Instant Vortex for 10 minutes at 360 F on Bake function. Serve.

RECIPE 802: BROCCOLI AND MUSHROOM BEEF

Serve: 4 | Total Time: 30 minutes

1 lb sirloin strip steak, cubed
1 cup sliced cremini mushrooms
2 tbsp potato starch
½ cup beef broth
1 tsp soy sauce
2 ½ cups broccoli florets
1 onion, chopped
1 tbsp grated fresh ginger
1 cup cooked quinoa

Add potato starch, broth, and soy sauce to a bowl and mix, then add in the beef and coat thoroughly. Marinate for 5 minutes. Preheat Air Fryer to 400°F. Set aside the broth and move the beef to a bowl. Add broccoli, onion, mushrooms, and ginger and transfer the bowl to the Air Fryer. Bake for 12-15 minutes until the beef is golden brown and the veggies soft. Pour the reserved broth over the beef and cook for 2-3 more minutes until the sauce is bubbling. Serve warm over cooked quinoa.

RECIPE 803: BROCCOLI CHEDDAR QUICHE

Serve: 8 | Total Time: 60 minutes

1 cup milk
6 eggs
1 tsp garlic, minced
¼ tsp cayenne
1 cup cheddar, grated
3 cups broccoli florets, chopped
½ tsp salt

Prepare a pie pan by greasing it and setting it aside. Whisk milk, eggs, garlic, cayenne, and salt in a bowl until well combined. Add in the cheese. Place the broccoli florets in the bottom of the pie pan and press down firmly. Add egg mixture over the broccoli. Position the oven rack in Rack Position 1 and place the pan on top. Select the Bake setting. Preheat the oven to temperature of 350 degrees Fahrenheit set the timer to 45 minutes. Cool for 5 minutes and serve.

RECIPE 804: BRUSCHETTA WITH BASIL PESTO

Serve: 4 | Total Time: 21 minutes

8 slices French bread, ½ inch thick
2 tbsp softened butter
1 cup shredded Mozzarella cheese
½ cup basil pesto
1 cup chopped grape tomatoes
2 green onions, thinly sliced

Place the butter-side up bread in the Air Fryer basket. 3–5 minutes at 350°F (177°C) until the bread is light golden brown. Remove the bread from the basket and cover with cheese. Then bake at 350°F (177°C) for 1–3 minutes, or until the cheese melts. Meanwhile, mix pesto, tomatoes, and green onions. Take the bread out of the Air Fryer and place it on a serving tray to cool. Serve with a tbsp of pesto on each piece of spaghetti.

RECIPE 805: BUFFALO CHICKEN MEATBALLS

Serve: 4 | Total Time: 20 minutes

1 lb. ground chicken
1 egg, beaten

1 celery stalk, trimmed and finely diced
1 cup buffalo wing sauce
1 tsp black pepper
1 tsp pink sea salt
1 tsp garlic powder
1 tsp onion powder
1 tbsp mayonnaise
1 tbsp almond flour
2 sprigs of green onion, finely chopped

Place the baking pan in Air Fryer and spray with olive oil. In a bowl, combine all ingredients, except buffalo sauce. Mix well. Use your hands to form 2-inch balls. Place the meatballs in Air Fryer and bake at 350°Fahrenheit for 15-minutes. Remove the meatballs from the Air Fryer. Place them in a low-heat pan. Coat meatballs with buffalo sauce and stir cooking in pan for 5-minutes. Serve.

RECIPE 806: BUTTER BAKED MUSSELS

Serve: 2 | Total Time: 30 minutes

15 mussels
10 grape tomatoes, halved
1/3 cup unsalted butter
1/8 cup parsley, chopped
¼ tsp crushed red peppers
¼ tsp kosher salt

Mussels should be soaked for 10 minutes in cold salted water. Insert the wire rack at mid-position in the COSORI Air Fryer Toaster Oven. Select the Bake function, set the timer to 15 minutes, then press Start/Cancel to preheat. In a glass baking dish, combine the mussels, tomatoes, butter, parsley, crushed red peppers, and salt. Place the baking dish on top of the wire rack in the prepared Air Fryer toaster oven and bake for 15 minutes. Press Start/Cancel. Remove when done and serve immediately.

RECIPE 807: BUTTER WALNUT AND RAISIN COOKIES

Serve: 8 | Total Time: 15 minutes

½ tsp pure almond extract
½ tsp pure vanilla extract
2 tbsp rum
½ cup almond flour
1 stick butter, room temperature
1/3 cup corn flour
2 tbsp Truvia
¼ cup raisins
1/3 cup walnuts, ground

In a small bowl, place rum and raisins and allow to sit for 15-minutes. In a mixing dish, beat the butter with Truvia, vanilla and almond extract until light and fluffy. Then, throw in both types of flour and ground almonds. Fold in the soaked raisins. Continue mixing until it forms a dough. Refrigerate for approximately 20 minutes after covering. Meanwhile, preheat the air-fryer to 330°Fahrenheit. Roll the dough into small cookies and place them in air-fryer cake pan; gently press each cookie with a spoon. Bake cookies for 15-minutes.

RECIPE 808: CAPRESE FLATBREAD

Serve: 2 | Total Time: 15 minutes

1 fresh mozzarella ball, sliced
1 flatbread
2 tsp olive oil
¼ garlic clove, minced
1 egg
⅛ tsp salt
¼ cup diced tomato
6 basil leaves
½ tsp dried oregano
½ tsp balsamic vinegar

Preheat Air Fryer to 380°F. Lightly brush the top of the bread with olive oil, then top with garlic. Crack the egg into a small bowl and sprinkle with salt. Place the bread into the frying basket and gently pour the egg onto the top of the pita. Top with tomato, mozzarella, oregano and basil. Bake for 6 minutes. When ready, remove the pita pizza and drizzle with balsamic vinegar. Let it cool for 5 minutes. Slice and serve.

RECIPE 809: CAULIFLOWER AND BACON BAKE

Serve: 2 | Total Time: 25 minutes

2 cups cauliflower florets
5 rashers bacon, chopped.
1 cup breadcrumbs
1/4 cup parmesan cheese, grated.
1/4 cup milk
1/4 cup onions, sliced.
1-tbsp. garlic, minced.
1/2-tsp. paprika

Preheat the Air Fryer to temperature of 350 degrees F. Mix the breadcrumbs, parmesan cheese and paprika and set aside. Whisk the milk with the minced garlic and set aside. Place the cauliflower florets in the Air Fryer Baking Pan. Add the onions and the garlic milk. Top with the breadcrumbs and chopped bacon. Place the Air Fryer Baking Pan in the Air Fryer Basket. Cook for 15 minutes. Serve and enjoy!

RECIPE 810: CAULIFLOWER CHICKEN CASSEROLE

Serve: 4 | Total Time: 40 minutes

1 lb. cooked chicken, shredded
4 oz cream cheese, softened
4 cups cauliflower florets
1/8 tsp black pepper
1/4 cup Greek yogurt
1 cup cheddar cheese, shredded
1/2 cup salsa
1/2 tsp kosher salt

Microwave the cauliflower florets for 10 minutes in the baking dish. Add cream cheese and microwave for 30 seconds more. Mix well. Add chicken, yogurt, cheddar cheese, salsa, pepper, and salt and stir everything well. Select Bake mode. Set time to 20 minutes and temperature 375 F then press START. The Air Fryer display will prompt you to ADD FOOD once the temperature is reached then place the baking dish in the Air Fryer basket. Serve and enjoy.

RECIPE 811: CAULIFLOWER COTTAGE PIE

Serve: 4 | Total Time: 40 minutes

Half a cup of bacon bits
2 cups cauliflower rice
1/4 cup tomato puree
1 tbsp coconut oil
1/2 white onion, chopped
2 lbs. lean ground beef
1 tbsp mixed spice blend

In the frying pan add coconut oil and onions cook for 2-minutes. Add the ground beef into pan and cook for an additional 5-minutes or until meat is browned. Add spices and stir to combine. Cook for another 10 minutes after completely mixing in the tomato puree. Transfer to Air Fryer baking dish. Top with cauliflower rice and bacon bits. Bake in Air Fryer at 350°Fahrenheit for 20-minutes. Serve warm.

RECIPE 812: CAULIFLOWER POPPERS

Serve: 6 | Total Time: 30 minutes

3 tbsp olive oil
1 tsp paprika
1/2 tsp ground cumin
1/4 tsp ground turmeric
Salt and ground black pepper, as required
1 medium head cauliflower, cut into florets

In a bowl, place all ingredients and toss to coat well. Place the cauliflower mixture in the greased baking pan. Select "Bake" of Iconites Air Fryer Toaster Oven and then adjust the temperature to 450 degrees F. Preheat the oven for 20 minutes by setting the timer for 20 minutes and pressing "Start." After preheating, insert the baking pan in the oven. Flip the cauliflower mixture once halfway through. After the cooking time, remove the pan from the oven, it will allow it to be served warm.

RECIPE 813: CHEESE AND CRAB STUFFED MUSHROOMS

Serve: 2 | Total Time: 30 minutes

6 oz lump crabmeat, shells discarded
6 oz mascarpone cheese, softened
2 jalapeño peppers, minced
1/4 cup diced red onions
2 tsp grated Parmesan cheese
2 portobello mushroom caps
2 tbsp butter, divided
1/2 tsp prepared horseradish
1/4 tsp Worcestershire sauce
1/4 tsp smoked paprika
Salt and pepper to taste
1/4 cup bread crumbs

30 seconds in a skillet with 1 tbsp butter. Add in onion and cook for 3 minutes until tender. Stir in mascarpone cheese, Parmesan cheese, horseradish, jalapeño peppers, Worcestershire sauce, paprika, salt and pepper and cook for 2 minutes until smooth. Fold in crabmeat. Spoon mixture into mushroom caps. Set aside. Preheat Air Fryer at 350ºF. Microwave the remaining butter until melted. Stir in breadcrumbs. Scatter over stuffed mushrooms. Place mushrooms in the greased frying basket and Bake for 8 minutes. Serve immediately.

RECIPE 814: CHEESE CAULIFLOWER MUFFINS

Serve: 4 | Total Time: 15 minutes

3 cups Cauliflower rice
1 cup shredded cheddar cheese
1/4 cup Almond flour
1 tsp Baking powder
1 tbsp Garlic powder
1 tbsp Parsley
1 tbsp Oregano
1 tbsp Paprika
1 large egg
Salt and pepper to taste
1/4 cup Crumbled feta

Put the cauliflower rice in a bowl and add all the dry ingredients, the bacon, and the cheese. Add two eggs and mix well until you can squeeze the dough with your hand

and keep its shape. Oiled a muffin container with muffins. Pour the batter into every cup of muffin, cover with feta cheese, Set the fryer to 350 degrees F. Check the muffins carefully for the correct baking time as each model bakes differently. Muffins should be cooked for between 11 and 15 minutes.

RECIPE 815: CHEESY BACON AND EGG HASH

Serve: 4 | Total Time: 45 minutes

7 oz. diced bacon, trimmed fat
24 oz. potatoes, scrubbed and peeled
2 tbsp olive oil
2 scallions, trimmed and sliced
¼ cup Mozzarella cheese, shredded
4 eggs
Salt, pepper, to taste

Cut potatoes into small cubes. Bake the potatoes for 30 minutes in a single layer on a baking sheet. Grease with cooking spray and position the baking pan in Rack Position. Select the Bake setting. Set the temperature to 30 and the time to 400F. Stir once halfway. Remove from the oven, add bacon and bake for 10 minutes. Make 4 wells in the hash and add an egg into each well. Add mozzarella around each egg. Add the pan back to the oven and bake until eggs are done. Serve.

RECIPE 816: CHEESY BREAKFAST CASSEROLE

Serve: 4 | Total Time: 24 minutes

6 slices bacon
6 eggs
Salt and pepper, to taste
Cooking spray
½ cup chopped green bell pepper
½ cup chopped onion
¾ cup shredded Cheddar cheese
Place the bacon in a skillet over medium-high heat and cook each side for about 4 minutes until evenly crisp. Remove from the heat to a paper towel-lined plate to

drain. Crumble it into small pieces and set aside. Whisk together the eggs, pepper, and salt in a medium mixing basin. Spritz a baking pan with cooking spray. Place the whisked eggs, crumbled bacon, green bell pepper, and onion in the prepared pan. Bake it in the Air Fryer for 6 minutes. Scatter the Cheddar cheese all over and bake at 400ºF (204ºC) for 2 minutes more. Allow to sit in for about 5 minutes and serve on plates.

RECIPE 817: CHEESY BROCCOLI CASSEROLE

Serve: 6 | Total Time: 35 minutes

16 oz frozen broccoli florets, defrosted and drained
1/2 tsp onion powder
15 oz can cream of mushroom soup
1 cup cheddar cheese, shredded
1/3 cup unsweetened almond milk
1 tbsp butter, melted
1/2 cup cracker crumbs

Pour the ingredients into a casserole dish, except the topping ingredients, and stir well to mix. In a medium-sized bowl, mix cracker crumbs and melted butter and sprinkle over the casserole dish mixture. Select bake mode and set the Omni to 350 F for 30 minutes, once the oven beeps, place the casserole dish into the oven. Serve and enjoy.

RECIPE 818: CHEESY BROCCOLI RICE

Serve: 8 | Total Time: 25 minutes

1 1/2 cups cooked brown rice
1 garlic clove, chopped
16 oz frozen broccoli florets
1 large onion, chopped
1 tbsp butter
3 tbsp parmesan cheese, grated
15 oz condensed cheddar cheese soup
1/3 cup unsweetened almond milk

In a medium-sized saucepan, melt the butter. Add onion and cook until tender. Add garlic and

broccoli and cook until broccoli is tender. Stir in rice, soup, and milk and cook until hot. Stir in cheese and pour broccoli mixture into the 11*8*2-inch baking dish. Select bake mode and set the Omni to 350 F for 20 minutes once the oven beeps, place the baking dish into the oven. Serve and enjoy.

RECIPE 819: CHEESY CHORIZO, CORN, AND POTATO FRITTATA

Serve: 4 | Total Time: 20 minutes

2 tbsp olive oil
1 chorizo, sliced
4 eggs
1/2 cup corn
1 large potato, boiled and cubed
1 tbsp chopped parsley
1/2 cup feta cheese, crumbled
Salt and ground black pepper, to taste

Stirring frequently, heat the olive oil until it shimmers. Cook for 4 minutes or until golden brown. Whisk the eggs in a bowl, then sprinkle with salt and ground black pepper. Mix the remaining ingredients in the egg mixture, then pour the chorizo and its fat into a baking pan. Pour in the egg mixture. Place the pan on the bake position. Select Bake, set temperature to 330ºF (166ºC) and set time to 8 minutes. Stir the mixture halfway through. When cooking is complete, the eggs should be set. Serve immediately.

RECIPE 820: CHEESY CRAB TOASTS

Serve: 6 | Total Time: 15 minutes

1 (6-ounce / 170-g) can flaked crab meat, well drained
3 tbsp light mayonnaise
¼ cup shredded Parmesan cheese
¼ cup shredded Cheddar cheese
1 tsp Worcestershire sauce
½ tsp lemon juice
1 loaf artisan bread, French bread, or baguette, cut into ⅜-inch-thick slices

Preheat the Air Fryer to temperature 360°F (182°C). Combine all of the specified ingredients, except the bread pieces, in a medium-sized mixing basin. On a clean work surface, lay the bread slices. Spread ½ tbsp of crab mixture onto each slice of bread. Arrange the bread slices in the Air Fryer basket in a single layer. You'll need to work in batches to avoid overcrowding. Bake for 5 minutes until the tops are lightly browned. Transfer to a plate and repeat with the remaining bread slices. Serve warm.

RECIPE 821: CHEESY CREAMY BROCCOLI CASSEROLE

Serve: 4 | Total Time: 35 minutes

4 cups broccoli florets
¼ cup heavy whipping cream
1/2 cup sharp Cheddar cheese, shredded
¼ cup ranch dressing
salt and black pepper, to taste

Combine all of the said ingredients above in a medium-sized bowl. Toss to coat well broccoli well. Pour the mixture into a baking pan. Place the pan on the bake position. Select Bake, set temperature to 375°F (190°C) and set time to 30 minutes. When cooking is complete, the broccoli should be tender. Remove the baking pan from the Air Fryer grill and serve immediately.

RECIPE 822: CHEESY GARLIC SWEET POTATOES

Serve: 8 | Total Time: 50 minutes

¼ cup garlic butter, melted
4 sweet potatoes, halved lengthwise
¾ cup Mozzarella cheese, shredded
½ cup Parmesan cheese, grated
2 tbsp parsley, chopped
½ tbsp salt and black pepper, to taste

Brush potatoes with garlic butter and season well with salt and pepper. Place cut side down on a greased baking pan. Position the baking pan in Rack Position 2 and select the Bake setting. Set the temperature to 425° F and the time to 30 minutes. Remove from the oven, flip and top with parsley, mozzarella and parmesan. Select the Broil setting. Set the temperature to Broil and the time to 2 minutes. Season well and serve.

RECIPE 823: CHEESY GREEN WONTON TRIANGLES

Serve: 10 | Total Time: 55 minutes

6 oz marinated artichoke hearts
6 oz cream cheese
¼ cup sour cream
¼ cup grated Parmesan
¼ cup grated cheddar
5 oz chopped kale
2 garlic cloves, chopped
Salt and pepper to taste
20 wonton wrappers

Microwave cream cheese in a bowl for 20 seconds. Combine with sour cream, Parmesan, cheddar, kale, artichoke hearts, garlic, salt, and pepper. Lay the wrappers out on the board. Scoop 1 ½ tsp of cream cheese mixture on top of the wrapper. Fold up diagonally to form a triangle. Bring together the two bottom corners. Squeeze out any air and press together to seal the edges. Preheat Air Fryer to 375°F. Place a batch of wonton in the greased frying basket and Bake for 10 minutes. Flip them and cook for 5-8 minutes until crisp and golden. Serve.

RECIPE 824: CHEESY ITALIAN MEATLOAF

Serve: 4 | Total Time: 50 minutes

1 pound ground beef
¾ cup mozzarella cheese, shredded
¼ cup fresh grated parmesan
1 tsp Italian seasoning
¼ tsp ground black pepper
¼ tsp salt
1 tbsp almond flour

1 tbsp tomato paste
1 tbsp monk fruit sweetener
1 tsp apple cider vinegar
1 tsp Dijon mustard

Preheat your Air Fryer at 350 degrees Fahrenheit and grease two loaf pans that will fit in the basket. Combine the meat, cheeses, Italian seasoning, pepper, salt, and almond flour in a large mixing basin. Blend together well and then place in a greased loaf pan. Bake for 35 minutes. While the meatloaf is baking, combine the tomato paste, monk fruit sweetener, vinegar and mustard. Mix well. Once the meatloaf is done, spoon the sauce over the top and then slice and serve.

RECIPE 825: CHEESY MUSHROOMS AND SPINACH FRITTATA

Serve: 2 | Total Time: 15 minutes

1 cup chopped mushrooms
2 cups spinach, chopped
4 eggs, lightly beaten
3 ounces (85 g) feta cheese, crumbled
2 tbsp heavy cream
A handful of fresh parsley, chopped
Salt and ground black pepper, to taste
Cooking spray

Spritz a baking pan with cooking spray. In a large bowl, combine all ingredients. Stir to mix well. Pour the created mixture in the prepared baking pan. Place the pan on the bake position. Select Bake, set temperature to 350°F (180°C) and set time to 8 minutes. Stir the mixture halfway through. When cooking is complete, the eggs should be set. Serve immediately.

RECIPE 826: CHEESY TUNA TOWER

Serve: 2 | Total Time: 15 minutes

½ cup grated mozzarella
1 (6-oz) can tuna in water
¼ cup mayonnaise
2 tsp yellow mustard

1 tbsp minced dill pickle
1 tbsp minced celery
1 tbsp minced green onion
Salt and pepper to taste
4 tomato slices
8 avocado slices

Preheat Air Fryer to 350ºF. In a bowl, combine tuna, mayonnaise, mustard, pickle, celery, green onion, salt, and pepper. Cut a piece of parchment paper to fit the bottom of the frying basket. Place tomato slices on paper in a single layer and top with 2 avocado slices. Share tuna salad over avocado slices and top with mozzarella cheese. Place the towers in the frying basket and Bake for 4 minutes until the cheese starts to brown. Serve warm.

RECIPE 827: CHICKEN CHEESE TAQUITOS

Serve: 5 | Total Time: 23 minutes

¾ pound (340 g) chicken breasts, boneless and skinless
Kosher salt and ground black pepper, to taste
½ tsp red chili powder
5 small corn tortillas
5 ounces (142 g) Cotija cheese, crumbled

Pat the chicken dry with kitchen towels. Toss the chicken breasts in a bowl with pepper, salt, and red chili powder to coat. Cook the chicken at 380ºF (193ºC) for 12 minutes, turning them over halfway through the cooking time. Place the shredded chicken and cheese on one end of each tortilla. Roll them up tightly and transfer them to a lightly oiled Air Fryer basket. Bake your taquitos at 360ºF (182ºC) for 6 minutes. Bon appétit!

RECIPE 828: CHICKEN CHEESE ZUCCHINI CASSEROLE

Serve: 4 | Total Time: 55 minutes

2 pounds ground chicken
2 7 oz cans tomato paste
3 cloves garlic

1 pint ricotta cheese
3 eggs
2 tbsp bragg's liquid aminos
½ small onion, diced
2 15 oz cans tomato sauce
a pinch of stevia
2 zucchini, cut into cubes
black pepper and sea salt to taste

Preheat the Air Fryer to 375F and grease a baking dish using oil. In a mixing bowl add the chicken. Add in the onion, liquid aminos, 2 eggs and liquid aminos. Add the ground chicken mix onto your baking dish. Add the zucchini cubes on top. In a bowl combine one egg with salt, pepper and cheese. Add the cheese mixture on top of the zucchinis. In another bowl combine the stevia, tomato sauce and mix well. Add on top of the cheese and bake in the Air Fryer for nearly 1 hour.

RECIPE 829: CHICKPEA AND BULGUR BAKED DINNER

Serve: 6 | Total Time: 55 minutes

1 cup bulgur
2 ¼ cups chicken stock
1 (15.5-oz) can chickpeas
½ cup diced carrot
½ cup green peas
1 tsp ground cumin
½ tsp ground turmeric
½ tsp ground ginger
½ tsp shallot powder
Salt and pepper to taste
¼ tsp ground cinnamon
¼ tsp garlic powder
2 tbsp cilantro, chopped

Preheat Air Fryer to 380ºF. Add the bulgur, stock, chickpeas, carrot, peas, cumin, turmeric, ginger, shallot powder, salt, cinnamon, garlic powder, and black pepper to a greased casserole dish and stir well to combine. Cover loosely with aluminum foil. Put the casserole dish into the Air Fryer and bake for 20 minutes. Stir well and uncover. Bake for 25 more minutes. Fluff with a spoon. Garnish with cilantro. Serve and enjoy!

RECIPE 830: CHIPOTLE PORK CHOPS

Serve: 4 | Total Time: 35 minutes

4 pork chops
1 lime, juiced
Salt and black pepper to taste
1 tsp garlic powder
2 cups white rice, cooked
1 can (14.5 oz) tomato sauce
1 onion, chopped
3 garlic cloves, minced
½ tsp dried oregano
1 tsp chipotle chili powder

Pork chops should be seasoned with salt, pepper, and garlic powder. In a bowl, mix onion, garlic, chipotle powder, oregano, and tomato sauce. Toss in the pork to coat. Let marinate for 1 hour. Remove the chops from the mixture and place them in a greased baking dish. Select Bake function, adjust the temperature to 380 F, and press Start. Cook for 25 minutes. Serve with rice.

RECIPE 831: CHOCOLATE AND NUT MIX BARS

Serve: 4 | Total Time: 20 minutes

1/4 cup walnuts
1/4 cup cashew nuts
1/4 cup almonds
1/4 cup coconut chips
1 egg, beaten1/2 cup butter, melted
1/4 cup dark chocolate chips
1/4 cup hemp seeds
Salt to taste
1 cup mixed dried berries

Preheat oven to a temperature of 350 F. Line a baking sheet with wax paper. In a food processor, pulse nuts until roughly chopped. Place in a bowl and stir in chocolate chips, egg, butter, hemp seeds, salt, and berries. Bake for 18 minutes after spreading the ingredients on the baking sheet. Let cool and cut into bars.

RECIPE 832: CHOCOLATE APRICOT MUFFINS

Serve: 6 | Total Time: 15 minutes

3 tsp cocoa powder
¾ dried apricots, roughly chopped
1 ¼ cups almond flour
1 tsp pure rum extract
1 ½ tbsp Truvia for baking
2 eggs
1 stick butter, room temperature
¼ cup maple syrup, sugar-free
1 cup rice milk
½ tsp baking soda
1 tsp baking powder
¼ tsp nutmeg, grated
½ tsp ground cinnamon
1/8 tsp salt

In a bowl, combine Truvia, almond flour, baking soda, baking powder, salt, nutmeg, cinnamon and cocoa powder. In another bowl, add butter and cream it, also add egg, rum extract, rice milk, sugar-free maple syrup; whisk to combine. Add next, your wet mixture to the dry mixture and fold in the apricots. Press the batter into a lightly greased muffin tin. Bake in air-fryer at 345°Fahrenheit for 15-minutes.

RECIPE 833: CHOCOLATE PEANUT BUTTER BREAD PUDDING

Serve: 8 | Total Time: 22 minutes

Nonstick baking spray with flour
1 egg
1 egg yolk
¾ cup chocolate milk
2 tbsp cocoa powder
3 tbsp brown sugar
3 tbsp peanut butter
1 tsp vanilla
5 slices firm white bread, cubed

Spray a 6-by-6-by-2-inch baking pan with nonstick spray. In a medium bowl, combine the egg, egg yolk, chocolate milk, cocoa, brown sugar, peanut butter, and vanilla, and mix until combined. Allow 10 minutes for the bread cubes to soak. Spoon this mixture into the prepared pan. Bake it for about 10-12 minutes or until the pudding is firm to the touch.

RECIPE 834: CHORIZO AND GARLIC VEGGIE BAKE

Serve: 4 | Total Time: 40 minutes

1 cup halved Brussels sprouts
1 lb baby potatoes, halved
1 cup baby carrots
1 onion, sliced
2 garlic cloves, sliced
2 tbsp olive oil
Salt and pepper to taste
1 lb chorizo sausages, sliced
2 tbsp Dijon mustard

Preheat the Air Fryer to 370°F. Put the potatoes, Brussels sprouts, baby carrots, garlic, and onion in the frying basket and drizzle with olive oil. Toss with salt and pepper. Bake for 15 minutes, shaking once, until crisp yet tender. Add the chorizo sausages to the fryer and cook for 8-12 minutes, shaking once until the sausages are hot and the veggies tender. Drizzle with the mustard to serve.

RECIPE 835: CHORIZO AND VEGETABLE BAKE

Serve: 4 | Total Time: 20 minutes

1/2-lb. Brussels sprouts, trimmed and halved
4 chorizo sausages
2 mixed bell peppers, sliced
1 red onion, sliced
1/2-tsp. dried thyme
Salt and black pepper to taste

Preheat the Air Fryer to temperature of 350 degrees F. Spray the Air Fryer basket with cooking spray. Take a bowl and, mix Brussels sprouts, bell peppers, red onion, thyme, salt and black pepper. Set aside. Arrange the chorizo sausages on the bottom of the Air Fryer basket. Cook for 6 minutes. Slide out the fryer basket, flip the chorizo and add the vegetable mixture; cook for another 8 minutes. Serve.

RECIPE 836: CINNAMON BANANA BREAD WITH PECANS

Serve: 6 | Total Time: 35 minutes

2 ripe bananas, mashed
1 egg
¼ cup Greek yogurt
¼ cup olive oil
½ tsp peppermint extract
2 tbsp honey
1 cup flour
¼ tsp salt
¼ tsp baking soda
½ tsp ground cinnamon
¼ cup chopped pecans

Preheat Air Fryer to 360°F. Add the bananas, egg, yogurt, olive oil, peppermint, and honey in a large bowl and mix until combined and mostly smooth. Sift the flour, salt, baking soda, and cinnamon into the wet mixture, then stir until just combined. Gently fold in the pecans. Spread to distribute evenly into a greased loaf pan. Place the loaf pan in the frying basket and Bake for 23 minutes or until golden brown on top and a toothpick inserted into the center comes out clean. Allow to cool for 5 minutes. Serve.

RECIPE 837: CINNAMON PEAR OAT MUFFINS

Serve: 6 | Total Time: 30 minutes

½ cup apple sauce
1 large egg
1/3 cup brown sugar
2 tbsp butter, melted
½ cup milk
11/3 cups rolled oats
1 tsp ground cinnamon
½ tsp baking powder
Pinch of salt
½ cup diced peeled pears

Preheat the Air Fryer to 350°F. Place the apple sauce, egg, brown sugar, melted butter, and milk into a bowl and mix to combine. Stir in the oats, cinnamon, baking powder, and salt and mix well, then fold in the pears. Grease 6 silicone muffin cups with baking spray, then spoon the batter in equal portions into the cups. Put the muffin cups in the frying basket and Bake for 13-18 minutes or until set. Leave to cool for 15 minutes. Serve.

RECIPE 838: CLASSIC BUTTER-BREAD PUDDING

Serve: 4 | Total Time: 28 minutes

1 tsp cloves, ground
1/3 cup half-and-half
1 cup milk
4 slices sweet raisin bread, torn into pieces
1 tbsp chocolate flavored liqueur
3 tbsp butter, softened
1 tsp bergamot extract
1/3 tsp ground ginger
3 eggs lightly beaten
1 tbsp Truvia for baking

In a bowl, add bread pieces. In another bowl, add the remaining ingredients and mix well. Scrape the mixture from second bowl, into bread bowl and allow it to soak for 15-minutes. Press with a wide spatula. Divide the bread pudding evenly between 2 mini loaf pans. Bake for 28-minutes at 305°Fahrenheit in air-fryer.

RECIPE 839: CLASSIC RAISIN BREAD PUDDING

Serve: 4 | Total Time: 28 minutes

1 tsp cloves, ground
1/3 cup half-and-half
1 cup milk
4 slices sweet raisin bread, torn into pieces
1 tbsp chocolate flavored liqueur
3 tbsp butter, softened
1 tsp bergamot extract
1/3 tsp ground ginger
3 eggs lightly beaten
1 tbsp Truvia for baking

In a bowl, add bread pieces. In another bowl, add the remaining ingredients and mix well. Scrape the mixture from second bowl, into bread bowl and allow it to soak for 15-minutes. Press with a wide spatula. Divide the bread pudding evenly between 2 mini loaf pans. Bake for 28-minutes at 305° Fahrenheit in air-fryer.

RECIPE 840: COATED ARTICHOKE FRIES

Serve: 4 | Total Time: 20 minutes

1 14-oz can artichoke hearts, quartered

For Wet Mix:
1 cup all-purpose flour
1 cup almond milk
½ tsp garlic powder¾ tsp salt
¼ tsp black pepper, or to taste

For Dry Mix:
1 ½ cup panko breadcrumbs
½ tsp paprika
¼ tsp salt

Preheat your Air Fryer to 370° Fahrenheit.
Combine the salmon, egg, celery, onion, dill, and garlic in a large mixing bowl.
Shape the mixture into golf ball size balls and roll them in the wheat germ.
In a small pan, warm olive oil over medium-low heat.
Add the salmon balls and slowly flatten them.
Transfer them to your Air Fryer and cook for 10-minutes.

RECIPE 841: COCKTAIL CHICKEN MEATBALLS

Serve: 4 | Total Time: 30 minutes

2 tsp olive oil
¼ cup onion, minced
¼ red bell pepper, minced
3 tsp grated Parmesan cheese
1 egg white
½ tsp cayenne pepper
½ tsp dried thyme
½ lb ground chicken

Preheat Air Fryer to 370°F. Combine the olive oil, onion, and red bell pepper in a baking pan, then transfer to the Air Fryer. Bake for 3-5 minutes until tender. Add the cooked vegetables, Parmesan cheese, egg white, ground chicken, cayenne pepper, and thyme to a bowl and stir. Form the mixture into small meatballs and put them in the frying basket. Air Fry for

10-15 minutes, shaking the basket once until the meatballs are crispy and brown on all sides. Serve warm.

RECIPE 842: COCONUT CHICKEN BAKE

Serve: 6 | Total Time: 20 minutes

2 large eggs, beaten
2-tbsp. garlic powder
1-tbsp. salt
1/2-tbsp. ground black pepper
3/4 cup breadcrumbs
3/4 cup shredded coconut
1-lb. chicken tenders
Cooking spray

Preheat the fryer to temperature of 400 degrees F. Spray a baking sheet with cooking spray. In a wide dish, whisk in garlic powder, eggs, pepper and salt. To make the breadcrumbs and coconut mixture, place it in a separate dish. Dip your chicken tenders in egg, then in the coconut mix; shake off any excess. Place the prepared chicken tenders in your Air Fryer's cooking basket and cook for 12-14 minutes until golden brown.

RECIPE 843: COCONUT CREAM ROLL-UPS

Serve: 4 | Total Time: 20 minutes

½ cup cream cheese, softened
1 cup fresh raspberries
¼ cup brown sugar
¼ cup coconut cream
1 egg
1 tsp corn starch
6 spring roll wrappers

Preheat Air Fryer to 350°F. Add the cream cheese, brown sugar, coconut cream, cornstarch, and egg to a bowl and whisk until all ingredients are completely mixed and fluffy, thick and stiff. Spoon even amounts of the creamy filling into each spring roll wrapper, then top each dollop of filling with several raspberries. Roll up the wraps around the creamy raspberry filling, and seal the seams with a few dabs of water. Place each roll on the foil-lined frying basket, seams facing down. Bake for 10 minutes, flipping them once until golden brown and perfect on the outside, while the raspberries and cream filling will have cooked together in a glorious fusion. Remove with tongs and serve hot or cold. Serve and enjoy!

RECIPE 844: COCONUT MINI TARTS

Serve: 2 | Total Time: 25 minutes

¼ cup almond butter
1 tbsp coconut sugar
2 tbsp coconut yogurt
½ cup oat flour
2 tbsp strawberry jam

Preheat Air Fryer to 350°F. Use 2 pieces of parchment paper, each 8-inches long. Draw a rectangle on one piece. Beat the almond butter, coconut sugar, and coconut yogurt in a shallow bowl until well combined. Mix in oat flour until you get a dough. Put the dough onto the undrawing paper and cover it with the other one, rectangle-side up. Using a rolling pin, roll out until you get a rectangle. Discard top paper. Cut it into 4 equal rectangles. Spread on 2 rectangles, 1 tbsp of strawberry jam each, then top with the remaining rectangles. Using a fork, press all edges to seal them. Bake in the fryer for 8 minutes. Serve right away.

RECIPE 845: COCONUT ORANGE CAKE

Serve: 6 | Total Time: 17 minutes

¾ cup shredded coconut
¼ tsp salt
1/3 tsp nutmeg, grated
½ tsp baking powder
1 ¼ cups almond flour
2 eggs
2 tbsp Truvia
1 stick butter
2 tbsp orange jam
1/3 coconut milk

Preheat your air-fryer to 355° Fahrenheit. Spritz the inside of your cake pan with cooking spray. Then, beat the butter with Truvia until fluffy. Fold in the eggs; continue mixing until smooth. Add nutmeg, salt, and flour; then, slowly pour in the coconut milk. Finally, add the shredded coconut and orange jam; mix to create cake batter. Then, press the batter into cake pan. Bake cake in air-fryer for 17-minutes, then transfer the cake to a cooling rack. Serve chilled.

RECIPE 846: COCONUT PIE

Serve: 4 | Total Time: 25 minutes

2 Eggs
1 1/2 cups Coconut milk
1/4 cup Butter
1 1/2 tsp Vanilla extract
1 cup shredded coconut
1/2 cup Granulated Monk Fruit
1/2 cup Coconut flour

Cover a 6-inch cake pan with a non-stick spray and fill it with batter. In a large bowl, add in all the ingredients and, using a wooden spoon, stir until well blended. Pour the batter into the pie dish that has been prepared and bake in the fryer for about 12 minutes at temperature of 350 degrees F. Check the cake halfway through the cooking process to make sure it's not burnt, turn the plate and use a toothpick to check that it's done.

RECIPE 847: CORN AND BELL PEPPER CASSEROLE

Serve: 4 | Total Time: 30 minutes

1 cup corn kernels
¼ cup bell pepper, finely chopped
1/2 cup low-fat milk
1 large egg, beaten
1/2 cup yellow cornmeal
1/2 cup all-purpose flour
1/2 tsp baking powder
2 tbsp melted unsalted butter
1 tbsp granulated sugar
Pinch of cayenne pepper

¼ tsp kosher salt
Cooking spray

Spritz a baking pan with cooking spray. In a big mixing basin, mix together all the ingredients. Stir to mix well. Pour the mixture into the baking pan. Place the pan on the bake position. Select Bake, set temperature to 330°F (166°C) and set time to 20 minutes. When cooking is complete, the casserole should be lightly browned and set. Remove the baking pan from the Air Fryer grill and serve immediately.

RECIPE 848: CORN DOG CUPCAKES

Serve: 6 | Total Time: 30 minutes

1 cup cornbread Mix
2 tsp granulated sugar
Salt to taste
3/4 cup cream cheese
3 tbsp butter, melted
1 egg
¼ cup minced onions
1 tsp dried parsley
2 beef hot dogs, sliced and cut into half-moons

Preheat Air Fryer at 350°F. Combine cornbread, sugar, and salt in a bowl. In another bowl, whisk cream cheese, parsley, butter, and egg. Pour wet ingredients to dry ingredients and toss to combine. Fold in onion and hot dog pieces. Transfer it into 8 greased silicone cupcake liners. Place it in the frying basket and Bake for 8-10 minutes. Serve right away.

RECIPE 849: CRAB CAKE BITES

Serve: 6 | Total Time: 20 minutes

8 oz lump crab meat
1 diced red bell pepper
1 spring onion, diced
1 garlic clove, minced
1 tbsp capers, minced
1 tbsp cream cheese
1 egg, beaten
¼ cup bread crumbs
¼ tsp salt
1 tbsp olive oil

1 lemon, cut into wedges

Preheat Air Fryer to 360°F. Combine the crab, bell pepper, spring onion, garlic, and capers in a bowl until combined. Stir in the cream cheese and egg. Mix in the bread crumbs and salt. Make 6 patties out of this mixture by dividing it into 6 equal parts. Put the crab cakes into the frying basket in a single layer. Drizzle the tops of each patty with a bit of olive oil and Bake for 10 minutes. Serve with lemon wedges on the side. Enjoy!

RECIPE 850: CRANBERRY CHICKEN CURRY

Serve: 4 | Total Time: 30 minutes

3 low-sodium boneless, skinless chicken breasts, 1 ½-inch cubes
2 tsp olive oil
2 tbsp cornstarch
1 tbsp curry powder
1 tart apple, chopped
½ cup low-sodium chicken broth
⅓ cup dried cranberries
2 tbsp freshly squeezed orange juice
Brown rice, cooked (optional)

Combine the chicken and olive oil in a medium mixing bowl. Sprinkle with the cornstarch and curry powder. Toss to coat. Stir in the apple and transfer to a metal pan. Bake in the Air Fryer at 380°F (193°C) for 8 minutes, stirring once during cooking. Add the chicken broth, cranberries, and orange juice. Bake it for about another 10 minutes, or until the sauce has thickened somewhat and the chicken has achieved an intended temperature of 165°F (74°C) on a meat thermometer. Serve with a hot cooked brown rice, if desired.

RECIPE 851: CRANBERRY CRUSTED SALMON

Serve: 4 | Total Time: 30 minutes

Olive oil cooking spray

4 salmon filets
Salt & pepper to taste
2 tbsp extra virgin olive oil
¼ cup dried cranberries, chopped
½ cup walnuts, chopped
1 tsp orange zest
1 tbsp Dijon mustard
2 tbsp parsley, chopped

Preheat your Air Fryer toast oven to 370°F. Lightly coat the basket of your Air Fryer toast oven with olive oil cooking spray. Generously season the fish filets with sea salt and pepper and arrange them on the baking sheet. In a small dish, combine the other ingredients until thoroughly combined. Spread the mixture across the filets and bake in the preheated fryer for approximately 15 minutes, or until the topping is gently browned on the edges. Remove from Air Fryer toast oven and serve.

RECIPE 852: CREAMY BAKED DORY

Serve: 2 | Total Time: 25 minutes

2 dory fillets
1/2 cup cheddar cheese, grated.
5 cloves garlic, sliced.
8 lemon slices
1/2 cup bacon bits
1 cup cream
1-tbsp. lemon juice
2-tbsp. rosemary, chopped.
1-tsp. garlic powder
1-tsp. paprika
salt and pepper, to taste

Attach the Air Fryer Grill Pan and preheat the Air Fryer to 350 degrees F. Season the dory fillets with salt, pepper, garlic powder and paprika. Arrange the fillets on the Air Fryer Grill Pan and cook for 10 minutes. While the fish fillets are cooking, make the cream sauce. To make the cream sauce: Mix the cream, cheese and garlic in a saucepan over medium heat. Season with salt, pepper, and rosemary leaves. Remove the fish from the Air Fryer. Drizzle over with the lemon juice and top with

the cream sauce, lemon slices and bacon bits. Serve and enjoy!

RECIPE 853: CREAMY CAULIFLOWER CASSEROLE

Serve: 4 | Total Time: 25 minutes

1 cauliflower head, cut into florets, and boil
2 cups cheddar cheese, shredded
2 tsp Dijon mustard
2 oz. cream cheese
1 cup heavy cream
1 tsp garlic powder
1/2 tsp pepper
1/2 tsp salt

Place the inner pot in the Air Fryer combo base. Add all ingredients into the inner pot and mix well. Cover the inner pot with an air frying lid. Select bake mode, then set the temperature to 375 °F and time for 15 minutes. Click start. When the countdown approaches zero, press the cancel button. Serve and enjoy.

RECIPE 854: CREAMY HORSERADISH ROAST BEEF

Serve: 6 | Total Time: 65 minutes

1 topside roast, tied
Salt to taste
1 tsp butter, melted
2 tbsp Dijon mustard
3 tbsp prepared horseradish
1 garlic clove, minced
2/3 cup buttermilk
2 tsp red wine
1 tbsp minced chives
Salt and pepper to taste

Preheat Air Fryer to 320°F. Mix salt, butter, half of the mustard, 1 tsp of horseradish, and garlic until blended. Rub all over the roast. Bake the roast in the Air Fryer for 30-35 minutes, flipping once until browned. Transfer to a cutting board and cover with foil. Let rest for 15 minutes. In a bowl, mix buttermilk, horseradish, remaining mustard, chives, wine, salt, and pepper until smooth. Refrigerate. When ready to serve, carve the roast into thin slices and serve with horseradish cream on the side.

RECIPE 855: CREAMY SPINACH-BROCCOLI DIP

Serve: 4 | Total Time: 24 minutes

½ cup low-fat Greek yogurt
¼ cup nonfat cream cheese
½ cup frozen chopped broccoli, thawed and drained
½ cup frozen chopped spinach, thawed and drained
⅓ cup chopped red bell pepper
1 garlic clove, minced
½ tsp dried oregano
2 tbsp grated low-sodium Parmesan cheese

Firstly, combine the cream cheese and yogurt in a mixing bowl until well blended. Stir in the broccoli, spinach, red bell pepper, garlic, and oregano. Transfer to a baking pan. Sprinkle with the Parmesan cheese. Close the cover and place the pan in the Air Fryer basket. Bake at 340°F (171°C) for 9 to 14 minutes, or until the dip is bubbly and the top starts to brown. Serve immediately.

RECIPE 856: CROISSANT MUSHROOM AND EGG

Serve: 1 | Total Time: 8 minutes

1 croissant, sliced in half crosswise
½ sprig rosemary, chopped
1 large egg
Salt and pepper to taste
3 cherry tomatoes, halved
1 ½ ounces of cheddar cheese, shredded
4 small button mushrooms, quartered
Handful of salad greens
Butter for greasing baking dish

Prepare baking dish by greasing it with butter. Arrange all the ingredients in two layers in baking dish except for salad greens and croissant. Crack egg into baking dish, add mushrooms and cheese on the top then season with salt, pepper, and rosemary. Preheat your

Air Fryer to 325°Fahrenheit. Bake for 8-minutes and then assemble your breakfast sandwich and enjoy!

RECIPE 857: CROISSANT MUSHROOM, TOMATOES AND EGG

Serve: 1 | Total Time: 8 minutes

1 croissant, sliced in half crosswise
½ sprig rosemary, chopped
1 large egg
Salt and pepper to taste
3 cherry tomatoes, halved
1 ½ ounces of cheddar cheese, shredded
4 small button mushrooms, quartered
Handful of salad greens
Butter for greasing baking dish

Prepare baking dish by greasing it with butter. Arrange all the Ingredients in two layers in baking dish except for salad greens and croissant. Crack egg into baking dish, add mushrooms and cheese on the top then season with salt, pepper, and rosemary. Preheat your Air Fryer to 325°Fahrenheit. Bake for 8-minutes and then assemble your breakfast sandwich and enjoy!

RECIPE 858: CRUNCHY GRANOLA MUFFINS

Serve: 4 | Total Time: 15 minutes

1 cup walnut pieces
1 cup sunflower seeds
1 cup coconut flakes
¼ cup granulated sugar
⅛ cup coconut flour
⅛ cup pecan flour
2 tsp ground cinnamon
2 tbsp melted butter
2 tbsp almond butter
⅛ tsp salt

Preheat Air Fryer to 300ºF. In a bowl, mix the walnuts, sunflower seeds, coconut flakes, sugar, coconut flour, pecan flour, cinnamon, butter, almond butter, and salt. Spoon the mixture into an

ungreased round 4-cup baking dish. Place it in the frying basket and Bake for 6 minutes, stirring once. Transfer to an airtight container, let cool for 10 minutes, then cover and store at room temperature until ready to serve.

RECIPE 859: CRUSTED SCALLOPS

Serve: 4 | Total Time: 30 minutes

1-1/2 lb Bay scallops, rinsed
3 garlic cloves, minced
1/2 cup panko crumbs
1 tsp onion powder
4 tbsp butter, melted
1/2 tsp cayenne pepper
1 tsp garlic powder
1/4 cup parmesan cheese, shredded

Mix everything in a bowl except scallops. Toss in scallops and mix well to coat them. Spread the scallops with the sauce on a baking tray. Press the "power button" of the Air Fryer and turn the dial to select the "bake" mode. Press the Time button and again turn the dial to set the cooking time to 20 minutes. Now push the temp button and rotate the dial to set the temperature at 400°F. Once preheated, place the scallop's baking tray in the oven and close its lid.

RECIPE 860: CRUSTLESS CHEESECAKE

Serve: 4 | Total Time: 15 minutes

16 oz. cream cheese softened to room temperature
3/4 cup monk fruit sweetener
2 Eggs
1 tsp vanilla extract
1/2 tsp lemon juice
2 tbsp sour cream

Preheat the Vortex Air Fryer to 350 degrees F. Mix the eggs, sweetener, vanilla, and lemon juice in a blender until creamy. Put sour cream and cream cheese and mix until the pieces are smooth and glossy. The more you beat, the richer the consistency will be. Pour the dough into two 4-inch spring form pans and bake for 8-10 minutes or until done. Let leave it to cool fully on the spring plate. Store in the fridge overnight or at least 1 to 2 hours. Enjoy it!

RECIPE 861: CURRIED CAULIFLOWER

Serve: 4 | Total Time: 25 minutes

2 lbs. cauliflower, cut into florets
1 1/2 tsp curry powder
1 tbsp olive oil
1 tbsp cilantro, chopped
2 tsp fresh lemon juice
1 tsp kosher salt

In a large mixing basin, toss the cauliflower florets with the olive oil. Sprinkle cauliflower florets with curry powder and salt. Spread cauliflower florets onto a cooking pan. Select bake mode and set the Omni to 425 degrees Fahrenheit for 15 minutes. When the oven beeps, put the baking pan in the oven and bake for another 15 minutes. Return roasted cauliflower florets into the bowl and toss with cilantro and lemon juice. Serve and enjoy.

RECIPE 862: DATE AND HAZELNUT COOKIES

Serve: 10 | Total Time: 20 minutes

3 tbsp sugar-free maple syrup
1/3 cup dated, dried
¼ cup hazelnuts, chopped
1 stick butter, room temperature
½ cup almond flour
½ cup corn flour
2 tbsp Truvia for baking
½ tsp vanilla extract
1/3 tsp ground cinnamon
½ tsp cardamom

Firstly, cream the butter with Truvia and maple syrup until mixture is fluffy. Sift both types of flour into bowl with butter mixture. Add remaining ingredients. Knead the ingredients to make a dough, then chill it for 20 minutes. To finish, shape the chilled dough into bite-size balls; arrange them on a baking dish and flatten balls with back of spoon. Bake the cookies for 20-minutes at 310°Fahrenheit.

RECIPE 863: DELICIOUS CLAFOUTIS

Serve: 6 | Total Time: 25 minutes

¼ tsp nutmeg, grated
½ tsp crystalized ginger
1/3 tsp ground cinnamon
½ tsp baking soda
½ tsp baking powder
2 tbsp Truvia for baking
½ cup coconut cream
¾ cup coconut milk
3 eggs, whisked
4 medium-sized pears, cored and sliced
1 ½ cups plums, pitted
¾ cup almond flour

Lightly grease 2 mini pie pans using a non-stick cooking spray. Lay the plums and pears on the bottom of pie pans. Warm the cream and coconut milk in a medium saucepan over medium heat. Remove from heat and whisk in flour, baking soda, and baking powder. In a bowl, mix the eggs, Truvia, spices until the mixture is creamy. Add the creamy milk mixture. Carefully spread this mixture over your fruit in pans. Bake at 320°Fahrenheit for 25-minutes.

RECIPE 864: DIJON SHRIMP CAKES

Serve: 4 | Total Time: 30 minutes

1 cup cooked shrimp, minced
¾ cup saltine cracker crumbs
1 cup lump crabmeat
3 green onions, chopped
1 egg, beaten
¼ cup mayonnaise
2 tbsp Dijon mustard
1 tbsp lemon juice

Preheat the Air Fryer to 375°F. Combine the crabmeat, shrimp, green onions, egg, mayonnaise, mustard, ¼ cup of cracker crumbs, and the lemon juice in a bowl and mix gently. Make 4 patties, sprinkle with the rest of the cracker crumbs on both sides, and spray with cooking oil. Line the frying basket with a round parchment paper with holes poked in it. Coat the paper with cooking spray and lay the patties on it. Bake for 10-14 minutes or until the patties are golden brown. Serve warm.

RECIPE 865: EFFORTLESS TOFFEE ZUCCHINI BREAD

Serve: 6 | Total Time: 30 minutes

1 cup flour
½ tsp baking soda
½ cup granulated sugar
¼ tsp ground cinnamon
¼ tsp nutmeg
¼ tsp salt
1/3 cup grated zucchini
1 egg
1 tbsp olive oil
1 tsp vanilla extract
2 tbsp English toffee bits
2 tbsp mini chocolate chips
1/2 cup chopped walnuts

Preheat Air Fryer at 375°F. Combine the flour, baking soda, toffee bits, sugar, cinnamon, nutmeg, salt, zucchini, egg, olive oil, vanilla and chocolate chips in a bowl. Add the walnuts to the batter and mix until evenly distributed. Pour the mixture into a greased cake pan. Place the pan in the fryer and Bake for 20 minutes. Let sit for 10 minutes until slightly cooled before slicing. Serve immediately.

RECIPE 866: EGG AND BACON CUPS

Serve: 4 | Total Time: 23 minutes

4 bread slices
2 bacon slices, cooked and chopped
4 large eggs
Salt and black pepper to taste

Preheat the Air Fryer's oven in Bake mode at 400 F for 2–3 minutes. Fit each bread slice into each of 4 medium muffin cups to form cups and divide the bacon into each. Crack the eggs into the cups, season with salt, black pepper, and place the cups on the cooking tray. Insert the cooking tray onto the middle rack of the oven, close the Air Fryer, and bake in the oven 13 minutes. Once ready, remove from the oven, take the food out of the cups, and serve immediately.

RECIPE 867: EGG AND BACON TOASTS

Serve: 4 | Total Time: 25 minutes

4 French bread slices, cut diagonally
1 + tsp butter
4 eggs
2 tbsp milk
½ tsp dried thyme
Salt and pepper to taste
4 oz cooked bacon, crumbled
2/3 cup grated Colby cheese

Preheat the Air Fryer to 350°F. Spray each slice of bread with oil and Bake in the frying basket for 2-3 minutes until light brown; set aside. Beat together the eggs, milk, thyme, salt, and pepper in a bowl and add the melted butter. Transfer to a 6-inch cake pan and place the pan into the fryer. Bake for 7-8 minutes, stirring once or until the eggs are set. Transfer the egg mixture into a bowl. Top the bread slices with egg mixture, bacon, and cheese. Return to the fryer and Bake for 4-8 minutes or until the cheese melts and browns in spots. Serve.

RECIPE 868: EGGLESS BROWNIES

Serve: 8 | Total Time: 50 minutes

1/4 cup walnuts, chopped
1/3 cup cocoa powder
2 tsp baking powder
1 cup of sugar
1 cup all-purpose flour

1/2 cup chocolate chips
2 tsp vanilla
1 tbsp milk
3/4 cup yogurt
1/2 cup butter, melted
1/4 tsp salt

Fit the Air Fryer oven with the rack in position. In a large mixing bowl, sift flour, cocoa powder, baking powder, and salt. Mix well and set aside. In another bowl, add butter, vanilla, milk, and yogurt and whisk until well combined. Mix it altogether in flour mixture until it is barely blended with the butter mixture, about 30 seconds. Fold in walnuts and chocolate chips. Pour batter into the prepared baking dish. Set to bake at 350 F for 45 minutes. After 5 minutes place the baking dish in the preheated oven. Slice and serve.

RECIPE 869: EGGPLANT AND BELL PEPPERS WITH BASIL

Serve: 2 | Total Time: 36 minutes

1 small eggplant, halved and sliced
1 yellow bell pepper, thick strips
1 red bell pepper, thick strips
2 garlic cloves, quartered
1 red onion, sliced
1 tbsp extra-virgin olive oil
Salt and ground black pepper, to taste
½ cup chopped fresh basil, for garnish
Cooking spray

Grease a nonstick baking dish with cooking spray. Place the eggplant, bell peppers, garlic, and red onion in the greased baking dish. Drizzle with olive oil and stir. Spritz any uncoated surfaces with cooking spray. Select Bake. Set temperature to 350ºF (180ºC) and set time to 20 minutes. Press Start to begin preheating. Once preheated, place the baking dish into the oven. Flip the vegetables halfway through the cooking time. Remove from oven and season. Sprinkle the basil on top for garnish and serve.

RECIPE 870: ENGLISH PUMPKIN EGG BAKE

Serve: 2 | Total Time: 20 minutes

2 eggs
½ cup milk
2 cups flour
2 tbsp cider vinegar
2 tsp baking powder
1 tbsp sugar
1 cup pumpkin purée
1 tsp cinnamon powder
1 tsp baking soda
1 tsp olive oil

Preheat the Air Fryer to a heat temperature of 300ºF (149ºC). Crack the eggs into a bowl and beat with a whisk. Combine with the milk, flour, cider vinegar, baking powder, sugar, pumpkin purée, cinnamon powder, and baking soda, mixing well. Grease a baking tray with oil. Add the mixture and transfer into the Air Fryer. Bake for 10 minutes. Serve warm.

RECIPE 871: FARFALLE WITH WHITE SAUCE

Serve: 4 | Total Time: 30 minutes

4 cups cauliflower florets
1 medium onion, chopped
8 oz farfalle pasta
2 tbsp chives, minced
½ cup cashew pieces
1 tbsp nutritional yeast
2 large garlic cloves, peeled
2 tbsp fresh lemon juice
Salt and pepper to taste

Preheat Air Fryer to 390°F. Put the cauliflower in the fryer, spray with oil, and Bake for 8 minutes. Remove the basket, stir, and add the onion. Roast for 10 minutes, or until brown and soft. Cook the farfalle pasta according to the package directions. Set aside. Put the roasted cauliflower and onions along with the cashews, 1 ½ of cups water, yeast, garlic, lemon, salt, and pepper in a blender. Blend until creamy. Pour a large portion of the sauce on top of the warm pasta and add the minced scallions. Serve.

RECIPE 872: FETA AND MUSHROOM FRITTATA

Serve: 4 | Total Time: 30 minutes

1 red onion, thinly sliced
4 cups button mushrooms, thinly sliced
Salt to taste
6 tbsp feta cheese, crumbled
6 medium eggs
Non-stick cooking spray
2 tbsp olive oil

Sauté the mushrooms and onion in olive oil over medium heat until the vegetables are tender. Remove the vegetables from pan and drain on a paper towel-lined plate. In a mixing bowl, whisk eggs and salt. Coat all sides of baking dish with cooking spray. Preheat your Air Fryer to 325°Fahrenheit. Pour the beaten eggs into prepared baking dish and scatter the sautéed vegetables and crumble feta on top. Bake in the Air Fryer for 30-minutes. Allow to cool slightly and serve!

RECIPE 873: FILLED MUSHROOMS WITH CRAB

Serve: 4 | Total Time: 20 minutes

2 brown button mushroom caps
½ cup lump crab meat
1 green onion, minced
3 garlic cloves, minced
1 tbsp mayonnaise
1 tbsp olive oil
¼ cup breadcrumbs
Salt and pepper to taste
1 tbsp chopped parsley
¼ tsp dried oregano

Preheat Air Fryer to 350°F. A big dish of crab meat, mayonnaise and bread crumbs is mixed well with salt and pepper. Brush the mushroom caps with olive oil. Divide the crab mixture among the caps and place them on the greased frying basket. Bake 10 minutes. Serve topped with parsley warm.

RECIPE 874: FISH WITH VEGETABLES

Serve: 4 | Total Time: 35 minutes

1/2 lb. Cod fillet, cut into four pieces
1 cup cherry tomatoes
2 tbsp olive oil
1 cup baby potatoes, diced
Salt and Pepper

Line instant pot multi-level Air Fryer basket with aluminum foil. Toss potatoes with half olive oil and add into the Air Fryer basket and place basket into the instant pot. Seal pot with Air Fryer lid and select bake mode then set the temperature to 380 f and timer for 15 minutes. Add cod and cherry tomatoes in the basket. Drizzle with the excess oil and season with pepper and salt. Seal pot with Air Fryer lid and select bake mode then set the temperature to 380 f and timer for 10 minutes. Serve and enjoy.

RECIPE 875: FLANK STEAK WITH CARAMELIZED ONIONS

Serve: 2 | Total Time: 30 minutes

½ lb flank steak, cubed
1 tbsp mustard powder
½ tsp garlic powder
2 eggs
1 onion, sliced thinly
Salt and pepper to taste

Preheat Air Fryer to 360°F. Coat the flank steak cubes with mustard and garlic powders. Place them in the frying basket along with the onion and Bake for 3 minutes. Flip the steak over and gently stir the onions and cook for another 3 minutes. Push the steak and onions over to one side of the basket, creating space for heat-safe baking dish. Crack the eggs into a ceramic dish. Place the dish in the fryer. Cook for 15 minutes at 320°F until the egg white are set and the onion is caramelized. Season with salt and pepper. Serve warm.

RECIPE 876: FLAVORFUL BAKED HALIBUT

Serve: 4 | Total Time: 20 minutes

1 lb. halibut fillets
1/4 tsp garlic powder
1/4 tsp paprika
1/4 tsp smoked paprika
1/4 tsp pepper
1/4 cup olive oil
1 lemon juice
1/2 tsp salt

Fit the Air Fryer oven with the rack in position. Place fish fillets into the baking dish. Combine the lemon juice, oil, paprika, smoked paprika, garlic powder, and salt in a small mixing bowl. Brush lemon juice mixture over fish fillets. Set to bake at 425 F for 17 minutes. After 5 minutes place the baking dish in the preheated oven. Serve and enjoy.

RECIPE 877: FLUFFY VEGETABLE STRATA

Serve: 4 | Total Time: 30 minutes

½ red onion, thickly sliced
8 asparagus, sliced
1 baby carrot, shredded
4 cup mushrooms, sliced
½ red bell pepper, chopped
2 bread slices, cubed
3 eggs
3 tbsp milk
½ cup mozzarella cheese
2 tsp chives, chopped

Preheat Air Fryer to 330°F. Add the red onion, asparagus, carrots, mushrooms, red bell pepper, mushrooms, and 1 tbsp of water to a baking pan. Put it in the Air Fryer and Bake for 3-5 minutes, until crispy. Remove the pan, add the bread cubes, and shake to mix. Combine the eggs, milk, and chives and pour them over the veggies. Cover with mozzarella cheese. Bake for 12-15 minutes. The strata should puff up and set, while the top should be brown. Serve hot.

RECIPE 878: FRUITY BAKED OATMEAL

Serve: 9 | Total Time: 60 minutes

2 eggs, lightly beaten
3 cups quick-coating oats
1 cup packed brown sugar
2 tsps baking powder
½ tsp ground cinnamon
1 cup fat-free milk
¾ cup tart apple, peeled and chopped
½ cup butter, melted
1/3 cup peaches, chopped
1/3 cup blueberries
1 tsp salt

Mix brown sugar, oats, baking powder, cinnamon, and salt in a bowl. Mix milk, eggs, and butter in a separate bowl and add to the dry ingredients. Add peaches, apple, and blueberries. Add the mixture to a baking dish coated with cooking spray. Position the oven rack in Rack Position 1 and place the dish on top. Select the Bake setting. Preheat the oven to temperature of 350 degrees Fahrenheit set the timer to 40 minutes. Cut into squares. Serve.

RECIPE 879: FULL BAKED TROUT EN PAPILLOTE WITH HERBS

Serve: 2 | Total Time: 30 minutes

3/4-lb. whole trout, scaled and cleaned
1/4 bulb fennel, sliced.
1/2 brown onion, sliced.
3-tbsp. chopped parsley
3-tbsp. chopped dill
2-tbsp. olive oil
1 lemon, sliced.
Salt and pepper to taste

Take a bowl and, add the onion, parsley, dill, fennel and garlic. Mix and drizzle the olive oil over. Preheat your Air Fryer to temperature of 350 degrees F. Open the cavity of the fish and fill with the fennel mixture. Wrap the fish completely in parchment paper and then in foil. In a fryer basket, place the fish and cook for 10 minutes on each side. Remove the paper and foil and top with lemon slices. Serve with cooked mushrooms.

RECIPE 880: GARLICKY VEGGIE BAKE

Serve: 3 | Total Time: 25 minutes

3 turnips, sliced
1 large red onion, cut into rings
1 large zucchini, sliced
Salt and black pepper to taste
2 cloves garlic, crushed
1 bay leaf, cut in 6 pieces
1 tbsp olive oil

Place the turnips, onion, and zucchini in a bowl. Toss with olive oil, salt, and pepper. Preheat Instant Vortex on Air Fry function to 380 F. Place the veggies into a baking pan. Slip the bay leaves in the different parts of the slices and tuck the garlic cloves in between the slices. Cook for 15 minutes. Serve warm with as a side to a meat dish or salad.

RECIPE 881: GINGER TURKEY MEATBALLS

Serve: 4 | Total Time: 25 minutes

¼ cup water chestnuts, chopped
¼ cup panko bread crumbs
1 lb ground turkey
½ tsp ground ginger
2 tbsp fish sauce
1 tbsp sesame oil
1 small onion, minced
1 egg, beaten

Preheat Air Fryer to 400°F. Place the ground turkey, water chestnuts, ground ginger, fish sauce, onion, egg, and bread crumbs in a bowl and stir to combine. Form the turkey mixture into 1-inch meatballs. Arrange the meatballs in the baking pan. Drizzle with sesame oil. Bake until the meatballs are cooked through, 10-12 minutes, flipping once. Serve and enjoy!

RECIPE 882: GOAT CHEESE STUFFED TURKEY ROULADE

Serve: 4 | Total Time: 55 minutes

1 (2-lb) boneless turkey breast, skinless
Salt and pepper to taste
4 oz goat cheese
1 tbsp marjoram
1 tbsp sage
2 garlic cloves, minced
2 tbsp olive oil
2 tbsp chopped cilantro

Preheat Air Fryer to 380°F. Butterfly the turkey breast with a sharp knife and season with salt and pepper. Mix together the goat cheese, marjoram, sage, and garlic in a bowl. Spread the cheese mixture over the turkey breast, then roll it up tightly, tucking the ends underneath. Put the turkey breast roulade onto a piece of aluminum foil, wrap it up, and place it into the Air Fryer. Bake for 30 minutes. Turn the turkey breast, brush the top with oil, and then continue to cook for another 10-15 minutes. Slice and serve sprinkled with cilantro.

RECIPE 883: GOLDEN PORK QUESADILLAS

Serve: 2 | Total Time: 50 minutes

¼ cup shredded Monterey jack cheese
2 tortilla wraps
4 oz pork shoulder, sliced
1 tsp taco seasoning
½ white onion, sliced
½ red bell pepper, sliced
½ green bell pepper, sliced
½ yellow bell pepper, sliced
1 tsp chopped cilantro

Preheat Air Fryer to 350°F. Place the pork, onion, bell peppers, and taco seasoning in the greased frying basket. Air Fry for 20 minutes, stirring twice; remove. Sprinkle half the shredded Monterey jack cheese over one of the tortilla wraps, cover with the pork mixture, and scatter with the remaining cheese and cilantro. Top with the second tortilla wrap. Place in the frying basket. 12 minutes, flipping halfway, until golden crisp. Let cool before slicing. Serve and enjoy!

RECIPE 884: GREEK COD WITH ASPARAGUS

Serve: 2 | Total Time: 26 minutes

1 lb. cod, cut into 4 pieces
8 asparagus spears
1 leek, sliced
1 onion, quartered
2 tomatoes, halved
1/2 tsp oregano
1/2 tsp red chili flakes
1/2 cup olives, chopped
1 tbsp olive oil
1/4 tsp pepper
1/4 tsp salt

Fit the Air Fryer oven with the rack in position. Arrange fish pieces, olives, asparagus, leek, onion, and tomatoes in a baking dish. Season with oregano, chili flakes, pepper, and salt and drizzle with olive oil. Set to bake at 400 F for 25 minutes. After 5 minutes place the baking dish in the preheated oven. Serve and enjoy.

RECIPE 885: GREEK GYROS WITH CHICKEN AND RICE

Serve: 4 | Total Time: 25 minutes

1 lb chicken breasts, cubed
¼ cup cream cheese
2 tbsp olive oil
1 tsp dried oregano
1 tsp ground cumin
1 tsp ground cinnamon
¼ tsp ground nutmeg
Salt and pepper to taste
¼ tsp ground turmeric
2 cups cooked rice
1 cup Tzatziki sauce

Preheat Air Fryer to 380°F. Combine all of the listed ingredients in a large mixing basin until the chicken is well covered. Spread the chicken mixture in the frying basket, then Bake for 10 minutes. Stir the chicken mixture

and Bake for an additional 5 minutes. Serve with rice and tzatziki sauce.

RECIPE 886: GREEK PITA POCKETS

Serve: 4 | Total Time: 30 minutes

2 pita breads, halved crosswise
1 peeled eggplant, chopped
1 red bell pepper, sliced
½ cup red onion, diced
1 baby carrot, shredded
1 tsp olive oil
1/3 cup hummus
6 Kalamata olives, sliced

Preheat Air Fryer to 390°F. Put the eggplant, red bell pepper, red onion, carrot, and olive oil in a baking pan and mix, then put the pan into the frying basket and Bake for 7-9 minutes. Cook until the veggies are soft, making sure to stir once. Spread the hummus inside the pita bread pockets. Add the vegetables and olives. Put the sandwiches in the Air Fryer and Bake for 2-3 minutes, until the bread is browned to your taste. Serve warm.

RECIPE 887: GREEN STRATA

Serve: 4 | Total Time: 35 minutes

5 asparagus, chopped
4 eggs
3 tbsp milk
1 cup baby spinach, torn
2 bread slices, cubed
½ cup grated Gruyere cheese
2 tbsp chopped parsley
Salt and pepper to taste

Preheat Air Fryer to 340°F. Add asparagus spears and 1 tbsp water in a baking pan. Place the pan into the Air Fryer. Bake until crisp and tender, 3-5 minutes. Remove. Wipe to basket clean and spray with cooking spray. Return asparagus to the pan and arrange the bread cubes. Beat the eggs and milk in a bowl. Then mix in baby spinach and Gruyere cheese, parsley, salt, and pepper. Pour over the asparagus and bread. Return to the

fryer and Bake until eggs are set, and the tops browned, 12-14 minutes. Serve warm.

RECIPE 888: HALIBUT QUESADILLAS

Serve: 2 | Total Time: 30 minutes

¼ cup shredded cheddar
¼ cup shredded mozzarella
1 tsp olive oil
2 tortilla shells
1 halibut fillet
½ peeled avocado, sliced
1 garlic clove, minced
Salt and pepper to taste
½ tsp lemon juice

Preheat Air Fryer to 350°F. Brush the halibut fillet with olive oil and sprinkle with salt and pepper. Bake in the Air Fryer for 12-14 minutes, flipping once until cooked through. Combine the avocado, garlic, salt, pepper, and lemon juice in a bowl and, using a fork, mash lightly until the avocado is slightly chunky. Add and spread the resulting guacamole on one tortilla. Top with the cooked fish and cheeses, and cover with the second tortilla. Bake in the Air Fryer 6-8, flipping once until the cheese is melted. Serve immediately.

RECIPE 889: HAM AND CORN MUFFINS

Serve: 4 | Total Time: 16 minutes

¾ cup yellow cornmeal
¼ cup flour
1½ tsp baking powder
¼ tsp salt
1 egg, beaten
2 tbsp canola oil
½ cup milk
½ cup shredded sharp Cheddar cheese
½ cup diced ham

Preheat the Air Fryer to a heat temperature of 390ºF (199ºC). In a medium bowl, stir together the cornmeal, flour, baking powder, and salt. Add the egg, oil, and milk to dry ingredients and mix well. Stir in shredded cheese and diced ham. Divide batter among 8 parchment paper-lined muffin cups. Put 4 filled muffin cups in Air Fryer basket and bake for 5 minutes. Reduce temperature to 330°F (166°C) and bake for 1 minute or until a toothpick inserted in center of the muffin comes out clean. Repeat steps 6 and 7 to bake remaining muffins. Serve warm.

RECIPE 890: HEALTHY BROCCOLI CASSEROLE

Serve: 4 | Total Time: 40 minutes

15 oz. broccoli florets
10 oz. can cream of mushroom soup
1 cup mozzarella cheese, shredded
1/3 cup milk
1/2 tsp onion powder
For topping:
1 tbsp. butter, melted
1/2 cup crushed crackers

Place the inner pot in the Air Fryer combo base. Add all ingredients except topping ingredients into the inner pot. Combine the melted butter and the cracker crumbs in a shallow dish, then sprinkle over the inner pot mixture. Cover the inner pot with an air frying lid. Select bake mode then set the temperature to 350 °F and time for 30 minutes. Click start. When the countdown approaches zero, press the cancel button. Serve and enjoy.

RECIPE 891: HERBED CHEDDAR CHEESE FRITTATA

Serve: 4 | Total Time: 30 minutes

1/2 cup shredded Cheddar cheese
1/2 cup half-and-half
4 large eggs
2 tbsp chopped scallion greens
2 tbsp chopped fresh parsley
1/2 tsp kosher salt
1/2 tsp ground black pepper
Cooking spray

Preheat your Air Fryer to 370°Fahrenheit. Combine the salmon, egg, celery, onion, dill, and garlic in a large mixing bowl. Shape the mixture into golf ball size balls and roll them in the wheat germ. In a small pan, warm olive oil over medium-low heat. Add the salmon balls and slowly flatten them. Transfer them to your Air Fryer and cook for 10-minutes.

RECIPE 892: HERBY CHEESY NUTS

Serve: 4 | Total Time: 35 minutes

1 egg white
4 tsp yeast extract
1 tsp swerve brown sugar
1 1/2 cups mixed nuts
1/2 cup sunflower seeds
Salt and black pepper to taste
3 tbsp grated Parmesan
1/2 tsp dried mixed herbs

Preheat oven to 350 F. In a bowl, beat egg white, yeast extract, and swerve brown sugar. Add in mixed nuts and sunflower seeds; combine and spread onto a lined baking sheet. Bake for 10 minutes. In a bowl, mix salt, pepper, Parmesan cheese, and herbs. Remove the nuts and toss with the cheese mixture. Bake for 5 minutes until sticky and brown. Let cool for 5 minutes and serve.

RECIPE 893: HERBY PARMESAN PITA

Serve: 2 | Total Time: 15 minutes

1 whole-wheat pita
2 tsp olive oil
¼ sweet onion, diced
¼ tsp garlic, minced
1 egg
¼ tsp dried tarragon
¼ tsp dried thyme
⅛ tsp salt
3 tsp grated Parmesan cheese

Preheat Air Fryer to 380°F. Lightly brush the top of the pita with olive oil, then top with onion and garlic. Crack the egg into a small bowl and sprinkle it with tarragon, thyme, and salt. Place the pita in the frying basket and gently pour the egg onto the top of the pita. Sprinkle with cheese over the top. Bake for 6 minutes. Leave to cool for 5 minutes. Cut into pieces and serve.

RECIPE 894: HERBY PRAWN AND ZUCCHINI BAKE

Serve: 4 | Total Time: 30 minutes

1 ¼ lb prawns, peeled and deveined
2 zucchini, sliced
2 tbsp butter, melted
½ tsp garlic salt
1 ½ tsp dried oregano
⅛ tsp red pepper flakes
½ lemon, juiced
1 tbsp chopped mint
1 tbsp chopped dill

Preheat Air Fryer to 350°F. Combine prawns, zucchini, butter, garlic salt, oregano, and pepper flakes in a large bowl. Toss to coat. Put the prawns and zucchini in the greased frying basket and Air Fry for about 6-8 minutes, shaking the basket once until the zucchini is golden and the shrimp are cooked. Remove the shrimp to a serving plate and cover with foil. Serve hot topped with lemon juice, mint, and dill. Enjoy!

RECIPE 895: HONEY OATMEAL

Serve: 6 | Total Time: 35 minutes

2 cups rolled oats
2 cups oat milk
¼ cup honey
½ cup Greek yogurt
1 tsp vanilla extract
½ tsp ground cinnamon
¼ tsp salt
1 ½ cups diced mango

Preheat Air Fryer to 380°F. Stir together the oats, milk, honey, yogurt, vanilla, cinnamon, and salt in a large bowl until well combined. Fold in ¾ cup of the mango and then pour the mixture into a greased cake pan. Sprinkle the remaining mango across the top of the oatmeal mixture. Bake in the

Air Fryer for 30 minutes. Leave to set and cool for 5 minutes. Serve and enjoy!

RECIPE 896: ITALIAN BAKED CHICKEN

Serve: 6 | Total Time: 75 minutes

2 lbs. boneless chicken breast
Salt and pepper to taste
2 tsp dry oregano
1 tsp fresh thyme
1 tsp sweet paprika
4 garlic cloves, minced
3 tbsp olive oil
Juice from ½ lemon
1 medium red onion, chopped
6 tomatoes, chopped
Handful chopped parsley
Handful basil leaves

Preheat the Air Fryer to 4000F for 5 minutes. Season the chicken with salt, pepper, oregano, thyme, paprika, and garlic cloves. In a mixing bowl, whisk together the lemon juice and olive oil until well combined. Place the onions in the bottom of a casserole dish. Pour in the tomatoes. Add the seasoned chicken slices on top. Place inside the Air Fryer. Select the Bake setting and adjust the cooking time to 60 minutes. Garnish with parsley and basil leaves.

RECIPE 897: ITALIAN BAKED GRAPE TOMATOES

Serve: 4 | Total Time: 35 minutes

12 ounces grape tomatoes
3 sprigs thyme
2 tbsp olive oil
3 cloves garlic, minced
¼ tsp oregano
¼ tsp red pepper flakes
¼ tsp kosher salt
¼ tsp cracked black pepper

To warm the COSORI Air Fryer Toaster Oven, choose the Bake function and set the timer to 30 minutes. Then click Start/Cancel to begin the preheat process. In a medium-sized mixing bowl, combine altogether the listed ingredients and put aside. Line a food tray with parchment paper and then equally distribute the tomatoes on top of it. Insert the food tray at a low position in the preheated Air Fryer toaster oven, then press Start/Cancel. Remove tomatoes when done, then serve.

RECIPE 898: ITALIAN BAKED TOFU

Serve: 2 | Total Time: 15 minutes

1 tbsp soy sauce
1 tbsp water
⅓ tsp garlic powder
⅓ tsp onion powder
⅓ tsp dried oregano
⅓ tsp dried basil
Black pepper, to taste
6 ounces (170 g) extra firm tofu, pressed and cubed

In a large mixing bowl, whisk together the soy sauce, water, garlic powder, onion powder, oregano, basil, and black pepper. Add the tofu cubes, stirring to coat, and let them marinate for 10 minutes. Preheat the Air Fryer to temperature 390°F (199°C). Arrange the tofu in the Air Fryer basket and bake for 10 minutes until crisp. Halfway through the cooking period, turn the tofu over and repeat the process. Transfer the contents of the basket to a platter and serve.

RECIPE 899: ITALIAN CHICKEN PESTO BAKE

Serve: 6 | Total Time: 35 minutes

¾ lbs. chicken breasts
2 tbsp pesto sauce
½ (14 oz) can tomatoes, diced
1 cup Mozzarella cheese, shredded
2 tbsp fresh basil, chopped

Place the flattened chicken breasts in a baking pan and top them with pesto. Add tomatoes, cheese, and basil on top of each chicken piece. Press "Power Button" of Air Fry Oven and turn the dial to select the "Bake" mode. Press the Time button and again turn the dial to

set the Cooking Time to 25 minutes. Now push the Temp button and rotate the dial to set the temperature at 355 degrees F. Once preheated, place the baking dish inside and close its lid. Serve warm.

RECIPE 900: ITALIAN SAUSAGE ROLLS

Serve: 4 | Total Time: 20 minutes

1 red bell pepper, cut into strips
4 Italian sausages
1 zucchini, cut into strips
½ onion, cut into strips
1 tsp dried oregano
½ tsp garlic powder
5 Italian rolls

Preheat Air Fryer to 360°F. Place all sausages in the Air Fryer. Bake for 10 minutes. While the sausages are cooking, season the bell pepper, zucchini and onion with oregano and garlic powder. When the time is up, flip the sausages, then add the peppers and onions. Cook for another 5 minutes or until the vegetables are soft and the sausages are cooked through. Put the sausage on Italian rolls, then top with peppers and onions. Serve.

RECIPE 901: ITALIAN STUFFED BELL PEPPERS

Serve: 4 | Total Time: 35 minutes

1 link sweet Italian pork sausage
12 turkey pepperoni slices, halved
1 ½ cups shredded mozzarella
4 red bell peppers
1 cup passata sauce
2 tbsp fresh basil, picked

Preheat Air Fryer to 370°F. Bake sausage in the frying basket for 10 minutes, flipping once until cooked. Remove and let cool. Chop into small pieces. Cut the peppers in half lengthwise. Remove the seeds and membranes. Lower the Air Fryer to 350°F. Put the peppers in the greased frying basket and Bake for 6-8, flipping once until just softened. Set aside. Add 2 tbsp of passata to the pepper halves. Top with 3 tbsp of mozzarella, some sausage pieces, and 3 pepperoni halves. Sprinkle with basil. Place the stuffed peppers in the greased frying basket and Bake until the cheese has melted and the passata is warmed through, 7 minutes. Serve.

RECIPE 902: ITALIAN STYLE STUFFED MUSHROOMS

Serve: 4 | Total Time: 30 minutes

4 portobello mushroom caps
2 tbsp cream cheese, softened
3 tsp grated Parmesan cheese
1 tsp olive oil
2 cups fresh baby spinach
1 red bell pepper, chopped
1/3 cup chopped leeks
2 tsp fresh thyme, chopped
Preheat Air Fryer to 390°F. Coat the mushrooms in olive oil and put them in the frying basket, hole side up, and Air Fry for 3 minutes. Take them out carefully and set aside. Combine the spinach, red bell pepper, leeks, thyme, cream cheese, and Parmesan cheese in a bowl and stir together. Then, stuff the mushroom caps with a fourth of the mix and put them back in the fryer. Bake for 6-9 minutes until the mix is hot and the caps are softened.

RECIPE 903: LAMB POTATO CHIPS BAKED

Serve: 4 | Total Time: 35 minutes

½ lb. minced lamb
1 tbs parsley chopped
2 tsp curry powder
1 pinch salt and black pepper
1 lb. potato cooked, mashed
1 oz. cheese grated
1 ½ oz. potato chips crushed

Mix lamb, curry powder, seasoning and parsley. Spread this lamb mixture in a casserole dish. Top the lamb mixture with potato mash, cheese, and potato chips. Press "Power Button" of Air Fry Oven

and turn the dial to select the "Bake" mode. Press the Time button and again turn the dial to set the cooking time to 20 minutes. Now push the Temp button and rotate the dial to set the temperature at 350 degrees F. Once preheated, place casserole dish in the oven and close its lid. Serve warm.

RECIPE 904: LAMB TOMATO BAKE

Serve: 6 | Total Time: 45 minutes

25 oz. potatoes, boiled
14 oz. lean lamb mince
1 tsp cinnamon
23 oz. jar tomato pasta
12 oz. white sauce
1 tbsp olive oil

Mash the potatoes in a bowl and stir in white sauce and cinnamon. Sauté lamb mince with olive oil in a frying pan until brown. Layer a casserole dish with tomato pasta sauce. Top the sauce with lamb mince. Spread the potato mash over the lamb in an even layer. Choose "Power Button" of Air Fry Oven and turn the dial to select the "Bake" mode. Choose the Time button and again turn the dial to set the cooking time to 35 minutes. Now press the Temp button and rotate the dial to set the temperature at 350 degrees F. Once preheated, place casserole dish in the oven and close its lid. Serve warm.

RECIPE 905: LAVA CAKES

Serve: 4 | Total Time: 15 minutes

5 tbsp Self-Rising Flour
5 tbsp Stevia
5 oz Unsalted Butter
5 oz Dark Chocolate (Pieces or Chopped)
2 Eggs
Grease 4 standard baking pans and sprinkle with flour. Take a microwave-safe bowl and melt the dark chocolate and butter at speed 7 for 3 minutes and mix well. Remove from microwave and stir

evenly. Whisk eggs and stevia until foam. Put the melted chocolate into the egg mixture. Add the flour. Use a spoon to mix everything smoothly. Fill the molds to three by four with the mixer and bake in a 375F preheated Air Fryer oven for 10 minutes. Remove from fryer and let cool in pan for 2 minutes. Carefully turn the shells over and tap the bottom with a butter knife to detach the corners.

RECIPE 906: LEMON MINI PIES WITH COCONUT

Serve: 8 | Total Time: 5 minutes

1 box of lemon instant pudding filling mix (4-serving size)
½ tsp ground star anise
1/8 tsp salt
1 tsp pure vanilla extract
1 ¼ cups cream cheese, room temperature
1/3 cup coconut, shredded
18 wonton wrappers
1 tsp lemon peel, grated

Spray muffin pan with olive oil. Press the wonton wrappers evenly into cups. Transfer them into your Air Fryer and bake for 5-minutes at 350°Fahrenheit. When the edges are golden in color they are ready. Meanwhile, blend all remaining Ingredients using blender. Place the prepared cream in the fridge until ready to serve. Lastly, divide prepared cream among wrappers and keep refrigerated until ready to eat.

RECIPE 907: LEMON PIES WITH VANILLA AND COCONUT

Serve: 8 | Total Time: 10 minutes

1 box of lemon instant pudding filling mix (4-serving size)
½ tsp ground star anise
1/8 tsp salt
1 tsp pure vanilla extract
1 ¼ cups cream cheese, room temperature
1/3 cup coconut, shredded
18 wonton wrappers
1 tsp lemon peel, grated

Spray muffin pan with olive oil. Press the wonton wrappers evenly into cups. Transfer them into your Air Fryer and bake for 5-minutes at 350°Fahrenheit. When the edges are golden in color they are ready. Meanwhile, blend all remaining ingredients using blender. Place the prepared cream in the fridge until ready to serve. Lastly, divide prepared cream among wrappers and keep refrigerated until ready to eat.

RECIPE 908: LEMONY APPLE BUTTER

Serve: 2 | Total Time: 75 minutes

Cooking spray
2 cups unsweetened applesauce
⅔ cup packed light brown sugar
3 tbsp fresh lemon juice
½ tsp kosher salt
¼ tsp ground cinnamon
⅛ tsp ground allspice

Spray a metal cake pan with cooking spray. Whisk together all the ingredients in a bowl until smooth, then pour into the greased pan. Set the pan in the Air Fryer and bake at 340°F (171°C) until the apple mixture is caramelized, reduced to a thick purée, and fragrant, about 1 hour.
Remove the pan from the Air Fryer, stir to combine the caramelized bits at the edge with the rest, then let cool completely to thicken.
Serve immediately.

RECIPE 909: LENTILS AND DATES BROWNIES

Serve: 8 | Total Time: 25 minutes

28 oz canned lentils, rinsed and drained
12 dates
1 tbsp honey
1 banana, peeled and chopped
½ tsp baking soda
4 tbsp almond butter
2 tbsp cocoa powder

In your food processor, mix lentils with butter, banana, cocoa, baking soda and honey and blend really well. Add dates, pulse a few more times, pour this into a greased pan that fits your Air Fryer, spread evenly, introduce in the fryer at 360 degrees F and bake for 15 minutes. Take brownies mix out of the oven, cut, arrange on a platter and serve. Enjoy!

RECIPE 910: LOW CARB PEANUT BUTTER COOKIES

Serve: 27 | Total Time: 30 minutes

2 large eggs
½ cup erythritol
1 ¼ cup creamy peanut butter
¾ cup peanuts
¼ tsp. Salt

Crush the peanuts and set aside. Preheat the oven to 350 degrees and use a cookie sheet covered with parchment paper. Combine eggs, sweetener, salt, and creamy peanut butter in a blender or food processor. Manage until smooth and clean offsides when mixture sticks. Toss in crushed peanuts and join with other ingredients. Leave some crunch for texture. Scoop the dough into spheres and place them on a baking sheet. Press the dough using a fork to create a crosshatch top. Wipe fork with water before using it again. Bake for 20 minutes or wait until golden brown and crunchy.

RECIPE 911: LOW CARB SNICKERDOODLE COOKIES

Serve: 6 | Total Time: 30 minutes

2 cups superfine almond flour
½ tsp baking soda
¾ cup erythritol sweetener
1 tsp ground cinnamon
2 tbsp erythritol

Switch on the oven to 350 degrees. Combine all the fixings until you form a stiff dough. Then roll the cookie dough into 16 equal-sized balls, about 1 ½ inches wide.

Blend the sweetener and cinnamon in a small bowl to create the coating. Then roll the balls generously in the cinnamon coating. Place the covered cookie balls on a cookie sheet covered in parchment paper and bake. Then gently smash with a flat round surface.

RECIPE 912: LUSCIOUS TRIPLE BERRY COBBLER

Serve: 6 | Total Time: 32 minutes

3 tbsp melted butter
1/4 cup flour
1/2 cup quick oats
1/2 cup raspberries or blackberries
1/2 cup strawberries
1 cup blueberries
2-1/8 cups of white sugar, divided
1 tsp lemon juice
1/4 cup brown sugar
1 tsp vanilla

Combine berries, 1/8 cup white sugar, and lemon juice in a large mixing bowl. In a separate bowl, mix flour, vanilla, oats, melted butter, brown sugar, and the other 1/8 cup of white sugar. Mix well. Coat pan with non-stick cooking spray. Put the oats mixture in first. Then add the berries. Choose the bake function in your Air Fryer oven. Bake for 12 minutes at 390°F.

RECIPE 913: MARBLE CHEESECAKE

Serve: 8 | Total Time: 20 minutes

1 cup graham cracker crumbs
2 tbsp softened butter
10 Oz. Cream cheese, softened
1/3 cup sugar
2 organic eggs
1 tbsp flour
1 tsp vanilla extract
1/3 cup chocolate syrup

First, take a bowl and combine graham cracker and butter. Mix well. Press this mixture into a 6-by-6 baking pan and freeze it for a few hours. Next, combine the cream cheese and sugar in a bowl. Mix well. Add in the beaten eggs. Next, add the flour and vanilla. Stir in the chocolate syrup until combined. Pour this filling into the pan with the crust. Bake it for 20 minutes at 320 degrees or until it sets. Cool, and then serve.

RECIPE 914: MARGHERITA PIZZA

Serve: 4 | Total Time: 48 minutes

1 whole-wheat pizza crust
1/2 cup mozzarella cheese, grated
1/2 cup can tomatoes
2 tbsp olive oil
3 Roma tomatoes, sliced
10 basil leaves

Fit the Air Fryer oven with the rack in position. Roll out whole wheat pizza crust using a rolling pin. Make sure the crust is ½-inch thick. Sprinkle olive oil on top of pizza crust. Spread can tomatoes over pizza crust. Arrange sliced tomatoes and basil on pizza crust. Sprinkle grated cheese on top. Place pizza on top of the oven rack and set to bake at 425 F for 23 minutes. Slice and serve.

RECIPE 915: MARMALADE-ALMOND TOPPED BRIE

Serve: 6 | Total Time: 35 minutes

1 cup almonds
1 egg white, beaten
⅛ tsp ground cumin
⅛ tsp cayenne pepper
1 tsp ground cinnamon
¼ tsp powdered sugar
1 (8-oz) round Brie cheese
2 tbsp orange marmalad

Preheat Air Fryer to 325°F. In a bowl, mix the beaten egg white and almonds. In another bowl, mix the spices and sugar. Stir in almonds, drained of excess egg white. Transfer the almonds to the frying basket and Bake for 12 minutes, tossing once. Let cool for 5 minutes. When cooled, chop into smaller bits. Adjust the Air Fryer's temperature to 400°F. Place the

Brie on a parchment-lined pizza pan and Bake for 10 minutes. Transfer the Brie to a serving plate, spread orange marmalade on top, and garnish with spiced walnuts. Serve and enjoy!

RECIPE 916: MASCARPONE MUSHROOMS

Serve: 4 | Total Time: 25 minutes

Vegetable oil spray
4 cups sliced mushrooms
1 medium yellow onion, chopped
2 cloves garlic, minced
¼ cup heavy whipping cream or half-and-half
8 ounces (227 g) mascarpone cheese
1 tsp dried thyme
1 tsp kosher salt
1 tsp black pepper
½ tsp red pepper flakes
4 cups cooked konjac noodles, for serving
½ cup grated Parmesan cheese

350°F (177°C) Air Fryer preheat and spray a heatproof pan with oil. Melt the butter in a large skillet over medium-high heat. Mix well. Pour the mixture into the pan. Place in Air Fryer basket. Bake for 15 minutes, stirring halfway. 4 small bowls of spaghetti Distribute mushroom mixture over spaghetti. Serve with Parmesan cheese.

RECIPE 917: MASCARPONE MUSHROOMS WITH PASTA

Serve: 4 | Total Time: 25 minutes

Vegetable oil spray
4 cups sliced mushrooms
1 medium yellow onion, chopped
1 cloves garlic,
1/4 cup heavy whipping cream
8 ounces (227 g) mascarpone cheese
1 tsp dried thyme
1 tsp kosher salt
1 tsp black pepper
1/2 tsp red pepper flakes
2 cups cooked konjac noodles, for serving
1/2 cup grated Parmesan cheese

Spray a pan with vegetable oil spray. In a medium bowl, merge the mushrooms, onion, garlic, cream, mascarpone, thyme, salt, black pepper, and red pepper flakes. Stir to combine. Transfer the mixture to the prepared pan. Placing the pan in the Air Fryer basket and covering it with the lid is a good idea. Bake at 350F (177C) for 15 minutes, stirring halfway through the baking time. Set the pasta among four bowls. Scoop the mushroom mixture evenly over the pasta. Sprinkle with Parmesan cheese and serve.

RECIPE 918: MATCHA GRANOLA

Serve: 4 | Total Time: 15 minutes

2 tsp matcha green tea
½ cup slivered almonds
½ cup pecan pieces
½ cup sunflower seeds
½ cup pumpkin seeds
1 cup coconut flakes
¼ cup coconut sugar
⅛ cup flour
⅛ cup almond flour
1 tsp vanilla extract
2 tbsp melted butter
2 tbsp almond butter
⅛ tsp salt

Preheat Air Fryer to 300°F. Mix the green tea, almonds, pecan, sunflower seeds, pumpkin seeds, coconut flakes, sugar, and flour, almond flour, vanilla extract, butter, almond butter, and salt in a bowl. Spoon the mixture into an ungreased round 4-cup baking dish. Place it in the fryer and Bake for 6 minutes, stirring once. Transfer to an airtight container, let cool for 10 minutes, then cover and store at room temperature until ready to serve.

RECIPE 919: MEATBALL AND CABBAGE BAKE

Serve: 4 | Total Time: 30 minutes

2 cups chopped green cabbage
1 shallot, chopped
2 tbsp olive oil

16 pre-cooked meatballs
1 cup cooked rice
2 tomatoes, chopped
2 tbsp parsley, chopped
Salt and pepper to taste

Preheat Air Fryer to 370°F. Combine shallot and olive oil in a metal bowl. Place the bowl in the Air Fryer and Bake until the shallot is crispy and tender, 2-4 minutes. Stir in cabbage, meatballs, rice, tomatoes, parsley, salt and pepper. Bake for 6-8 minutes. Stir the contents in the bowl, and then continue baking for another 6-8 minutes or until the meatballs are hot, the rice is warm, and the veggies tender. Serve warm.

RECIPE 920: MEDITERRANEAN GRANOLA

Serve: 6 | Total Time: 40 minutes

1 cup rolled oats
¼ cup dried cherries, diced
¼ cup almond slivers
¼ cup hazelnuts, chopped
¼ cup pepitas
¼ cup hemp hearts
3 tbsp honey
1 tbsp olive oil
1 tsp ground cinnamon
¼ tsp ground nutmeg
¼ tsp salt
2 tbsp dark chocolate chips
3 cups Greek yogurt
Preheat Air Fryer to 260°F. Toss the oats with the dried fruit and nuts in a large bowl. Pour the mixture onto the parchment-lined frying basket and spread it into a single layer. Bake for 25-30 minutes, shaking twice. Let the granola cool completely. Stir in the chocolate chips. Divide between 6 cups. Top with Greek yogurt and remaining honey to serve.

RECIPE 921: MINI MOLTEN LAVA CAKES

Serve: 4 | Total Time: 20 minutes

4 ramekins
3 1/2 tbsps self-rising flour

3 1/2 ounces unsalted butter
3 1/2 ounces dark chocolate pieces
2 eggs

Spray the ramekins and set them aside. Thaw the chocolate and butter in a dish for thirty 30 at a time, mixing after each time. Beat the eggs and mix in the sugar. Stir egg and chocolate mixtures together, then add flour and mix well. Preheat your fryer to 375 degrees. Fill each ramekin with the batter about 3/4 of the way. Bake in your fryer for 10 minutes, then serve warm.

RECIPE 922: MINT LAMB WITH ROASTED HAZELNUTS

Serve: 2 | Total Time: 35 minutes

¼ cup hazelnuts, toasted
2/3 lb. shoulder of lamb cut into strips
1 tbsp hazelnut oil
2 tbsp fresh mint leaves chopped
½ cup frozen peas
¼ cup of water
½ cup white wine
Salt and black pepper to taste

Toss lamb with hazelnuts, spices, and all the ingredients in a baking pan. Press "Power Button" of Air Fry Oven and turn the dial to select the "Bake" mode. Press the Time button and again turn the dial to set the cooking time to 25 minutes. To adjust the temperature, press the Temp button and crank the dial to 370 degrees F. After the baking pan has warmed, place it in the oven and close the lid. Slice and serve warm.

RECIPE 923: MIXED BERRY DUTCH BABY PANCAKE

Serve: 4 | Total Time: 26 minutes

1 tbsp unsalted butter, at room temperature
1 egg
2 egg whites
½ cup 2% milk
½ cup whole-wheat pastry flour
1 tsp pure vanilla extract

1 cup sliced fresh strawberries
½ cup fresh raspberries
½ cup fresh blueberries

Preheat the Air Fryer to 330°F (166°C). Grease a baking pan with the butter. Combine the egg, egg whites, milk, pastry flour, and vanilla in a medium mixing dish. Bake for 12-16 minutes, or until the centre puffs up and the edges are golden brown, after pouring the mixture into the pan. Allow the pancake to cool for 5 minutes and serve topped with the berries.

RECIPE 924: MIXED SEED CRACKERS

Serve: 6 | Total Time: 20 minutes

1/3 cup sesame seed flour
1/3 cup pumpkin seeds
1/3 cup sunflower seeds
1/3 cup sesame seeds
1/3 cup chia seeds
1 tbsp psyllium husk powder
1 tsp salt
1/4 cup butter, melted

Preheat oven to 300 F. Combine sesame seed flour with pumpkin, chia and sunflower seeds, psyllium husk powder, and salt. Pour in butter and 1 cup of boiling water and mix until a dough forms with a gel-like consistency. Bake on a parchment-lined baking sheet. Cover with another parchment paper and with a rolling pin to flatten into the baking sheet. Remove the parchment paper on top. Bake for 25 minutes. Turn off and allow the crackers to cool and dry in the oven, 10 minutes. Break and serve.

RECIPE 925: MUSHROOM AND TURKEY BREAD PIZZA

Serve: 4 | Total Time: 35 minutes

10 cooked turkey sausages, sliced
1 cup shredded mozzarella cheese
1 cup shredded Cheddar cheese
1 French loaf bread
2 tbsp butter, softened
1 tsp garlic powder

1 1/3 cups marinara sauce
1 tsp Italian seasoning
2 scallions, chopped
1 cup mushrooms, sliced

Preheat the Air Fryer to 370°F. Cut the bread in half crosswise, then split each half horizontally. Combine butter and garlic powder, then spread on the cut sides of the bread. Bake the halves in the fryer for 3-5 minutes or until the leaves start to brown. Set the toasted bread on a work surface and spread marinara sauce over the top. Sprinkle the Italian seasoning, then top with sausages, scallions, mushrooms, and cheeses. Set the pizzas in the Air Fryer and Bake for 8-12 minutes or until the cheese is melted and starting to brown. Serve hot.

RECIPE 926: NORDIC SALMON QUICHE

Serve: 4 | Total Time: 30 minutes

¼ cup shredded mozzarella cheese
¼ cup shredded Gruyere cheese
1 refrigerated pie crust
2 eggs
¼ cup milk
Salt and pepper to taste
1 tsp dry dill
5 oz cooked salmon
1 large tomato, diced

Preheat Air Fryer to 360°F. In a baking dish, add the crust and press firmly. Trim off any excess edges. Poke a few holes. Beat the eggs in a bowl. Stir in the milk, dill, tomato, salmon, half of the cheeses, salt, and pepper. Mix well as break the salmon into chunks, mixing it evenly among other ingredients. Transfer the mix to the baking dish. Bake in the fryer for 15 minutes until firm and almost crusty. Slide the basket out and top with the remaining cheeses. Cook further for 5 minutes, or until golden brown. Let cool slightly and serve.

RECIPE 927: OAT MUFFINS WITH BLUEBERRIES

Serve: 6 | Total Time: 25 minutes

¾ cup old-fashioned rolled oats
1 ½ cups flour
½ cup evaporated cane sugar
1 tbsp baking powder
1 tsp ground cinnamon
¼ tsp ground chia seeds
¼ tsp ground sesame seeds
½ tsp salt
1 cup vanilla almond milk
4 tbsp butter, softened
2 eggs
1 tsp vanilla extract
1 cup blueberries
2 tbsp powdered sugar

Preheat Air Fryer to 350°F. Combine flour oats, sugar, baking powder, chia seeds, sesame seeds, cinnamon, and salt in a bowl. Mix the almond milk, butter, eggs, and vanilla in another bowl until smooth. Pour in dry ingredients and stir to combine. Fold in blueberries.Fill 12 silicone muffin cups about halfway and place them in the frying basket. Bake for 12-15 minutes until just browned, and a toothpick in the center comes out clean. Cool for 5 minutes. Serve topped with powdered sugar.

RECIPE 928: ONION OMELET

Serve: 2 | Total Time: 22 minutes

3 eggs
Salt and ground black pepper, to taste
½ tsp soy sauce
1 large onion, chopped
2 tbsp grated Cheddar cheese
Cooking spray

Firstly, whisk together the eggs, pepper, salt, and soy sauce. Spritz a small pan with cooking spray. Spread the chopped onion across the bottom of the pan, then transfer the pan to the Air Fryer. Bake in the Air Fryer at temperature 355ºF (179ºC) for 6 minutes or until the onion is translucent. Add the egg mixture on top of the onions to coat well. Add the cheese on top, then continue baking for another 6 minutes. Allow to cool before serving.

RECIPE 929: ORANGE CHICKEN RICE

Serve: 4 | Total Time: 56 minutes

3 tbsps olive oil
1 medium onion, chopped
1 3/4 cups chicken broth
1 cup brown basmati rice
Zest and juice of 2 oranges
Salt to taste
4 boneless, skinless chicken thighs
Black pepper, to taste
2 tbsps fresh mint, chopped
2 tbsps pine nuts, toasted

Spread the rice in a casserole dish and place the chicken on top. Toss the rest of the ingredients in a bowl and liberally pour over the chicken. Press "Power Button" of Air Fry Oven and turn the dial to select the "Bake" mode. Press the Time button and again turn the dial to set the cooking time to 55 minutes. Now push the Temp button and rotate the dial to set the temperature at 350 degrees F. Once preheated, place the casserole dish inside and close its lid. Serve warm.

RECIPE 930: PAPRIKA MUSHROOM AND BUCKWHEAT PILAF

Serve: 4 | Total Time: 45 minutes

8 oz button mushrooms, diced
2 tbsp cilantro, chopped
2 tbsp olive oil
½ onion, diced
2 garlic cloves, minced
1 cup buckwheat
2 cups vegetable broth
1 tbsp thyme, chopped
½ tsp salt
¼ tsp smoked paprika

Preheat Air Fryer to 380°F. A medium skillet with olive oil Add the mushrooms, garlic, and onion and cook, stirring occasionally, until tender, about 5 minutes. Remove the vegetables to a large bowl. Stir in the buckwheat, broth, thyme, salt, and paprika. Air fry the ingredients in a greased casserole dish. Bake for 25-30 minutes. Allow to rest for 5 minutes. Fluf with a fork and sprinkle with cilantro.

RECIPE 931: PARMA HAM AND EGG TOAST CUPS

Serve: 4 | Total Time: 25 minutes

4 crusty rolls
4 Gouda cheese thin slices
5 eggs
2 tbsp heavy cream
½ tsp dried thyme
3 Parma ham slices, chopped
Salt and pepper to taste

Preheat Air Fryer to 330°F. Slice off the top of the rolls, then tear out the insides with your fingers, leaving about ½-inch of bread to make a shell. Press one cheese slice inside the roll shell until it takes the shape of the roll. Beat eggs with heavy cream in a medium bowl. Next, mix in the remaining ingredients. Spoon egg mixture into the rolls lined with cheese. Place rolls in the greased frying basket and Bake until eggs are puffy and brown, 8-12 minutes. Serve warm.

RECIPE 932: PARMESAN BAKED CHICKEN BREAST

Serve: 2 | Total Time: 25 minutes

1 lb. skinless and boneless chicken breast
1 ½ tbsp garlic powder
2 tbsp lemon juice
Salt and ground black pepper to taste
3 dashed cayenne pepper
½ cup grated parmesan cheese
Cooking spray
Lemon wedges for garnish

Preheat the Air Fryer to 3500F for 5 minutes. Season the chicken with garlic powder, lemon juice, salt, pepper, and cayenne pepper. Dredge in the parmesan cheese then spray with cooking oil. Place the chicken on the crisper tray. Select the Air Fry setting and adjust the cooking time to 20 minutes.

RECIPE 933: PARMESAN, GARLIC, LEMON ROASTED ZUCCHINI

Serve: 4 | Total Time: 10 minutes

1 ½ lbs. zucchini (about 4 small zucchini)
Salt and pepper to taste
¾ cup parmesan cheese, finely shredded
2 cloves garlic, minced
Zest of 1 lemon
2 tbsp olive oil

Zucchini should be chopped into thick wedges or halves (cut each zucchini in half, then half again, for a total of four wedges). Combine the olive oil, garlic, and lemon zest in a mixing bowl. Arrange zucchini in an Air Fryer, spacing them out evenly. Brush the zucchini tops with the olive oil mixture. Season gently with salt and pepper and top with parmesan cheese. Bake in Air Fryer at 375°Fahrenheit for 10-minutes. Serve warm.

RECIPE 934: PARMESAN SAUSAGE EGG MUFFINS

Serve: 4 | Total Time: 25 minutes

6 ounces (170 g) Italian sausage, sliced
6 eggs
⅛ cup heavy cream
Salt and ground black pepper, to taste
3 ounces (85 g) Parmesan cheese, grated
Cooking spray

Cooking spray should be sprayed onto a muffin pan. Fill the muffin tin halfway with the cut sausage. In a medium-sized mixing bowl, combine the eggs and cream. Season with salt and pepper. Half of the mixture should be poured over the sausages in the pan. Cheese and the leftover egg mixture should be sprinkled on top. Bake for 20 minutes at 350oF (177oC) in an Air Fryer or in a conventional oven until set. Serve as soon as possible.

RECIPE 935: PARSNIP AND POTATO BAKE

Serve: 8 | Total Time: 30 minutes

28 oz. potato, cubed
3-tbsp. pine nuts
28 oz. parsnips, chopped.
1 ¾ oz. coarsely chopped Parmesan cheese
6 ¾ oz. crème fraiche
1 slice bread
2 tbsp sage
4 tbsp butter
4 tsp mustard

Preheat your Air Fryer to temperature of 360 degrees F. Put salted water in a pot over medium heat. Add potatoes and parsnips. Bring to a boil for 15 minutes. Take a bowl and, mix mustard, crème fraiche, sage, salt and pepper. Drain the potatoes and parsnips and mash them with butter using a potato masher. Add mustard mixture, bread, cheese and nuts to the mash and mix. Add the batter to your Air Fryer's basket and cook for 15 minutes, shaking once. Serve.

RECIPE 936: PEACH CAKE

Serve: 6 | Total Time: 35 minutes

½ lb. peaches, pitted and mashed
½ tsp baking powder
1 ¼ cups almond flour
½ tsp orange extract
¼ tsp nutmeg, freshly grated
2 eggs
2 tbsp Truvia for baking
1/3 cup ghee
¼ tsp ground cinnamon
1 tsp pure vanilla extract

Preheat your air-fryer to 310°Fahrenheit. Spritz the cake pan with olive oil cooking spray. In a mixing bowl, beat the ghee with Truvia until creamy. Fold in the egg, mashed peaches and honey. Then, make the cake batter by mixing the remaining ingredients; now, stir in the peach mixture in with rest of ingredients. Pour batter into cake pan and level the surface of batter. Bake 35-minutes and enjoy!

RECIPE 937: PEACH FRENCH TOAST

Serve: 6 | Total Time: 70 minutes

5 eggs
1 ½ cups whole milk
1 cup packed brown sugar
½ cup butter, cubed
2 tbsp water
1 tbsp vanilla extract
12 slices day-old French bread
29 oz. can slice peaches, drained
½ tbsp Ground cinnamon

Add butter, water, and brown sugar to a pan and bring to boil. Reduce the heat and simmer for 10 minutes, stirring often. Add to a greased baking dish and add peaches on top. Add bread over the peaches. Whisk milk, eggs, and vanilla in a bowl and pour over the bread. Cover and refrigerate overnight. Preheat the oven to temperature of 350 degrees Fahrenheit set the timer to 40 minutes. Add cinnamon on top. Position the oven rack in Rack Position 1 and place the pan on top. Select the Bake setting. Preheat the oven to temperature of 350 degrees Fahrenheit and set the timer for 50 minutes. Serve.

RECIPE 938: PEACH PIE

Serve: 2 | Total Time: 15 minutes

2 cups sliced peaches
2 tbsp of maple syrup
1 tbsp sugar
1 tsp vanilla extract
1 tbsp liquefied coconut oil
1 pie crust

Preheat the Airfryer to 360 degrees F. Combine the peaches, syrup, sugar, vanilla in a bowl and mix by hand. Put the pie crust into a safe oven form that fits in the Airfryer. Brush with the coconut oil. Put the peach mixture into the pie crust. Fold over any edges that hang out over the form. Bake for 15

minutes. Serve with ice cream or whipped cream. A garnish of mint adds a gourmet touch.

RECIPE 939: PEANUT BUTTER-CHOCOLATE BREAD PUDDING

Serve: 8 | Total Time: 20 minutes

1 egg
1 egg yolk
3/4 cup chocolate milk
3 tbsp brown sugar
3 tbsp peanut butter
2 tbsp cocoa powder
1 tsp vanilla
5 slices firm white bread, cubed
Nonstick cooking spray

Nonstick cooking spray a baking pan. Whisk together the egg, egg yolk, chocolate milk, brown sugar, peanut butter, cocoa powder, and vanilla until well combined. Stir in the bread cubes until everything is nicely combined. Allow the bread soak for 10 minutes. When ready, transfer the egg mixture to the prepared baking pan. Select Bake, set temperature to 330°F (166°C), and set time to 10 minutes. Select Start to begin preheating. Once the oven has preheated, slide the pan into the oven. When done, the pudding should be just firm to the touch. Serve at room temperature.

RECIPE 940: PECORINO DILL MUFFINS

Serve: 4 | Total Time: 25 minutes

¼ cup grated Pecorino cheese
1 cup flour
1 tsp dried dill
⅛ tsp salt
¼ tsp onion powder
2 tsp baking powder
1 egg
¼ cup Greek yogurt
Preheat Air Fryer to 350°F. In a bowl, combine dry the ingredients. Set aside. In another bowl, whisk the wet ingredients. Combine the wet components with the dry ones until everything is well-combined.

Transfer the batter to 6 silicone muffin cups lightly greased with olive oil. Place muffin cups in the frying basket and Bake for 12 minutes. Serve right away.

RECIPE 941: PESTO CHICKEN BAKE

Serve: 3 | Total Time: 45 minutes

3 chicken breasts
1 (6 oz.) jar basil pesto
2 medium fresh tomatoes, sliced
6 mozzarella cheese slices

Spread the tomato slices in a casserole dish and top them with chicken. Add pesto and cheese on top of the chicken and spread evenly. Press "Power Button" of Air Fry Oven and turn the dial to select the "Air Fry" mode. Press the Time button and again turn the dial to set the Cooking Time to 30 minutes. Now push the Temp button and rotate the dial to set the temperature at 350 degrees F. Once preheated, place the casserole dish inside and close its lid. After it is baked, switch the oven to broil mode and broil for 5 minutes. Serve warm.

RECIPE 942: PESTO EGG AND HAM SANDWICHES

Serve: 2 | Total Time: 20 minutes

4 sandwich bread slices
2 tbsp butter, melted
4 eggs, scrambled
4 deli ham slices
2 Colby cheese slices
4 tsp basil pesto sauce
¼ tsp red chili flakes
¼ sliced avocado

Preheat Air Fryer at 370°F. Brush 2 pieces of bread with half of the butter and place them, butter side down, into the frying basket. Divide eggs, chili flakes, sliced avocado, ham, and cheese on each bread slice. Spread pesto on the remaining bread slices and place them, pesto side-down, onto the sandwiches. Brush the remaining butter on the tops of the sandwiches and Bake for 6 minutes, flipping once. Serve immediately.

RECIPE 943: PESTO PEPPERONI PIZZA BREAD

Serve: 4 | Total Time: 25 minutes

2 eggs, beaten
2 tbsp flour
2 tbsp cassava flour
1/3 cup whipping cream
¼ cup chopped pepperoni
1/3 cup grated mozzarella
2 tsp Italian seasoning
½ tsp baking powder
⅛ tsp salt
3 tsp grated Parmesan cheese
½ cup pesto

Preheat Air Fryer to 300°F. Combine all of the listed ingredients above, except for the Parmesan and pesto sauce, in a bowl until mixed. Pour the batter into a pizza pan. Place it in the frying basket and Bake for 20 minutes. After, sprinkle Parmesan on top and cook for 1 minute. Let chill for 5 minutes before slicing. Serve with warmed pesto sauce.

RECIPE 944: PHILLY CHEESE STEAK STUFFED PEPPERS

Serve: 2 | Total Time: 40 minutes

8-ounces of roast beef, thinly sliced
8-slices of provolone cheese
2 large green bell peppers
1 medium sweet onion, diced
1 (6-ounce) package of baby Bella mushrooms
1 tbsp garlic, minced
2 tbsp olive oil
2 tbsp butter

Cut your peppers in half lengthwise, removing ribs and seeds. Slice onions and mushrooms. Sauté over medium heat with butter, olive oil, a dash of salt, pepper, and minced garlic. Cook for 20-minutes or until the mushrooms and onions are sweet

and caramelized. Slice the roast beef into thin strips and add to the onion/mushroom mixture. Allow cooking for 10-minutes. In the inside of each pepper line it with a slice of provolone cheese. Fill each pepper with meat mixture. Garnish top of each pepper with another slice of provolone cheese. Bake in the Air Fryer at 375°Fahrenhiet for 10-minutes.

RECIPE 945: PINTO BEAN CASSEROLE

Serve: 2 | Total Time: 15 minutes

1 (15-oz) can pinto beans
¼ cup tomato sauce
2 tbsp cornstarch
2 garlic cloves, minced
½ tsp dried oregano
½ tsp cumin
1 tsp smoked paprika
Salt and pepper to taste

Preheat Air Fryer to 390°F. Stir the beans, tomato sauce, cornstarch, garlic, oregano, cumin, smoked paprika, salt, and pepper in a bowl until combined. Pour the bean mix into a greased baking pan. Bake in the fryer for 4 minutes. Remove, stir, and Bake for 4 minutes or until the mix is thick and heated through. Serve hot.

RECIPE 946: PISTACHIO CRUSTED SALMON

Serve: 4 | Total Time: 25 minutes

1 lb. salmon or 1 large filet
¼ cup parmesan cheese, grated
1/3 cup pistachios, crushed or chopped
Pepper and salt as desired
¼ panko breadcrumbs

Switch oven to 400 degrees. Crush or finely chop the pistachios if necessary. Mix the pistachios, breadcrumbs, and cheese in a bowl. Arrange foil to a sizeable pan and smear the foil with oil. Then place salmon on greased foil, skin side down. Sprinkle pepper and salt as desired. Top the salmon with

pistachio mixture, pressing firmly, so the mixture adheres. Then bake with the pan exposed for 15-20 minutes, or until the seasoned salmon easily flakes.

RECIPE 947: PITA AND PEPPERONI PIZZA

Serve: 1 | Total Time: 16 minutes

1 tsp olive oil
1 tbsp pizza sauce
1 pita bread
6 pepperoni slices
¼ cup grated Mozzarella cheese
¼ tsp garlic powder
¼ tsp dried oregano

Olive oil should be used to grease the Air Fryer basket. Spread the pizza sauce on top of the pita bread. Put the pepperoni slices over the sauce, followed by the Mozzarella cheese. Season with garlic powder and oregano. Put the pita pizza inside the Air Fryer and place a trivet on top. Bake at 350ºF (177ºC) for 6 minutes and serve.

RECIPE 948: PIZZA PUFFS

Serve: 6 | Total Time: 15 minutes
6 oz crescent roll dough
1/2 cup mozzarella cheese, shredded
3 oz pepperoni
3 oz mushrooms, chopped
1 tsp oregano
1 tsp garlic powder
1/4 cup Marina sauce, for dipping

Unroll the crescent dough. Set out the dough using a rolling pin; cut into 6 pieces. Place the cheese, pepperoni, and mushrooms in the center of each pizza puff. Sprinkle with oregano and garlic powder. Fold each corner over the filling using wet hands. Press together to cover the filling entirely and seal the edges. Now, spritz the bottom of the Air Fryer basket with cooking oil. Lay the pizza puffs in a single layer in the cooking basket. Work in batches. Bake at 370 degrees F for 5 to 6 minutes or until golden brown. Serve with the marinara sauce for dipping.

RECIPE 949: PLUM CAKE

Serve: 8 | Total Time: 56 minutes

7 ounces flour
1 package dried yeast
1 ounce butter, soft
1 egg, whisked
5 tbsp sugar
3 ounces warm milk
1 and ¾ pounds plums, pitted and cut into quarters
Zest from 1 lemon, grated
1 ounce almond flakes

In a bowl, mix yeast with butter, flour and 3 tbsps sugar and stir well. Add milk and egg and whisk for 4 minutes until you obtain a dough. Arrange the dough in a spring form pan that fits your Air Fryer and which you've greased with some butter, cover and leave aside for 1 hour. Arrange plumps on top of the butter, sprinkle the rest of the sugar, introduce in your Air Fryer at 350 degrees F, bake for 36 minutes, cool down, sprinkle almond flakes and lemon zest on top, slice and serve. Enjoy!

RECIPE 950: POTATO CASSEROLE

Serve: 6 | Total Time: 40 minutes

5 eggs
1/2 cup cheddar cheese, shredded
2 medium potatoes, 1/2-inch cubes
1 green bell pepper, diced
1 onion, chopped
1 tbsp olive oil
3/4 tsp pepper
3/4 tsp salt
Spray 9x9-inch casserole dish with cooking spray and set aside. Heat olive oil in a large pan over medium heat. Add onion and sauté for 1 minute. Add potatoes, bell peppers, ½ tsp black pepper, and 2 tsp salt and sauté for 4 minutes more or until onions are softened. Transfer sautéed vegetables to the prepared casserole dish and spread evenly. In a bowl, whisk eggs and remaining pepper and salt. Pour

egg mixture into the casserole dish and sprinkle cheddar cheese on top. Select bake mode and set the Omni to 350 °F for 35 minutes, once the oven beeps, place the casserole dish into the oven. Serve and enjoy.

RECIPE 951: PUMPKIN BREAD WITH WALNUTS

Serve: 6 | Total Time: 30 minutes

½ cup canned pumpkin purée
1 cup flour
½ tsp baking soda
½ cup granulated sugar
1 tsp pumpkin pie spice
¼ tsp nutmeg
¼ tsp salt
1 egg
1 tbsp vegetable oil
1 tbsp orange juice
1 tsp orange zest
¼ cup crushed walnuts

Preheat Air Fryer at 375°F. Combine flour, baking soda, sugar, nutmeg, pumpkin pie spice, salt, pumpkin purée, egg, oil, orange juice, orange zest, and walnuts in a bowl. Bake in a greased cake pan. Place cake pan in the frying basket and Bake for 20 minutes. Let sit for 10 minutes until slightly cooled before slicing. Serve.

RECIPE 952: PUMPKIN CAKE

Serve: 10 | Total Time: 30 minutes

1 tbsp pumpkin pie spice
12 oz. evaporated milk
3 large room temperature eggs
1 cup walnuts, diced
1 package yellow cake mix
1 cup granulated sugar
15 oz. pumpkin puree
3/4 cup melted unsalted butter
8 tbsp room temperature butter for frosting
1 tsp ground cinnamon
8 oz. room temperature cream cheese
1 cup powdered sugar
2 tbsp vanilla extract

Combine pumpkin puree, eggs, sugar, milk, ground cinnamon, and pumpkin spice in a large bowl. Next add the cake mix, diced walnuts, and melted unsalted butter. Mix well. Pour batter on greased pan or skillet. Choose the bake function. Bake for 15 minutes at 320°F. In a separate bowl create frosting by combining cream cheese, butter, sugar, vanilla extract, and walnuts.

RECIPE 953: PUMPKIN EMPANADAS

Serve: 4 | Total Time: 30 minutes

1 (15-oz) can pumpkin purée
¼ cup white sugar
2 tsp cinnamon
1 tbsp brown sugar
½ tbsp cornstarch
¼ tsp vanilla extract
2 tbsp butter
4 empanada dough shells

Place the puree in a pot and top with white and brown sugar, cinnamon, cornstarch, vanilla extract, 1 tbsp of water and butter and stir thoroughly. Bring to a boil over medium heat. Simmer for 4-5 minutes. Allow to cool. Preheat Air Fryer to 360°F. Lay empanada shells flat on a clean counter. Spoon the pumpkin mixture into each of the shells. Fold the empanada shells over to cover completely. Water the edges and fasten with a fork. Place the empanadas on the greased frying basket and Bake for 15 minutes, flipping once halfway through until golden. Serve hot.

RECIPE 954: PUMPKIN PUDDING AND VANILLA WAFERS

Serve: 4 | Total Time: 25 minutes

1 cup canned no-salt-added pumpkin purée
¼ cup packed brown sugar
3 tbsp all-purpose flour
1 egg, whisked
2 tbsp milk
1 tbsp unsalted butter, melted
1 tsp pure vanilla extract

4 low-fat vanilla wafers, crumbled
Cooking spray

Coat a baking pan with cooking spray. Set aside. Mix the pumpkin purée, brown sugar, flour, whisked egg, milk, melted butter, and vanilla in a medium bowl and whisk to combine. Transfer the mixture to the baking pan. Select Bake, set temperature to 350°F (180°C), and set time to 15 minutes. Select Start to begin preheating. Once the oven has preheated, slide the pan into the oven. When cooking is complete, the pudding should be set. Remove the pudding from the oven to a wire rack to cool. Divide the pudding into four bowls and serve with the vanilla wafers sprinkled on top.

RECIPE 955: QUICK PAELLA

Serve: 4 | Total Time: 22 minutes

(10-ounce) package frozen cooked rice, thawed
1 (6-ounce) jar artichoke hearts, drained and chopped
¼ cup vegetable broth
½ tsp turmeric
½ tsp dried thyme
1 cup frozen cooked small shrimp
½ cup frozen baby peas
1 tomato, diced

Preparing the ingredients. In a 6-by-6-by-2-inch pan, combine the rice, artichoke hearts, vegetable broth, turmeric, and thyme, and stir gently. Air Frying Place in the Air Fryer oven and bake for 8 to 9 minutes or until the rice is hot. Remove the shrimp, peas, and tomato from the Air Fryer and carefully toss them in. Cook it for about 5-8 minutes or until the shrimp and peas are hot and the paella is bubbling.

RECIPE 956: RICH SALMON BURGERS WITH BROCCOLI SLAW

Serve: 4 | Total Time: 25 minutes

1 lb salmon fillets
1 egg
¼ cup dill, chopped
1 cup bread crumbs
Salt to taste
½ tsp cayenne pepper
1 lime, zested
1 tsp fish sauce
4 buns
3 cups chopped broccoli
½ cup shredded carrots
¼ cup sunflower seeds
2 garlic cloves, minced
1 cup Greek yogurt

Preheat Air Fryer to 360°F. Blitz the salmon fillets in your food processor until they are finely chopped. Remove to a large bowl and add egg, dill, bread crumbs, salt, and cayenne. Stir to combine. Form the mixture into 4 patties. Put them into the frying basket and Bake for 10 minutes, flipping once. Combine broccoli, carrots, sunflower seeds, garlic, salt, lime, fish sauce, and Greek yogurt in a bowl. Serve the salmon burgers onto buns with broccoli slaw. Enjoy!

RECIPE 957: RICOTTA AND BROCCOLI CANNELLONI

Serve: 4 | Total Time: 35 minutes

1 cup shredded mozzarella cheese
½ cup cooked broccoli, chopped
½ cup cooked spinach, chopped
4 cooked cannelloni shells
1 cup ricotta cheese
½ tsp dried marjoram
1 egg
1 cup passata
1 tbsp basil leaves

Preheat Air Fryer to 360°F. Then beat the egg till frothy. Add the ricotta, marjoram, half of the mozzarella, broccoli, and spinach and stir to combine. Cover the base of a baking dish with a layer of passata. Fill the cannelloni with the cheese mixture and place them on top of the sauce. Spoon the remaining passata over the tops and top with the rest of the mozzarella cheese. Put the dish in the frying basket and Bake for 25 minutes until the cheese is melted and golden. Top with basil.

RECIPE 958: ROSEMARY BAKED CASHEWS

Serve: 2 | Total Time: 8 minutes

2 sprigs of rosemary
1 tsp olive oil
1 tsp kosher salt
½ tsp honey
2 cups roasted and unsalted whole cashews
Cooking spray

Preheat the Air Fryer to temperature 300 degrees Fahrenheit (180 degrees Celsius) (149 degrees Celsius). Whisk together the rosemary, olive oil, kosher salt, and honey in a medium mixing bowl until thoroughly blended. Remove from the equation. Cook for 3 minutes after spraying the Air Fryer basket with frying spray and adding the cashews and entire rosemary sprig. Remove the cashews and rosemary from the Air Fryer, discarding the rosemary before tossing the cashews in the olive oil mixture to coat. Allow 15 minutes for cooling before serving.

RECIPE 959: RUSSET POTATOES WITH YOGURT AND CHIVES

Serve: 4 | Total Time: 40 minutes

4 (7-ounce / 198-g) russet potatoes, rinsed
Olive oil spray
1/2 tsp kosher salt, divided
1/2 cup 2% plain Greek yogurt
¼ cup minced fresh chives
Freshly ground black pepper, to taste

Dry the potatoes and puncture them with a fork all over. Spritz the potatoes with olive oil spray. Sprinkle with ¼ tsp of the salt. Place the potatoes in the air fry basket to cook. Place the basket on the bake position. Select Bake, set temperature to 400°F (205°C), and set time to 35 minutes. When cooking is complete, the potatoes should be fork-tender. Remove from the Air Fryer grill and split open the potatoes. Top with the chives, yogurt, the remaining ¼ tsp of salt, and finish with the black pepper. Serve immediately.

RECIPE 960: SALMON AND GREEK YOGURT SAUCE

Serve: 2 | Total Time: 30 minutes

2 medium salmon fillets
1 tbsp basil, chopped
6 lemon slices
Sea salt and black pepper to the taste
1 cup Greek yogurt
2 tsp curry powder
A pinch of cayenne pepper
1 garlic clove, minced
½ tsp cilantro, chopped
½ tsp mint, chopped

Place each salmon fillet on a parchment paper piece, make 3 splits in each and stuff them with basil. Season with pepper, and salt, then top each fillet with 3 lemon slices, fold parchment, seal edges, and bake for 20 minutes at 400 degrees F. Meanwhile, in a bowl, mix yogurt with cayenne pepper, salt to the taste, garlic, curry, mint and cilantro and whisk well. Transfer fish to plates, drizzle the yogurt sauce you've just prepared on top and serve right away! Enjoy!

RECIPE 961: SALMON BAKED CHEESE AND BROCCOLI

Serve: 2 | Total Time: 20 minutes

3 cups broccoli, cut into small florets.
1/4 cup fresh parsley, chopped.
1 cup salmon flakes in olive oil
1/2 cup cream
1/4 cup cream cheese, softened.
1/2 cup cheddar cheese, grated.
1/2 cup mozzarella, grated.
1/2-tsp. pepper

Preheat the Air Fryer to temperature of 350 degrees F.

Place the broccoli florets in the Air Fryer Baking Pan. Season the salmon flakes with pepper and top them over the broccoli. Whisk together the cream and cream cheese in a bowl. Fold in the cheddar cheese, mozzarella cheese and fresh parsley. Add the cheese/cream mixture to the Air Fryer Baking Pan. Cook for 15 minutes or until the cheese is melted. Serve and enjoy!

RECIPE 962: SAUSAGE FRITTATA WITH PARMESAN

Serve: 1 | Total Time: 15 minutes

1/2 sausage, chopped.
1 slice bread
4 cherry tomatoes, halved
1 slice bread
3 whole eggs
1-tbsp. olive oil
2-tbsp. Parmesan cheese, shredded for garnish
Salt and pepper to taste
A bunch of parsley, chopped

Preheat the Air Fryer to temperature of 360 degrees F. Place tomatoes and sausages in your Air Fryer's cooking basket and cook for 5 minutes. Take a bowl and, mix baked tomatoes, sausages, eggs, salt, parsley, Parmesan cheese, oil and pepper. Add the bread to the Air Fryer cooking basket and cook for 5 minutes. Add the frittata mixture over baked bread and top with Parmesan cheese. Serve and enjoy!

RECIPE 963: SCALLOPED POTATOES

Serve: 4 | Total Time: 55 minutes

4 sweet potatoes, peeled
1/4 cup olive oil
1/2 tsp paprika
1 tbsp. maple syrup
1/2 cup fresh orange juice
1/2 tsp orange zest
1 tsp salt

Slice sweet potatoes 1/16-inch thick using a slicer. Arrange sweet

potato slices into the greased baking dish. Combine the other ingredients in a basin and pour over the sweet potatoes. Place the inner pot in the Air Fryer combo base. Place baking dish into the inner pot. Cover the inner pot with an air frying lid. Select bake mode, then set the temperature to 350 °F and time for 45 minutes. Click start. When the countdown approaches zero, press the cancel button. Serve and enjoy.

RECIPE 964: SICILIAN-STYLE VEGETARIAN PIZZA

Serve: 2 | Total Time: 20 minutes

1 pizza pie crust
¼ cup ricotta cheese
½ tbsp tomato paste
½ white onion, sliced
½ tsp dried oregano
¼ cup Sicilian olives, sliced
¼ cup grated mozzarella

Preheat Air Fryer to 350°F. Lay the pizza dough on a parchment paper sheet. Spread the tomato paste evenly over the pie crust, allowing at least ½ inch border. Sprinkle with oregano and scatter the ricotta cheese on top. Cover with onion and Sicilian olive slices and finish with a layer of mozzarella cheese. Bake it for about 10 minutes long until the cheese has melted and lightly crisped, and the crust is golden brown. Serve sliced and enjoy!

RECIPE 965: SIMPLE GREEN BAKE

Serve: 4 | Total Time: 15 minutes

1 cup asparagus, chopped
2 cups broccoli florets
1 tbsp olive oil
1 tbsp lemon juice
1 cup green peas
2 tbsp honey mustard
Salt and pepper to taste

Preheat Air Fryer to 330°F. Add asparagus and broccoli to the frying basket. Drizzle with olive oil and lemon juice and toss. Bake for 6 minutes. Remove the basket and add peas. Allow the veggies to steam for a further 3 minutes, or until they are hot and tender. Pour the vegetables into a serving dish. Drizzle with honey mustard and season with salt and pepper. Toss and serve warm.

RECIPE 966: SMOKED SALMON CROISSANT SANDWICH

Serve: 1 | Total Time: 30 minutes

1 croissant, halved
2 eggs
1 tbsp guacamole
1 smoked salmon slice
Salt and pepper to taste

Preheat Air Fryer to 360°F. Place the croissant, crusty side up, in the frying basket side by side. Whisk the eggs in a small ceramic dish until fluffy. Place in the Air Fryer. Bake for 10 minutes. Gently scramble the half-cooked egg in the baking dish with a fork. Flip the croissant and cook for another 10 minutes until the scrambled eggs are cooked, but still fluffy, and the croissant is toasted. Place one croissant on a serving plate, then spread the guacamole on top. Scoop the scrambled eggs onto guacamole, then top with smoked salmon. Sprinkle with salt and pepper. Top with the second slice of toasted croissant, close sandwich, and serve hot.

RECIPE 967: SMOOTH WALNUT-BANANA LOAF

Serve: 4 | Total Time: 40 minutes

1/3 cup peanut butter, melted
2 tbsp butter, melted and cooled
¾ cup flour
½ tsp salt
¼ tsp baking soda
2 ripe bananas
2 eggs
1 tsp lemon juice
½ cup evaporated cane sugar
½ cup ground walnuts
1 tbsp blackstrap molasses
1 tsp vanilla extract

Preheat Air Fryer to 310°F. In a small mixing basin, combine the flour, salt, and baking soda. A big bowl with mashed bananas, eggs, sugar, peanut butter and vanilla. When it is well incorporated, stir in the flour mixture until just combined. Transfer the batter to a parchment-lined baking dish and make sure it is even. Bake in the Air Fryer for 30 to 35 minutes until a toothpick in the middle comes out clean, and the top is golden. Serve and enjoy.

RECIPE 968: SPAGHETTI SQUASH LASAGNA

Serve: 6 | Total Time: 70 minutes

2 large spaghetti squash, cooked
4 pounds ground beef
1 large jar Marinara sauce
25 slices Mozzarella cheese
30 ounces whole-milk ricotta cheese

Slice the spaghetti squash and place it face down inside a baking dish. Fill with water until covered. Bake in the Air Fryer at 375°F (191ºC) for 45 minutes until skin is soft. Sear the ground beef in a skillet over medium-high heat for 5 minutes or until browned, then add the marinara sauce and heat until warm. Set aside. Scrape the flesh off the cooked squash to resemble strands of spaghetti. Layer the lasagna in a large greased pan in alternating layers of spaghetti squash, beef sauce, Mozzarella, ricotta. Do this until you've used all of the ingredients. Bake for 30 minutes and serve!

RECIPE 969: SPICY HONEY ORANGE CHICKEN

Serve: 4 | Total Time: 20 minutes

1 ½-lb. chicken breast, washed and sliced
3/4 cup breadcrumbs
2 whole eggs, beaten
1/4 cup honey
1/2 cup orange marmalade
1/2 cup flour
1 cup coconut, shredded
1-tbsp. red pepper flakes
3-tbsp. Dijon mustard
1/2-tsp. pepper
Salt to taste

Preheat your Air Fryer to temperature of 400 degrees F. In a mixing bowl, combine coconut, flour, salt and pepper. In another bowl, add the beaten eggs. Place breadcrumbs in a third bowl. Dredge chicken in egg mix, flour and finally in the breadcrumbs. Place the chicken in the Air Fryer cooking basket and bake for 15 minutes. In a separate bowl, mix honey, orange marmalade, mustard and pepper flakes. Cover chicken with marmalade mixture and fry for 5 more minutes.

RECIPE 970: SPICY SPINACH DIP

Serve: 4 | Total Time: 40 minutes

10 oz. frozen spinach, thawed and drained
1/2 cup onion, diced
2 tsp garlic, minced
1/2 cup mozzarella cheese, shredded
1/2 cup Monterey jack cheese, shredded
2 tsp jalapeno pepper, minced
1/2 cup cheddar cheese, shredded
8 oz. cream cheese
1/2 tsp salt

In a mixing bowl, add all of the ingredients and stir until thoroughly blended. Pour mixture into the greased baking dish. Place the inner pot in the Air Fryer combo base. Place baking dish into the inner pot. Cover the inner pot with an air frying lid. Select bake mode then set the temperature to 350 °F and time for 30 minutes. Click start. When done, serve and enjoy.

RECIPE 971: SPINACH FRITTATA

Serve: 2 | Total Time: 15 minutes

1 small red onion, minced
1/3 pack of spinach

3 eggs, whisked
Salt and ground black pepper to taste
Mozzarella cheese

Ensure that your Air Fryer is preheated to 360 F. Let the oil in the baking pan stay for a minute before adding minced onions. Allow staying for another 2-3 minutes or until the onions become translucent. Add spinach and fry until it is half-cooked (for about 3-5 minutes). Do not worry if the spinach appears dry, just continue frying. Season the whisked eggs and add cheese. Finally, pour the seasoned mixture into the pan and bake until cooked - it takes about 8 minutes.

RECIPE 972: SRIRACHA SALMON MELT SANDWICHES

Serve: 4 | Total Time: 20 minutes

2 tbsp butter, softened
2 (5-oz) cans pink salmon
2 English muffins
1/3 cup mayonnaise
2 tbsp Dijon mustard
1 tbsp fresh lemon juice
1/3 cup chopped celery
½ tsp sriracha sauce
4 slices tomato
4 slices Swiss cheese

Preheat the Air Fryer to 370°F. Fork-split the English muffins and butter each half. Put the halves in the basket and Bake for 3-5 minutes, or until toasted. Remove and set aside. Combine the salmon, mayonnaise, mustard, lemon juice, celery, and sriracha in a bowl. Divide among the English muffin halves. Top each sandwich with tomato and cheese and put in the frying basket. Bake for 4-6 minutes or until the cheese is melted and starts to brown. Serve hot.

RECIPE 973: STRIP STEAK WITH POTATOES

Serve: 6 | Total Time: 60 minutes

2 lbs. New York Strop steak, cut into 1-inch pieces
2 russet potatoes, halved
Salt and pepper to taste
2 tbsp Worcestershire sauce
Canola oil for brushing
Fresh chives for garnish

Preheat the Air Fryer to 4000 degrees Fahrenheit for 5 minutes. Place all ingredients in a bake tray and toss using your hands to coat potatoes and steaks with the seasonings. Place in the Air Fryer and select the Air Fry setting. Adjust the cooking time to 60 minutes. Halfway through the cooking time, stir the potatoes and beef.

RECIPE 974: STUFFED PEPPER

Serve: 4 | Total Time: 35 minutes

4 eggs
1/4 cup baby broccoli florets
1/4 cup cherry tomatoes
1 tsp dried sage
2.5 oz. cheddar cheese, grated
7 oz. almond milk
2 bell peppers, halved
Pepper
Salt

In a bowl, whisk together eggs, milk, broccoli, cherry tomatoes, sage, pepper, and salt. Pour egg mixture into the bell pepper halves. Sprinkle cheese on top of bell pepper. Place the inner pot in the Air Fryer combo base. Place stuffed peppers into the inner pot. Cover the inner pot with an air frying lid. Select bake mode, then set the temperature to 390 °F and time for 25 minutes. Click start. When done, serve and enjoy.

RECIPE 975: STUFFED TOMATOES AND BROCCOLI

Serve: 2 | Total Time: 25 minutes

¼ cup cheddar cheese, grated
¼ cup broccoli, chopped
1 organic tomato (preferably big size)
4-5 florets broccoli

Butter (unsalted)
Pinch of natural country herbs

Ensure that your Air Fryer is preheated to 360 F. Get a clean small bowl and in it, mix the grated Cheddar cheese and the chopped broccoli. Remove the pulps and seeds from the tomato. Stuff the empty tomato with the cheddar and broccoli mixture. Transfer the stuffed tomato into the Air Fryer basket, add the florets of the broccoli, and finally some butter on top. Allow the tomato to air bake for 12 or 15 minutes. Sprinkle some herbs on the melted cheese. Serve.

RECIPE 976: SUMPTUOUS TURKEY AND CAULIFLOWER MEATLOAF

Serve: 6 | Total Time: 65 minutes

2 pounds lean ground turkey
1 ⅓ cups riced cauliflower
2 large eggs, lightly beaten
¼ cup almond flour
⅔ cup chopped white onion
1 tsp ground dried turmeric
1 tsp ground cumin
1 tsp ground coriander
1 tsp minced garlic
1 tsp salt
1 tsp black pepper
Cooking spray

Spritz a loaf pan with cooking spray. In a big bowl, mix everything. Stir to mix well. Pour half of the mixture in the prepared loaf pan and press with a spatula to coat the bottom evenly. Spritz the mixture with cooking spray. Arrange the loaf pan in the Air Fryer and bake at 350°F for 25 minutes or just until the meat is well browned and the internal temperature reaches at least 165°F. Repeat with remaining mixture. Serve the loaf pan straight from the Air Fryer.

RECIPE 977: SWEET ROASTED PUMPKIN ROUNDS

Serve: 4 | Total Time: 35 minutes

1 (2-lb) pumpkin
1 tbsp honey
1 tbsp melted butter
¼ tsp cardamom
¼ tsp sea salt

Preheat the Air Fryer to 370°F. Remove the seeds from the pumpkin by cutting it in half lengthwise. Slice each half crosswise into 1-inch-wide half-circles, then cut each half-circle in half again to make quarter rounds. Combine the honey, butter, cardamom, and salt in a bowl and mix well. Toss the pumpkin in the mixture until coated, then put into the frying basket. Bake for 15-20 minutes, shaking once during cooking until the edges start to brown and the squash is tender.

RECIPE 978: SWEET SQUARES

Serve: 6 | Total Time: 40 minutes

1 cup flour
½ cup butter, soft
1 cup sugar
¼ cup powdered sugar
2 tsp lemon peel, grated
2 tbsp lemon juice
2 eggs, whisked
½ tsp baking powder
In a bowl, mix flour with powdered sugar and butter, stir well, press on the bottom of a pan that fits your Air Fryer, introduce in the fryer and bake at 350 degrees F for 14 minutes. In another bowl, mix sugar with lemon juice, lemon peel, eggs and baking powder, stir using your mixer and spread over baked crust. Bake for 15 minutes more, leave aside to cool down, cut into medium squares and serve cold. Enjoy!

RECIPE 979: SWEETY BLUEBERRY MUFFINS

Serve: 4 | Total Time: 40 minutes

3 oz flour
1 egg
3 oz milk
2 oz butter, melted
4 oz dried blueberries

1 tsp cinnamon
3 tbsps brown sugar

In the large bowl sift the flour, add cinnamon, sugar and stir to combine. In another bowl whisk one egg with milk and add melted butter. Mix well and stir this mixture in the flour. Add dried blueberries to the mixture. Put the batter into the muffin cups. Preheat the Air Fryer to 380°F. Carefully place filled muffin cups to the Air Fryer basket and set the timer to 15 minutes. Bake muffins until they become golden brown. Cool and serve.

RECIPE 980: TACO CRUNCH WRAP

Serve: 2 | Total Time: 15 minutes

1 regular size of gluten free tortilla
2 tbsp. of grated cheese
2 small corn of tortillas
2 tbsp. of refried pinto beans
2 tbsp. of guacamole
Iceberg lettuce

First preheat your Air Fryer to temperature of 350°F. Assemble each crunch wrap by stacking in the following order, large regular tortilla, cheese, small corn tortilla, beans, guacamole, lettuce, and the second small corn tortilla. Carefully fold and turn the wrap with your hands more cheese to seal. Set your Air Fryer to cook the taco crunch wrap for about 6 minutes at 350°F. Bake it at 325°F for about 5 to 8 minutes, or until it has warmed through and slightly crispy. After baking, serve immediately with dairy free sour cream and guacamole for dipping. Make use of the mashed avocado, lemon juice and sea salt to prepare the guacamole. Serve and enjoy!

RECIPE 981: TACO PIE WITH MEATBALLS

Serve: 4 | Total Time: 40 minutes

1 cup shredded quesadilla cheese
1 cup shredded Colby cheese
10 cooked meatballs, halved

1 cup salsa
1 cup canned refried beans
2 tsp chipotle powder
½ tsp ground cumin
4 corn tortillas

Preheat the Air Fryer to 375°F. Combine the meatball halves, salsa, refried beans, chipotle powder, and cumin in a bowl. In a baking pan, add a tortilla and top with one-quarter of the meatball mixture. Sprinkle one-quarter of the cheeses on top and repeat the layers three more times, ending with cheese. Put the pan in the fryer. Baking time: 15-20 minutes, until the cheese has melted. Let cool on a wire rack for 10 minutes. Remove the sides of the pan with a knife and serve in wedges.

RECIPE 982: TILAPIA ROAST IN GARLIC AND OLIVE OIL

Serve: 4 | Total Time: 23 minutes

4 (4 ounces) tilapia fillets
4 cloves garlic
3 tbsp extra-virgin olive oil
2 chopped onions
1/4 tsp salt

Rub the tilapia fillets with garlic and arrange them on a large plate. Drizzle the fish with olive oil until well coated and top with onion. Refrigerate the fish, covered, for at least 8 hours or overnight to soak in the marinade. When ready, preheat your Air Fryer toast oven to 350 degrees F. Transfer the fish fillets to the basket of your Air Fryer toast oven; Reserve the marinade for basting. Bake for 8 minutes, four minutes per side, and baste with the marinade halfway through cook time. Enjoy!

RECIPE 983: TOFU SCRAMBLE

Serve: 4 | Total Time: 35 minutes

2 tbsp soy sauce
1 tofu block, cubed
1 tsp turmeric, ground
1 tbsp extra virgin olive oil
2 cups broccoli florets

1/2 tsp onion powder
1/2 tsp garlic powder
2 and 1/2 cup red potatoes, cubed
1/2 cup yellow onion, chopped
Salt and black pepper

Merge tofu with 1 tbsp oil, salt, pepper, soy sauce, garlic powder, onion powder, turmeric and onion in a bowl, stir and leave aside. In a separate bowl, merge potatoes with the rest of the oil, a pinch of salt and pepper and toss to coat. Set potatoes in your Air Fryer at 350 degrees F and bake for 15 minutes, shaking once. Add tofu and its marinade to your Air Fryer and bake for 15 minutes. Attach broccoli to the fryer and cook everything for 5 minutes more. Serve right away.

RECIPE 984: TOMATO AND HALLOUMI BRUSCHETTA

Serve: 4 | Total Time: 20 minutes

2 tbsp softened butter
8 French bread slices
1 cup grated halloumi cheese
½ cup basil pesto
12 chopped cherry tomatoes
2 green onions, thinly sliced

Preheat Air Fryer to 350°F. Butter should be put on one side of the bread. Place butter-side up in the frying basket. Bake until the bread is slightly brown, 3-5 minutes. Remove the bread and top it with halloumi cheese. Melt the cheese on the bread in the Air Fryer for another 1-3 minutes. Meanwhile, mix pesto, cherry tomatoes, and green onions in a small bowl. When the cheese has already melted, take the bread out of the fryer and arrange on a plate. Top with pesto mix and serve.

RECIPE 985: TOMATO MUSHROOM FRITTATA

Serve: 4 | Total Time: 30 minutes

1 cup egg white
2 tbsp whole milk
¼ cup sliced tomato
¼ cup sliced mushrooms

2 tbsp chopped fresh chives
Salt and black pepper to taste

Preheat the Air Fryer on Bake mode at 320 F for 3 to 4 minutes with the drip pan on the bottom rack. Lightly grease a 6-inch casserole dish with olive oil, add all the ingredients, and whisk until well distributed. Place the dish on top of the cooking tray on the center rack of the oven. Close the oven and bake until the frittata is set, about 15 minutes. Remove from the oven, allow cooling for 2 to 3 minutes, and serve the frittata.

RECIPE 986: TRI-COLOR FRITTATA

Serve: 4 | Total Time: 30 minutes

8 eggs, beaten
1 red bell pepper, diced
Salt and pepper to taste
1 garlic clove, minced
½ tsp dried oregano
½ cup ricotta

Preheat Air Fryer to 360°F. Place the beaten eggs, bell pepper, oregano, salt, black pepper, and garlic and mix well. Fold in ¼ cup half of ricotta cheese. Pour the egg mixture into a greased cake pan and top with the remaining ricotta. Place into the Air Fryer and Bake for 18-20 minutes or until the eggs are set in the center. Let the frittata cool for 5 minutes. Serve sliced.

RECIPE 987: TUNA BAKE

Serve: 6 | Total Time: 55 minutes

1 ½ cups, sweet peas, frozen
1 tsp. seasoned salt
1 ½ cups, evaporated milk
2 4/5 oz. onion, French fried
4 cups, egg noodles, wide uncooked
10 ¾ oz. soup, cream of celery, condensed
1 tbsp. onion, dried, minced
10 oz. tuna, water-packed, drained, flaked

Follow package directions in cooking noodles. Add peas at last

minute. Drain and set aside. Preheat Air Fryer at 325 degrees Fahrenheit. Combine soup with milk, seasoned salt, and dried onion in an ungreased casserole (2-quart). Add cooked noodles and toss to combine. Cover dish and air-fry for thirty minutes. Give dish a stir, add French fried onions on top, and return to Air Fryer to cook for another five minutes.

RECIPE 988: TUNA MELTS WITH ENGLISH MUFFINS

Serve: 4 | Total Time: 15 minutes

1 (6-oz) can tuna, drained
¼ cup mayonnaise
2 tsp mustard
1 tbsp lime juice
½ red onion, minced
2 English muffins, halved
2 tbsp butter, softened
4 Muenster cheese slices

Preheat Air Fryer to 390°F. Mix together tuna, mayonnaise, mustard, lime juice, and red onion in a small bowl. Set aside. Butter the English muffins' cut side. Place into the Air Fryer with the butter side up. Bake until lightly golden, 3 minutes. Remove from the Air Fryer. 1 cheese slice per muffin. Bake in the Air Fryer for another 2-4 minutes until the cheese melts. Remove the muffins to a serving plate. Top with tuna mixture and serve.

RECIPE 989: TUNA SANDWICHES

Serve: 4 | Total Time: 15 minutes

16 oz canned tuna, drained
¼ cup mayonnaise
2 tbsp mustard
1 tbsp lemon juice
2 green onions, chopped
3 English muffins, halved
3 tbsp butter
6 provolone cheese
In a bowl, mix tuna with mayo, lemon juice, mustard and green onions and stir. Grease muffin halves with the butter, place them in preheated Air Fryer and bake

them at 350 degrees F for 4 minutes. Spread tuna mix on muffin halves, top each with provolone cheese, return sandwiches to Air Fryer and cook them for 4 minutes, divide among plates and serve for breakfast right away. Enjoy!

RECIPE 990: TURKEY AND LEEK HAMBURGER

Serve: 4 | Total Time: 30 minutes

1 cup leftover turkey, cut into bite-sized chunks
1 leek, sliced
1 Serrano pepper, deveined and chopped
2 bell peppers, deveined and chopped
2 tbsp Tabasco sauce
½ cup sour cream
1 tbsp fresh cilantro, chopped
1 tsp hot paprika
¾ tsp kosher salt
½ tsp ground black pepper
4 hamburger buns
Cooking spray

Spritz a baking pan with cooking spray. In a large mixing basin, combine all of the ingredients except the buns. Toss to combine well. Place it in the baking pan in the Air Fryer and pour the contents in. Bake at 385°F (196°C) for 20 minutes or until the turkey is well browned and the leek is tender. Assemble the hamburger buns with the turkey mixture and serve immediately.

RECIPE 991: TURKEY CHEESE TAQUITOS

Serve: 6 | Total Time: 29 minutes

1 pound (454 g) turkey breasts, boneless and skinless
Kosher salt and freshly ground black pepper, to taste
1 clove garlic, minced
1 habanero pepper, minced
4 ounces (113 g) Mexican cheese blend, shredded
6 small corn tortillas
½ cup salsa

Pat the turkey breasts dry with kitchen towels. Toss the turkey breasts with the salt and black pepper. Cook the turkey breasts at 380°F (193°C) for 18 minutes, turning them over halfway through the cooking time. Place the shredded chicken, garlic, habanero pepper, and cheese on one end of each tortilla. Roll them up tightly and transfer them to a lightly oiled Air Fryer basket. Bake your taquitos at 360°F (182°C) for 6 minutes. Serve your taquitos with salsa and enjoy!

RECIPE 992: TURKEY, MUSHROOM AND EGG CASSEROLE

Serve: 4 | Total Time: 15 minutes

6 eggs
1 ½ cups spinach
1 ¼ cups shredded cheddar cheese
2 onions, chopped
¼ cup cooked turkey, diced
4 mushrooms, diced
Pinch of onion powder
Salt and pepper to taste
Pinch of garlic powder
¼ green bell pepper, chopped

Preheat your Air Fryer to 400°Fahrenheit. Whisk the eggs in mixing bowl. Add mushrooms, garlic powder, bell pepper, onion powder, onions, 1 cup cheese and cooked diced turkey. Mix well and add mixture to casserole dish. Sprinkle the top of mixture with remaining cheese. Add spinach on top. Bake in Air Fryer for 15-minutes. Serve hot!

RECIPE 993: TURKEY TACO CASSEROLE

Serve: 6 | Total Time: 45 minutes

8 oz shredded cheese
1 ½ - 2 lbs ground turkey
1 cup salsa
2 tbsp. taco seasoning
16 oz. cottage cheese

Switch on the oven to 400 degrees. In a sizeable casserole dish, put in the ground meat and mix in the taco seasoning—Bake for 20 minutes. While ground turkey is baking, mix 1 cup of shredded cheese, cottage cheese, and salsa. Take the casserole from the oven and strain out any leftover juices from the ground meat. Pound and crush the meat into smaller pieces and then layer the cottage cheese and salsa combo over the meat. Sprinkle remaining cheese on top of the ground meat. Put the casserole back into the oven and bake for 15-20 minutes until the meat cooks all the way through. And the cheese is melted and bubbling.

RECIPE 994: TUSCAN SALMON

Serve: 4 | Total Time: 15 minutes

2 tbsp olive oil
4 salmon fillets
½ tsp salt
¼ tsp red pepper flakes
1 tsp chopped dill
2 tomatoes, diced
¼ cup sliced black olives
4 lemon slices

Preheat Air Fryer to 380°F. Lightly spray the olive oil on both sides of the salmon fillets and season with salt, red pepper flakes, and dill before grilling or baking. Using a frying basket, arrange the fish fillets in a single layer, then top with the tomatoes and black olives. Top each fillet with a lemon slice. Bake for 8 minutes. Serve and enjoy!

RECIPE 995: VEGETARIAN QUINOA CUPS

Serve: 6 | Total Time: 25 minutes

1 carrot, chopped
1 zucchini, chopped
4 asparagus, chopped
¾ cup quinoa flour
2 tbsp lemon juice
¼ cup nutritional yeast
¼ tsp garlic powder
Salt and pepper to taste

Preheat Air Fryer to 340°F. Combine the vegetables, quinoa flour, water, lemon juice, nutritional yeast, garlic powder, salt, and pepper in a medium bowl, and mix well.Divide the mixture between 6 cupcake molds. Place the filled molds into the Air Fryer and Bake for 20 minutes, or until the tops are lightly browned and have a toothpick inserted into the center that comes out clean. Serve cooled.

RECIPE 996: VIETNAMESE GINGERED TOFU

Serve: 4 | Total Time: 25 minutes

1 (8-oz) package extra-firm tofu, cubed
4 tsp shoyu
1 tsp onion powder
½ tsp garlic powder
½ tsp ginger powder
½ tsp turmeric powder
Black pepper to taste
2 tbsp nutritional yeast
1 tsp dried rosemary
1 tsp dried dill
2 tsp cornstarch
2 tsp sunflower oil
Sprinkle the tofu with shoyu and toss to coat. Add the onion, garlic, ginger, turmeric, and pepper. Gently toss to coat. Add the yeast, rosemary, dill, and cornstarch. Toss to coat. Dribble with the oil and toss again. Preheat Air Fryer to 390°F. Spray the fryer basket with oil, put the tofu in the basket and Bake for 7 minutes. Remove, shake gently, and cook for another 7 minutes or until the tofu is crispy and golden. Serve warm.

RECIPE 997: VIKING TOAST

Serve: 2 | Total Time: 20 minutes

2 tbsp minced green chili pepper
1 avocado, pressed
1 clove garlic, minced
¼ tsp lemon juice
Salt and pepper to taste
2 bread slices
2 plum tomatoes, sliced
4 oz smoked salmon

¼ diced peeled red onion

Preheat Air Fryer at 350°F. Combine the avocado, garlic, lemon juice, and salt in a bowl until you reach your desired consistency. Spread avocado mixture on the bread slices. Top with tomato slices and sprinkle with black pepper. Place bread slices in the frying basket and Bake for 5 minutes. Transfer to a plate. Top each bread slice with salmon, green chili pepper, and red onion. Serve.

RECIPE 998: WINTER VEGETABLES WITH HERBS

Serve: 2 | Total Time: 30 minutes

1/2 lb broccoli florets
2 celery root, peeled and cut into pieces
1 onion, cut into wedges
2 tbsp unsalted butter, melted
1/2 cup chicken broth
1/4 cup tomato sauce
1 tsp parsley
1 tsp rosemary
1 tsp thyme

Start by preheating your Air Fryer to temperature of 380 degrees F. Place all ingredients in a lightly greased casserole dish. Stir to combine well. Bake in the preheated Air Fryer for 10 minutes. Gently stir the vegetables with a large spoon and cook for 5 minutes more. Serve in individual bowls with a few drizzles of lemon juice. Bon appétit!

RECIPE 999: YOGURT BAKED POTATOES

Serve: 4 | Total Time: 40 minutes

4 (7-ounce / 198-g) russet potatoes, rinsed
Olive oil spray
½ tsp kosher salt, divided
½ cup 2% plain Greek yogurt
¼ cup minced fresh chives
Freshly ground black pepper, to taste

Dry the potatoes and puncture them with a fork all over. Spritz the potatoes with olive oil spray. Sprinkle with ¼ tsp of the salt. Bake the potatoes for 35 minutes at 400°F (204°C) in the Air Fryer basket, or until a knife can effortlessly be inserted into the center of the potatoes. Remove from the basket and split open the potatoes. Top with the yogurt, chives, the remaining ¼ tsp of salt, and finish with the black pepper. Serve immediately.

RECIPE 1000: ZUCCHINI EGG BAKE

Serve: 4 | Total Time: 35 minutes

6 eggs
1/2 tsp dill
1/2 tsp oregano
1/2 tsp basil
1/2 tsp baking powder
1/2 cup almond flour
1 cup cheddar cheese, shredded
1 cup kale, chopped
1 onion, chopped
1 cup zucchini, shredded and squeezed out all liquid
1/2 cup milk
1/4 tsp salt

Grease 9x9-inch baking dish and set aside. In a large mixing basin, whisk together the eggs and milk. In a separate medium-sized mixing dish, add the remaining ingredients. Transfer the egg mixture into the baking dish that has been prepared. Select bake mode and set the Omni to 375 °F for 30 minutes once the oven beeps, place the baking dish into the oven. Serve and enjoy.

RECIPE 1001: ZUCCHINI MANICOTTI

Serve: 4 | Total Time: 15 minutes

2 tbsp fresh basil, chopped
1 ½ cups mozzarella, shredded
1 cup marinara sauce
4 medium zucchinis, sliced ¼-inch
Salt and pepper to taste
½ tsp Italian seasoning

1 clove garlic, minced
1 large egg, lightly beaten
1 cup parmesan cheese, grated
1 ½ cups ricotta

In a mixing bowl, combine ½ cup parmesan, ricotta, egg, garlic and Italian seasoning. Season with salt and pepper and mix well. On a clean working surface place three slices of zucchini so they are slightly overlapping. Add a spoonful of ricotta mixture on top. Roll up and transfer to a greased Air Fryer baking dish. Repeat with remaining zucchini and ricotta mixture. On top of the zucchini manicotti, sprinkle with the remaining 12 cup parmesan and mozzarella. Bake in the Air Fryer at 350°Fahrenheit for 15-minutes. Use fresh basil as garnish and serve right away.